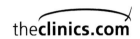

HAND CLINICS

Nerve Transfers

GUEST EDITORS
Susan E. Mackinnon, MD
Christine B. Novak, PT, MS, PhD(c)

November 2008 • Volume 24 • Number 4

SAUNDERS

An Imprint of Elsevier, Inc.
PHILADELPHIA   LONDON   TORONTO   MONTREAL   SYDNEY   TOKYO

W.B. SAUNDERS COMPANY

A Division of Elsevier Inc.

1600 John F. Kennedy Blvd. • Suite 1800 • Philadelphia, Pennsylvania 19103

http://www.theclinics.com

HAND CLINICS	**Volume 24, Number 4**
November 2008	**ISSN 0749-0712**
Editor: Debora Dellapena	**ISBN-13: 978-1-4160-6304-9**
	ISBN-10: 1-4160-6304-8

Hand Clinics (ISSN 0749-0712) is published quarterly by Elsevier Inc., 360 Park Avenue South, New York, NY 10010-1710. Months of publication are February, May, August, and November. Business and Editorial Offices: 1600 John F. Kennedy Blvd., Suite 1800, Philadelphia, PA 19103-2899. Customer Service Office: 11830 Westline Industrial Drive, St. Louis, MO 63146. Periodicals postage paid at New York, NY, and additional mailing offices. Subscription price is $282.00 per year (domestic individuals), $446.00 per year (domestic institutions), $144.00 per year (domestic students/residents), $321.00 per year (Canadian individuals), $510.00 per year (Canadian institutions), $383.00 per year (international individuals), $510.00 per year (international institutions), and $189.00 per year (international and Canadian students/residents). Foreign air speed delivery is included in all *Clinics* subscription prices. All prices are subject to change without notice. **POSTMASTER:** Send address changes to *Hand Clinics*, 11830 Westline Industrial Drive, St. Louis, MO 63146. Customer Service (orders, claims, online, change of address): Elsevier Periodicals Customer Service, 11830 Westline Industrial Drive, St. Louis, MO 63146. Tel: 1-800-654-2452 (U.S. and Canada). Fax: 314-523-5170. E-mail: journalscustomerservice-usa@elsevier.com (for print support); journalsonlinesupport-usa@elsevier.com (for online support).

Reprints. For copies of 100 or more of articles in this publication, please contact the Commercial Reprints Department, Elsevier Inc., 360 Park Avenue South, New York, NY 10010-1710. Tel.: 212-633-3812; Fax: 212-462-1935; E-mail: reprints@elsevier.com.

Hand Clinics is covered in *MEDLINE/PubMed (Index Medicus), Current Contents/Clinical Medicine, EMBASE/Excerpta Medica*, and *ISI/BIOMED.*

Printed in the United States of America.

GUEST EDITORS

SUSAN E. MACKINNON, MD, Schoenberg Professor of Surgery and Chief, Division of Plastic and Reconstructive Surgery, Department of Surgery, Washington University School of Medicine, St. Louis, Missouri

CHRISTINE B. NOVAK, PT, MS, PhD(c), Research Associate, University Health Network, Toronto, Ontario, Canada

CONTRIBUTORS

DIMITRI J. ANASTAKIS, MD, MHPE, MHCM, FRCSC, FACS, Associate Professor and Chair, Division of Plastic Surgery, University of Toronto, Toronto, Ontario, Canada

KEITH A. BENGTSON, MD, Department of Physical Medicine and Rehabilitation, Mayo Clinic, Rochester, Minnesota

ALLEN T. BISHOP, MD, Department of Orthopaedic Surgery, Division of Hand Surgery, Mayo Clinic, Rochester, Minnesota

JUSTIN M. BROWN, MD, Assistant Professor, Department of Neurological Surgery, Washington University School of Medicine, St. Louis, Missouri

PAUL S. CEDERNA, MD, Department of Surgery, Section of Plastic and Reconstructive Surgery, University of Michigan, Ann Arbor, Michigan

ROBERT CHEN, MBBChir, MSc, FRCPC, Professor, Division of Neurology, University of Toronto, Toronto, Ontario, Canada

DAVID CHWEI-CHIN CHUANG, MD, Professor, Department of Plastic Surgery, Chang Gung Memorial Hospital, Chang Gung University, Taipei-Linkou, Taiwan

STEPHEN H. COLBERT, MD, Assistant Professor of Surgery, Division of Plastic Surgery, University of Missouri School of Medicine, Columbia, Missouri

KRISTA COLEMAN-WOOD, PhD, Department of Orthopaedic Surgery, Division of Hand Surgery, Mayo Clinic, Rochester, Minnesota

KAREN D. DAVIS, PhD, Professor and Canada Research Chair (Brain and Behavior), Division of Neurosurgery, Institute of Medical Science, University of Toronto; Senior Scientist and Head, Division of Brain, Imaging and Behaviour — Systems Neuroscience, Toronto Western Research Institute, University Health Network, Toronto, Ontario, Canada

LINDA T. DVALI, MD, Assistant Professor, Division of Plastic and Reconstructive Surgery, University of Toronto, University Health Network, Toronto Western Division, Toronto, Ontario, Canada

KENTON R. KAUFMAN, PhD, Department of Orthopaedic Surgery, Division of Hand Surgery, Mayo Clinic, Rochester, Minnesota

MICHELLE F. KIRCHER, RN, Department of Orthopaedic Surgery, Division of Hand Surgery, Mayo Clinic, Rochester, Minnesota

ZINON T. KOKKALIS, MD, Orthopaedic Surgeon and Senior Fellow, Microsurgery Program, Department of Surgery, Eastern Virginia Medical School, Norfolk, Virginia

EPAMINONDAS KOSTOPOULOS, MD, Plastic Surgeon and Fellow, Microsurgery Program, Department of Surgery, Division of Plastic and Reconstructive Surgery, Eastern Virginia Medical School, Norfolk, Virginia

SCOTT H. KOZIN, MD, Associate Professor, Department of Orthopaedic Surgery, Temple University; Director, Upper Extremity Center of Excellence, Shriners Hospitals for Children, Philadelphia, Pennsylvania

WILLIAM M. KUZON, Jr, MD, PhD, Department of Surgery, Section of Plastic and Reconstructive Surgery, University of Michigan, Ann Arbor, Michigan

SAMUEL C. LIEN, BS, Department of Surgery, Section of Plastic and Reconstructive Surgery, University of Michigan, Ann Arbor, Michigan

SUSAN E. MACKINNON, MD, Schoenberg Professor of Surgery and Chief, Division of Plastic and Reconstructive Surgery, Department of Surgery, Washington University School of Medicine, St. Louis, Missouri

MARTIJN J.A. MALESSY, MD, Department of Neurosurgery, Leiden University Medical Centre, Leiden, The Netherlands

DAVID MIKULIS, MD, Professor, Department of Medical Imaging, University of Toronto, Toronto, Ontario Canada

HANNO MILLESI, MD, Professor, Millesi Center, Vienna Private Clinic, Vienna, Austria

TERENCE M. MYCKATYN, MD, Assistant Professor, Division of Plastic and Reconstructive Surgery, Washington University School of Medicine, St. Louis, Missouri

CHRISTINE B. NOVAK, PT, MS, PhD(c), Research Associate, University Health Network, Toronto, Ontario, Canada

ROBERT SCHMIDHAMMER, MD, Assistant Professor, Millesi Center, Vienna Private Clinic; Austrian Cluster for Tissue Regeneration, Ludwig Boltzmann Institute for Experimental and Clinical Traumatology, Research Center for Traumatology, Austrian Workers' Compensation Board, Vienna, Austria, European Union, Austria

ALEXANDER Y. SHIN, MD, Department of Orthopaedic Surgery, Division of Hand Surgery, Mayo Clinic, Rochester, Minnesota

ROBERT J. SPINNER, MD, Department of Neurosurgery, Mayo Clinic, Rochester, Minnesota

JULIA K. TERZIS, MD, PhD, Professor, Department of Surgery, Division of Plastic and Reconstructive Surgery, Eastern Virginia Medical School, Norfolk, Virginia

CONTENTS

> In the forearm, vital and expendable functions have been identified, and tendon transfers use these conventions to maximize function and minimize disability. Using similar concepts, distal nerve transfers offer a reconstruction that often is superior to reconstruction accomplished by traditional grafting. The authors present nerve transfer options for restoring motor and sensory deficits within each nerve distribution on the forearm and hand.

> Brachial plexus injuries result in devastating loss of function for patients and present incredible challenges for peripheral nerve surgeons. Recently, nerve transfers have produced superior results compared with traditional interposition nerve grafts for brachial plexus reconstruction. The authors present a review of current surgical options for treatment of partial and complete adult brachial plexus injuries using nerve transfers.

> The advent of nerve transfers has greatly increased surgical options for children who have brachial plexus birth palsies. Nerve transfers have considerable advantages, including easier surgical techniques, avoidance of neuroma resection, and direct motor and sensory reinnervation. Therefore, any functioning nerve fibers within the neuroma are preserved. Furthermore, a carefully selected donor nerve results in little or no clinical deficit. However, some disadvantages and unanswered questions remain. Because of a lack of head-to-head comparison between nerve transfers and nerve grafting, the window of opportunity for nerve grafting may be missed, which may degrade the ultimate outcome. Time will tell the ultimate role of nerve transfer or nerve grafting.

recovery following a nerve transfer. Neurostimulation (transcranial magnetic stimulation), and neuroimaging (functional MRI, structural MRI, magnetoencephalography) measure different aspects of cortical physiology and when used together are powerful tools in the study of cortical plasticity. The mechanisms of cortical plasticity, according to current and widely accepted opinions, involve the unmasking of previously ineffective connections or the sprouting of intact afferents from adjacent cortical or subcortical territories. Although significant strides have been made in our understanding of cortical plasticity following nerve transfer and during motor relearning, a great deal remains that we do not understand. Cortical plasticity and its manipulation may one day become important contributors to improve functional outcome following nerve transfer.

FORTHCOMING ISSUES

RECENT ISSUES

ELSEVIER
SAUNDERS

Hand Clin 24 (2008) ix–xi

HAND
CLINICS

Dedication

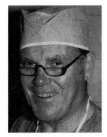

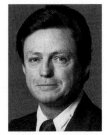

James F. Murray, MD, FRCS(C)   Alan A.R. Hudson, MD, FRCS(C)

Every year, more than one million people in the United States suffer peripheral nerve injuries resulting in significant neurologic morbidity [1]. The introduction of microsurgery and the popularization of nerve grafting techniques in the late 1970's and 1980's improved surgical results and patient outcome. In the 1990's, synthetic conduits found a role for the management of short nerve gaps in small diameter sensory nerves, and nerve allotransplantation found a limited role for devastating otherwise irreparable nerve injuries. However, for more than a decade, innovation in peripheral nerve surgery has "stalled" somewhat.

In 1991, within my own clinical practice, I began to expand the use of nerve transfers for several specific reasons. Early in my training, I was fortunate to work with Dr. Alan Hudson, past Chairman of Neurosurgery at the University of Toronto, who taught me about brachial plexus surgery. The clinical results of brachial plexus surgery were such that surgeons were eager for new surgical options that improved function and patient outcome; therefore, this patient population was ideal to introduce new endeavors, such as nerve transfers.

Dr. James F. Murray, Past President of the American Society for Surgery of the Hand, taught me about tendon transfer surgery, and I worked as his associate in the 1980's. He trained with Dr. William Littler in New York, who was trained by the "father" of hand surgery, Dr. Sterling Bunnell. I recognized that for every donor muscle available for a tendon transfer, there was a proximal donor nerve that would be expendable as well.

The third individual who was critical in bringing nerve transfers to such a prominent position in my practice was Dr. Christine Novak, coeditor of this issue of *Hand Clinics*. Christine used techniques of motor reeducation to maximize the results of nerve transfers.

Working with these fine individuals in the Canadian healthcare system also allowed me to focus on a large patient population that had peripheral nerve injuries. The introduction of nerve transfers into my clinical practice was advanced greatly by my postdoctoral research fellows (Appendix 1). Research work in the laboratory allowed me to ask and answer clinical questions and translate results from the laboratory directly to clinical practice. We found that sensory grafts actually inhibited nerve regeneration [2–4]. Thus, the avoidance of sensory graft interposition with direct motor-to-motor nerve repair not only decreases the time of muscle denervation, but also

doi:10.1016/j.hcl.2008.07.002

hand.theclinics.com

allows a more suitable environment for motor axon regeneration. Extensive work in the laboratory also demonstrated conclusively that end-to-side repairs would result only in limited sensory collateral sprouting and regeneration; and without injury, spontaneous motor collateral sprouting and regeneration did not occur [5,6].

Dr. Paul Guelinckx's work was critical in demonstrating the importance of maintaining the original muscle tendon configuration and demonstrating that a tenotomy had a more negative influence on overall motor functional recovery than appropriate end-to-end nerve repair [7]. Great advances in understanding the internal topography of the peripheral nerve showed me that operating within the nerve itself was not only possible, but also important in managing complex nerve injuries.

Key work by Dr. Tom Brushart showed that, while there was plexus formation between the fascicles in the proximal extremity, the topographical organization of the motor fibers specific to any given muscle was distinctly organized within the nerve [8]. Important work on the understanding of muscle denervation and reinnervation from Dr. Bill Kuzon's laboratory combined to provide the critical ingredients for the clinical introduction of nerve transfers.

I have kept a copy of *Hand Clinics* on tendon transfers published in 1974 in my bookcase for decades and refer to it frequently [9]. The authors of that issue, John A. Boswick, Paul W. Brown, William E. Burkhalter, Raymond M. Curtis, J. Leonard Goldner, George E. Omer, and Daniel C. Riordan, were all giants in tendon transfer technique. I hope that this issue of *Hand Clinics* on nerve transfers will be referred to with similar appreciation in years to come.

Appendix 1

Postdoctoral research fellows

1983: Victoria Bojanowski, University of Toronto, Toronto, Ontario, Canada
1984: James P. O'Brien, University of Toronto, Toronto, Ontario, Canada
1985–88: James R. Bain, University of Toronto, Toronto, Ontario, Canada
1986–89: Akiro Makino, Tokyo, Japan
1988–92: Peter J. Evans, University of Toronto, Toronto, Ontario, Canada
1989–91: Tomoo Maeda, Kobe University, Kobe, Japan
1989–91: Timothy J. Best, University of Toronto, Toronto, Ontario, Canada

1990: J.M. Weinberger, University of Toronto, Toronto, Ontario, Canada
1990: Cynthia Mizgala, University of Toronto, Toronto, Ontario, Canada
1990: Philip Narini, University of Toronto, Toronto, Ontario, Canada
1990–92: Raj Midha, University of Toronto, Toronto, Ontario, Canada
1990–92: Christine B. Novak, University of Toronto, Toronto, Ontario, Canada
1991–93: Yasushi Nakao, Keio University, Tokyo, Japan
1991–92: Gregory Hare, University of Toronto, Toronto, Ontario, Canada
1991–92: Douglas Ball, MA/MD Program, Washington University School of Medicine, St. Louis, MO
1992–94: Catherine Hertl, Washington University School of Medicine, St. Louis, MO
1992–95: Jun Kobayashi, Kyoto University, Kyoto, Japan
1993–1994: Paul Francel, Washington University School of Medicine, St. Louis, MO
1993–95: Osamu Watanabe, Keio University, Tokyo, Japan
1993–95: Suzanne Strasberg, Washington University School of Medicine, St. Louis, MO
1993–94: John Jensen, Washington University School of Medicine, St. Louis, MO
1994–95: Gregory Tarasidis, Washington University School of Medicine, St. Louis, MO
1995–96: Eric Genden, Washington University School of Medicine, St. Louis, MO
1996–97: Robert McDonald, Washington University School of Medicine, St. Louis, MO
1996–98: Vaishali Doolabh, Washington University School of Medicine, St. Louis, MO
1996–97: Arthur Atchabahian, Faculté De Médeciné Broussais-Hotel Dieu, Paris, France
1998–99: John Jensen. Washington University School of Medicine, St. Louis, MO
1999–2000: Aaron Grand, Washington University School of Medicine, St. Louis, MO
1999–2000: Terry Myckatyn, University of British Columbia, Vancouver, British Columbia, Canada
1999–2000: Barbara Robillard, Washington University School of Medicine, St. Louis, MO
2000–01: Subhro Sen, Northwestern University, Chicago, IL
2001–03: Michael Brenner, Washington University School of Medicine, St. Louis, MO
2002–04: Ida Fox, Rochester University, Rochester, NY

2003–05: Christopher Nichols, University of Florida–Gainsville, Gainsville, Florida

2004–2005: Jason Hess, Wright State School of Medicine

2005–2006: Ryan Lugenbuhl, Washington University in St. Louis, St. Louis, MO

2005–2007: Arash Moradzadeh, Washington University in St. Louis, St. Louis, MO

2006–2008: Christine Magill, Washington University in St. Louis, St. Louis, MO

2006–2007: David Kawamura, Washington University in St. Louis, St. Louis, MO

2007–2008: Nancy Solowski, Washington University in St. Louis, St. Louis, MO

2007–2008: Elizabeth Whitlock, Washington University in St. Louis, St. Louis, MO

2007–2009: Amy Moore, Washington University in St. Louis, St. Louis, MO

2008–2009: Rahul Kasukurthi, Washington University in St. Louis, St. Louis, MO

2008–2009: Zachary Ray, Washington University in St. Louis, St. Louis, MO

1981–Present: Daniel Hunter (Research Assistant), Washington University in St. Louis, St. Louis, MO

Susan E. Mackinnon, MD
Division of Plastic and Reconstructive Surgery
Department of Surgery
Washington University School of Medicine
660 South Euclid, Box 8238
St. Louis, MO 63110, USA

E-mail address: mackinnons@wustl.edu

References

[1] Noble J, Munro CA, Prasad VS, et al. Analysis of upper and lower extremity peripheral nerve injuries in a population of patients with multiple injuries. J Trauma 1998;45:116–22.

[2] Nichols CM, Brenner MJ, Fox IK, et al. Effects of motor versus sensory nerve grafts on peripheral nerve regeneration. Exp Neurol 2004;190:347–55.

[3] Lloyd BM, Luginbuhl RD, Brenner MJ, et al. Use of motor nerve material in peripheral nerve repair with conduits. Microsurgery 2007;27:138–45.

[4] Moradzadeh A, Borschel GH, Luciano JP, et al. The impact of motor and sensory nerve architecture on nerve regeneration. Experimental Neurology 2008; 212:370–6.

[5] Pannucci C, Myckatyn TM, Mackinnon SE, et al. End-to-side nerve repair: Review of the literature. Restorative Neurology and Neuroscience 2007; 25(1):45–63.

[6] Hayashi A, Pannucchi C, Moradzadeh A, et al. Axotomy or compression is required for axonal sprouting following end-to-side neurorrhaphy. Experimental Neurology 2008;211(2):539–50.

[7] Guelinckx PJ, Carlson BM, Faulkner JA. Morphologic characteristics of muscles grafted in rabbits with neurovascular repair. J Recons Microsurg 1992;8(6): 481–9.

[8] Brushart TM. Central course of digital axons within the median nerve of Macaca mulatta. J Comp Neurol 1991;311(2):197–209.

[9] Tendon transfers in the upper extremity. Orthop Clin North Am 1974;5(2).

ELSEVIER
SAUNDERS

Hand Clin 24 (2008) xiii

HAND
CLINICS

Preface

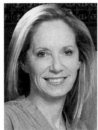
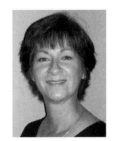

Susan E. Mackinnon, MD   Christine B. Novak, PT, MS, PhD(c)
Guest Editors

This issue of *Hand Clinics* introduces surgeons to the merits and virtues of nerve transfers, and much of what is presented here has yet to reach standard textbooks. We have invited a number of our colleagues to share their expertise and insight with the readers of *Hand Clinics*.

Drs. Anastakis, Malessy, Chen, Davis, and Mikulis describe the important central changes that occur with peripheral "re-wiring." Drs. Lien, Cederna, and Kuzon review important work on the effect of muscle denervation and the response to reinnervation. Drs. Bengston, Spinner, Bishop, Kaufman, Coleman-Wood, Kircher, and Shin present their experience with brachial plexus reconstruction and measuring outcomes. Dr. Terzis and coauthors Drs. Kokkalis and Kostopoulous provide a clinical review of using contralateral C7 transfers in adult plexopathies. Dr. Colbert and I review some of the nerve transfers that are used currently, and Dr. Kozin gives his perspective on nerve transfers in the obstetric and pediatric population. Drs. Dvali and Myckatyn contribute an update on end-to-side nerve regeneration.

We are fortunate to have several eminent international contributors. Dr. Millesi, a pioneer of nerve grafting, his coauthor, Dr. Schmidhammer from Austria and Dr. Chuang from Taiwan, have extraordinary experience with nerve reconstruction and have provided comprehensive reviews. Finally,

the important aspects of motor reeducation to maximize patient outcome are presented.

We sincerely thank all of the authors for their significant contributions to this extraordinary edition of *Hand Clinics*. Together, we have treated patients in clinical practice for decades, and it is our opinion that the use of nerve transfers has resulted in a positive paradigm shift in patient outcome and in the results obtainable for many peripheral nerve injuries. It is our hope that the readers of this publication will benefit from the expertise of the contributors and share our enthusiasm regarding the expanded use of nerve transfers in patients who have traumatic peripheral nerve injuries.

Susan E. Mackinnon, MD
Division of Plastic and Reconstructive Surgery
Department of Surgery
Washington University School of Medicine
660 South Euclid, Box 8238
St. Louis, MO 63110, USA

E-mail address: mackinnon@wustl.edu

Christine B. Novak, PT, MS, PhD(c)
Research Associate
University Health Network
8N-875, 200 Elizabeth Street
Toronto, Ontario M5G 2C4, Canada

E-mail address: christine.novak@utoronto.ca

Nerve Transfers in the Forearm and Hand

Justin M. Brown, MD[a],*, Susan E. Mackinnon, MD[b]

[a]Department of Neurological Surgery, Division of Plastic and Reconstructive Surgery, Washington University
School of Medicine, 660 South Euclid Avenue, Campus Box 8057, St. Louis, MO 63110-1093, USA
[b]Division of Plastic and Reconstructive Surgery, Department of Surgery, Washington University School of Medicine,
660 South Euclid, Box 8238, St. Louis, MO 63110, USA

Injuries to nerves that provide strength and sensation to the forearm and hand can result from a number of sources at a variety of locations. Transection, traction, contusion, gunshot wounds, ischemia and compression (including compartment syndromes), electrical injury, thermal injury, injection injury, irradiation injury, and iatrogenic injury are among those commonly listed [1]. The authors would add brachial plexus neuritis to this list because it seems to be a more frequently recognized cause that can result in injuries ranging from diffuse paralysis of the shoulder girdle and upper arm to discrete deficits within the forearm and hand [2]. Essentially any source of trauma or exposure, from the nerve roots at the cervical foramina to the digital nerves of the hand, has the potential to injure or disrupt a peripheral nerve and affect function at the level of the hand and wrist. When these injuries produce a Sunderland fourth- or fifth-degree injury, precluding the successful re-extension of axons, the only hope for recovery is surgical intervention [3].

A number of situations exist for which traditional nerve repairs offer little hope of useful neurologic recovery [4,5]. Alternative strategies must be considered for delayed presentation following injury, for very proximal injuries, including nerve-root avulsions, and for injuries that result in significant tissue loss or large neuromas-in-continuity [4,6–11]. In addition, injuries with excessive scarring at the primary injury site (exploration of which may endanger surrounding structures), in which the site of injury is unclear (as in an idiopathic neuritis or radiation injury), and which involve multiple levels of the nerve present similar challenges to the classic approach [5,7,11]. In the authors' experience, a patient who has a neurologic deficit is managed most appropriately with a functional goal rather in mind rather than an anatomic goal. In fact, nerve injuries with a discrete motor or sensory deficit usually are addressed best by a functionally targeted nerve transfer [12–15].

In the forearm, vital and expendable functions within each nerve distribution have been identified. Tendon transfers attempt to use these conventions to maximize function and minimize disability [16–18]. Although tendon transfers often can supply useful functional improvement, muscle reinnervation has the potential to provide a more physiologic and adaptive solution to these impairments [4].

During the past decade the central nervous system's ability to register effective function to even the most creative nerve transfers has been demonstrated [19–21]. Brachial plexus surgery has been revolutionized by this concept [6,8,22–24]. An understanding of the redundancy of innervation to particular muscle groups or movements has enabled the peripheral nerve surgeon to identify a number of options for donor nerves or fascicles within the forearm [4,5,7]. Timely use of these donor nerves for local nerve transfers offers a more reliable outcome in a shorter period of time than that provided by nerve grafting. A more natural, functional reconstruction than that provided by tendon transfers can be realized [25,26]. The authors now commonly use nerve transfers as the primary and definitive solution for many nerve injuries.

* Corresponding author.
E-mail address: brownjm@nsurg.wustl.edu
(J.M. Brown).

For a denervated distal stump, the best available donor nerve with which to restore axons and reverse the resulting deficit is selected. In the authors' algorithm, this selection is undertaken without bias for the original axon source unless it is the candidate most likely to provide a good result. Considerations for potential donor nerves include proximity to the target muscle, primary axon type, donor–recipient size match, axon number, and synergistic function of the original muscle compared with that of the recipient muscle [4,26]. A number of nerve transfers have been developed to address deficits in the forearm and hand that can simplify the approach to hand dysfunction and frequently provide a better clinical result than achieved with more traditional interventions.

Radial nerve deficits

Radial nerve injury results in the loss of finger and wrist extension, rendering the hand essentially useless [27,28]. With early grafting, this nerve is more amenable to successful repair than the median or ulnar nerves [28,29]. In many situations, however, nerve regeneration is precluded or inadequate for useful recovery [29,30]. In these cases a well-developed set of tendon transfers usually is proposed [27]. Although these tendon transfers are some of the most reliable available, they have been found by some to produce unnatural ergonomics and a lack of power grip [31,32]. In a review of 49 cases by Dunnet and colleagues [33], more than 80% of patients reported a loss of endurance, and more than 66% reported impaired coordination and dexterity.

The radial nerve's contribution to finger and wrist extension via the posterior interosseous nerve (PIN) and the extensor carpi radialis brevis (ECRB) are essential. Although it is only one of several muscles involved in wrist extension, the contribution of the ECRB alone is strong and functional. Therefore the PIN and ECRB are the authors' primary targets for restoration of radial nerve function.

In patients who have a radial nerve deficit but an intact median nerve, nerve transfers can be performed using branches to the flexor digitorum superficialis (FDS) (usually two branches are available), which are directed to the ECRB branch, and branches to the flexor carpi radialis (FCR) and palmaris longus (PL), which are redirected to the PIN (Fig. 1). Because strong wrist extension is essential for maximal grip, the ECRB should be the recipient of the strongest donor [10]. If possible, pairing the finger flexion from the FDS with wrist extension from the ECRB and wrist flexion from the FCR with finger extension via the PIN can provide complementarity. This strategy reproduces the tenodesis effect and can facilitate motor re-education [34]. Other potential sources of innervation are the branches of the ulnar nerve to the flexor carpi ulnaris (FCU), which can be identified via an additional incision in the forearm [11]. Pairing this branch of the ulnar nerve with the PIN should have the same complementary effect as produced by pairing the FCR with the PIN.

To provide some limited early hand function while the nerve is regenerating, the authors occasionally have used an internal splint to hold the wrist in extension using the familiar tenodesis of pronator teres to ECRB (Fig. 2) [10]. A recent study has indicated that this technique may limit effective active pronation of the extremity [35], but the authors have not encountered this problem, and they find this approach useful in appropriate patients.

The median to radial transfer: technique

With the patient under general anesthesia and an arm tourniquet in place, a lazy S incision is made over the proximal volar forearm, starting in the antecubital fossa and extending half the distance to the wrist crease. Care is taken to avoid the branches of the lateral antebrachial cutaneous nerve (LABC), which accompanies the cephalic or accessory cephalic vein. The lacertus fibrosus then is identified and incised.

The fascia is opened, and the radial vessels are found superficially between the pronator teres and the brachioradialis. Attention is directed to the radial side of these vessels within the distal half of the incision. Here the tendon of the superficial head of the pronator teres is identified by retracting the brachioradialis laterally and the radial vessels medially. A step-lengthening of this tendon is performed to release the superficial head of the pronator teres. The pronator teres muscle then is retracted medially, exposing the median nerve in the proximal aspect of the incision, deep and ulnar to the radial vessels (Fig. 3). To follow the median nerve distally, the deep head of the pronator teres is identified and divided. Likewise the tendinous arch of the FDS then is released (Fig. 4). The median nerve then is adequately exposed, and the major branches of the median nerve can be identified.

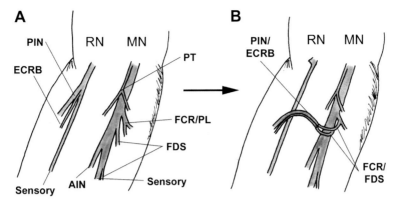

Fig. 1. Median to radial nerve transfer. (*A, B*) Depending on the integrity of other sources of wrist and finger flexion, median branches to FDS, FCR, and PL can be used to restore innervation to key wrist and finger extensors. AIN, anterior interosseous nerve; ECRB, branch to extensor carpi radialis brevis; FCR, branch to flexor carpi radialis; FDS, branches to flexor digitorum superficialis; MN, median nerve; PIN, posterior interosseous nerve; PL, branch to palmaris longus; RN, radial nerve.

The branch to the pronator teres is found most proximal and takes off from the volar surface of the nerve. It quickly divides into two branches. Next, the branches to the FCR and PL are found more distally on the ulnar side of the nerve followed by the branches to the FDS. At this

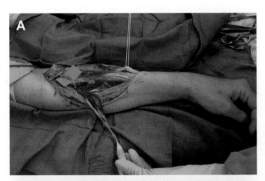

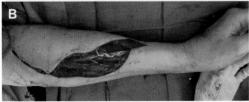

Fig. 2. Adjunctive internal splint: pronator teres to ECRB tendon transfer. (*A*) With a distal extension of the same incision, the pronator teres (mobilized and held in pickups) can be mobilized and tenodesed to the ECRB tendon (lifted with vessel loop) for early wrist extension. (*B*) The completed transfer allows for some early function during the interval between nerve transfer and successful reinnervation.

level, the larger-caliber anterior interosseous nerve (AIN) begins to deviate from the radial aspect of the median nerve (Fig. 5). It is the authors' practice to apply electrical stimulation (Veristim; Medtronic) to each of the branches to confirm their identity and innervation.

To expose the branches of the radial nerve, the brachioradialis is retracted, and the radial sensory nerve is found directly beneath the muscle. Once identified, this nerve is followed proximally to the main trunk of the PIN. As the radial sensory nerve is followed proximally, the crossing vessels of the leash of Henry are divided. At this level, the PIN and the branch to the ERCB can be visualized just deep and radial to the sensory branch (Fig. 6). The nerves are followed as far proximally as can be visualized safely and are transected at this level. The PIN then is followed distally and is released through the leading edge of the supinator. This release removes any compression on the nerve that could impede neural regeneration [36,37] and allows additional mobilization for a tension-free coaptation. Further dissection of the PIN to exclude the branch to the supinator muscle also may enhance the mobilization of the nerve. Removing the radial branch and the supinator should not affect supination, which still is provided effectively by the biceps. Removing the supinator muscle as a potential target allows all transferred axons to be directed to the primary functions of finger and wrist extension (Fig. 7).

With the recipient nerve mobilized and transposed, the donor nerve is identified and is followed

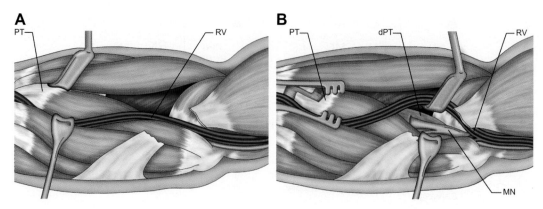

Fig. 3. Identification of the median nerve. Schematic of the right forearm. (*A*) Step-lengthening the tendon of the pronator teres provides effective retraction of this muscle. (*B*) This retraction facilitates identification of the proximal median nerve within the flexor-pronator muscle mass. dPT, deep head of pronator teres; MN, median nerve; PT, tendon of pronator teres muscle; RV, radial vessels.

distally into the muscle where it is transected with as much length as possible. Sufficient branches from the donor nerve to match the size of the recipient nerve should be included in the transfer. A tension-free coaptation of the donors (eg, FDS and FCR) to the recipients (PIN and ECRB) is undertaken using 9-0 nylon suture (Fig. 8).

Restoration of sensation to the radial sensory nerve distribution

The LABC is an excellent donor nerve for restoration of sensation to the dorsum of the hand via the radial sensory nerve. At the level of the mid-forearm these two nerves run essentially

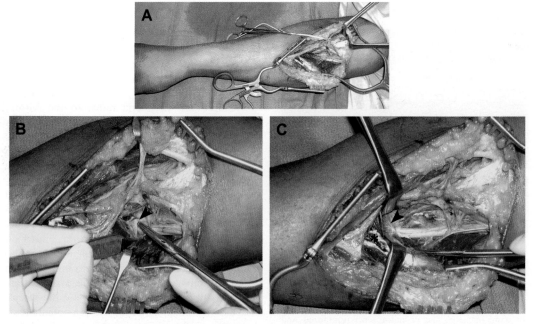

Fig. 4. Exposure of the median nerve. This technique provides exposure of all the branches that must be identified for this transfer. (*A*) Right volar forearm. (*B*) The median nerve exposure is carried distally by releasing the pronator teres (PT) through its deep head (*arrowhead*). (*C*) Following this, the exposure is completed by releasing the leading edge (*arrowhead*) of the flexor digitorum superficialis muscle fascia. The step-lengthened incision (*) on the PT tendon also is visible.

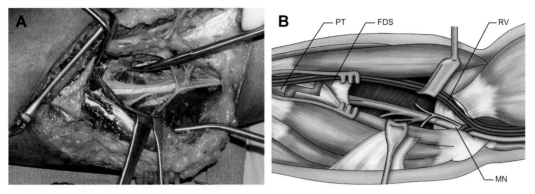

Fig. 5. Branches of the median nerve. (*A, B*) Volar forearm photograph and schematic. Moving proximal to distal or right to left, the sequence of branches is 1) pronator teres (PT) (*yellow*), 2) branch to flexor carpi radialis (FCR) and branch to palmaris longus (PL) (*green*), 3) flexor digitorum superficialis (FDS) (*blue*), and, to the radial side, 4) anterior interosseous nerve (AIN) (*pink*). The sequence remains consistent, although variations in the number of branches to each of these muscle groups are found. FDS, flexor digitorum superficialis; MN, median nerve; RN, radial vessels.

parallel. The radial sensory nerve courses under the brachioradialis, and the LABC runs within the fascia upon its medial surface. The size match is excellent for a direct end-to-end repair, which should restore a broad area of sensation to the dorsum of the hand at the expense of the less critical distal LABC distribution (Fig. 9). Because the quality of sensation is not critical in the radial-innervated dorsum of the hand, the authors also have used a strategy of end-to-side coaptation of the radial sensory branch to the median nerve distal to the takeoff of the AIN.

Although end-to-side nerve transfers have been used in a number of clinical scenarios [38–40], experimental data have shown that in the absence of some degree of injury to the donor nerve only

sensory axons traverse this repair [41–43]. The axons transmitted as a result of this technique are not expected to provide much more than protective sensation but do so via a method that prevents noticeable downgrading within the donor territory. As a result, the authors favor this technique for noncritical regions of the hand that would benefit from protective sensation, including the dorsum of the hand and the third and fourth web spaces.

Median nerve deficit

The median nerve provides the most important contribution to hand and finger flexion,

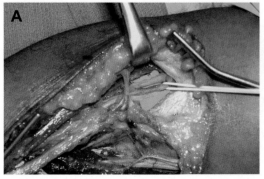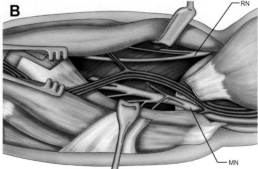

Fig. 6. (*A, B*) Branches of the radial nerve under the retracted brachioradialis. After following the radial sensory nerve proximally to the level of the elbow crease, the rest of the radial nerve can be identified. Superior to inferior are the posterior interosseous nerve (PIN) (*blue*), the nerve to the extensor carpi radialis brevis (ECRB) (*green*), which is looped and retracted, and the radial sensory branch (*yellow*). MN, median nerve; RN, radial nerve.

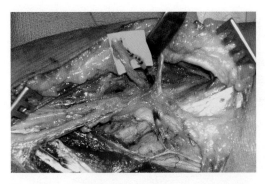

Fig. 7. Nerve to the supinator. After transecting the motor portion of the radial nerve, the nerve to the supinator (marked with purple dots) tethers most proximally as it enters the substance of the supinator muscle. This branch should be neurolysed away, if possible, or simply cut to release its tethering effect on the remainder of the bundle.

particularly to the radial three digits. In addition, it supplies forearm pronation, thumb opposition, and sensation to the regions of the hand, which are essential for fine manipulation (Fig. 10) [28,44]. The primary mechanical goal of any intervention to address a median nerve injury is to restore thumb opposition as well as innervation to the flexor pollicis longus and index finger flexor digitorum profundus (FDP) [45].

Thumb opposition

Loss of thumb opposition that is associated with thenar atrophy is the usual sequela of a median nerve injury of any level. Rarely, anomalous thenar innervation from the ulnar nerve will preserve opposition, and this innervation must be assessed carefully [45]. With denervation of the thenar muscles, direct repair of its motor fascicle or repair with an interposition graft remains the preferred intervention. When this anatomy is disrupted, however, anatomic repair

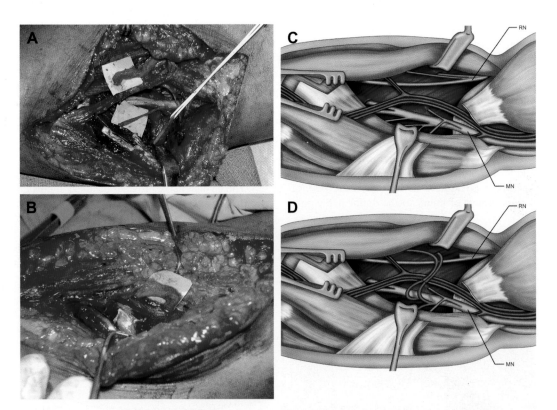

Fig. 8. The median to radial transfer. (*C*) following exposure of pertinent branches of the median and radial nerves, (*A*) the motor branches of the radial nerve are cut proximally and transposed toward the median nerve. This mobilization and transposition should include the release of the PIN through the supinator and exclusion of the branch to the supinator. (*B, D*) The median branches (*green*) are transected at their entry into the muscles that they supply and coapted to the proximal cut end of the ECRB and PIN branches of the radial nerve. MN, median nerve; RN, radial nerve.

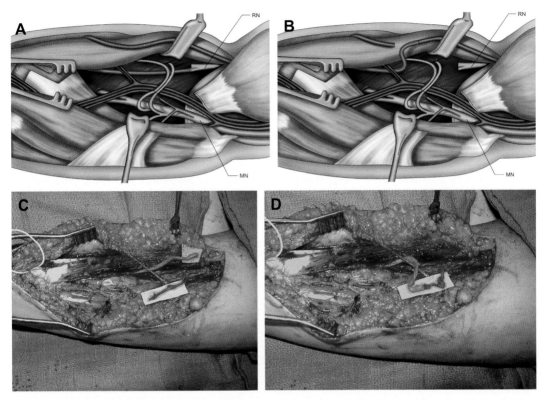

Fig. 9. Nerve transfer to restore radial sensation to the hand. (*A*) Freeing the LABC (*green*) from the fascia of the superficial surface of the brachioradialis (*B*) allows easy transposition to the radial sensory branch (*pink*), which runs parallel to it just underneath this muscle. (*C, D*) This anatomy allows ease of mobilization and effortless tension-free repair. MN, median nerve; RN, radial nerve.

may deliver less than desirable results because the nerve at this level is primarily sensory, and motor topography proximally becomes unclear [4,46,47]. In this situation nerve grafting can lead to aberrant regeneration of sensory fibers into the motor pathways, resulting in no thenar function.

Tendon transfers for thumb opposition are very effective, but these operative procedures require postoperative immobilization and produce unusual ergonomics. A nerve transfer from the terminal branch of the AIN supplying the pronator quadratus should be considered in

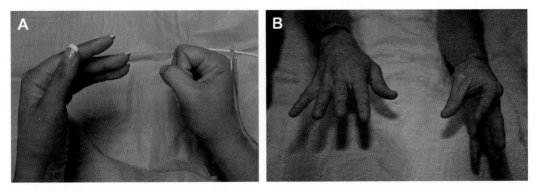

Fig. 10. Median nerve deficits. Median nerve injuries can result in (*A*) loss of flexion of the radial three digits and (*B*) loss of pronation, severely limiting the functionality of the extremity.

appropriate cases [47]. The nerve at this level is comprised of predominantly motor fibers with just a few sensory branches that innervate the wrist joint [48]. Although the number of axons in each of these nerves is comparable (about 900 in the distal AIN and about 1050 in the recurrent motor branch [47,49]), the necessary interposition graft downgrades the actual number of axons that reach the thenar muscles. Both animal studies and clinical evaluations have demonstrated the usefulness of such an intervention [50,51]. Transfer of this nerve is well tolerated with minimal donor-site morbidity [47,48]. If the median injury is discrete, and the AIN remains intact, this nerve transfer can be considered [47].

Anterior interosseous nerve to median recurrent motor branch transfer: technique

A carpal tunnel incision is extended approximately 2 inches proximal to the distal wrist crease. The median nerve is identified within the carpal tunnel and is followed distally to the takeoff of the recurrent motor branch toward the thenar eminence. Once this feature is identified, the branch is neurolysed from the remainder of the median nerve as proximally as possible until either its cut end is encountered or it forms a plexus precluding further mobilization. The flexor tendons then are retracted within the distal forearm to allow

exposure of both the median nerve and the pronator quadratus. The neurovascular bundle can be visualized entering the proximal edge of the pronator quadratus. The muscle belly is separated over the course of the nerve using tenotomy scissors. The nerve is followed as distally as possible until it arborizes fully into the muscle, usually just before its mid-portion. The nerve is transected at this point. An interposition graft (usually medial antebrachial cutaneous or sural) then is coapted to this nerve and is laid along the trajectory of the median nerve. The proximal end of the recurrent motor branch then is transected. If it has been divided already as a result of the original trauma, it must be trimmed back until soft, healthy-appearing nerve is encountered. This cut end then is coapted to the distal portion of the nerve graft in a tension-free manner. The wrist range of motion should be tested before trimming the graft to ensure that extension will not produce undue tension on the repair (Fig. 11).

In a high median nerve injury, the AIN will not be available for use as a donor nerve. Alternative nerve transfers have been described such as an ulnar to median nerve transfer in the hand using the third lumbrical motor branch [52] and a radial to median nerve transfer using the PIN branches to the extensor digiti quinti and extensor carpi ulnaris via an interposition nerve graft. In this

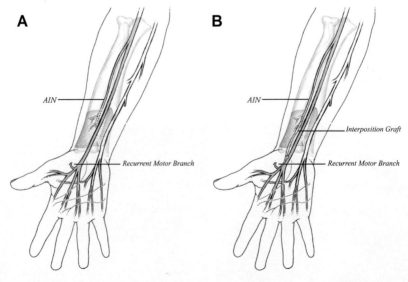

Fig. 11. Distal AIN to median recurrent motor branch transfer. (*A, B*) The axons of the distal AIN are redirected to the recurrent motor branch of the median nerve via a short interposition graft. Yellow = functional nerve; pink = region of dysfunction. (*Adapted from* Colbert SH, Mackinnon SE. Nerve transfers in the hand and upper extremity. Tech Hand Up Extrem Surg 2008;12:20–33; with permission.)

situation the authors prefer to use standard tendon transfers or the AIN transfer described earlier in the rare instance that its function is preserved.

Median nerve sensory restoration

Median nerve sensation is essential for fine motor tasks [53]. Many surgeons believe that the success of restoration of motor function following a median nerve injury is determined largely by the quality of hand sensation [45]. Additionally, some have proposed that restoring sensation is a prerequisite to restoring motor function [54].

Restoring sensation to the radial side of the index finger and the ulnar side of the thumb are priorities in median nerve palsy [4]. The median nerve–innervated third web space (when preserved, as in an upper trunk brachial plexus injury), the ulnar nerve–innervated fourth web space, and the radial nerve–innervated dorsum of the hand are less critical sensory distributions and therefore represent the sources from which local axon donors can be recruited [54,55].

Although the time to reinnervation is not as crucial in sensory restoration as in motor restoration, standard nerve grafting in proximal injuries can result in delays of more than a year until the recovery of even protective sensation. Function of the hand is severely limited during this period of sensory denervation, and the possibility of undetected injury and subsequent ulceration within this critical region of the hand remains a concern [13,45].

In a pure median nerve injury, the authors' preferred strategy for sensory restoration involves transfer of the ulnar-innervated fourth web space common digital nerve to the median-innervated first web space (radial aspect of the index finger and digital nerves to the thumb) via a direct end-to-end repair. Secondarily, restoration of sensation to the donor fourth web space and median-innervated third web space can be achieved using an end-to-side technique as described previously. In this case the ulnar digital nerve of the small finger is the axon source. This procedure can restore protective sensation to these digits without a noticeable downgrading of the ulnar sensation (Fig. 12).

Nerve transfers for median sensory deficit: technique

A carpal tunnel incision is used with Bruner-type zigzag extensions toward the first and fourth web spaces. Following division of the transverse carpal ligament, the branches of the median nerve can be followed to the first and the fourth web space (Fig. 13). The digital arteries and superficial palmar arch, which lie superficial to the plane of the nerves in the palm, must be protected. After the fourth web space branch is identified, this branch is transected at the level of the metacarpal heads and then is lifted and dissected free from the surrounding tissues. The nerves to the first web space, including the radial aspect of the index finger and the radial and ulnar aspect of the thumb, then are identified distally and followed proximally. This dissection involves careful separation of this branch from the main median nerve trunk. Once sufficient lengths of the donor and recipient nerves have been mobilized to allow a tension-free coaptation, the branch of the median nerve to the first web space is transected proximally and is mobilized to meet the cut end of the fourth web space. An end-to-end coaptation is performed with 9-0 nylon suture.

Upper plexus sensory restoration

In an upper trunk brachial plexus injury, sensation to the third web space is preserved and can be transferred using a similar approach. Because the innervation to this web space is comprised of a distinct fascicle of the nerve that can be neurolysed reliably quite proximally, this transfer can be performed within the distal forearm (Fig. 14) [56]. Nerve coaptations within the hand can be avoided by using a single incision that exposes both the donor and recipient nerves in close proximity [57]. In addition, more of the radial side of the nerve can be covered, restoring sensation to a greater area of the thumb, and the repair is simpler and faster to perform.

Intramedian nerve transfer for sensory loss caused by upper plexus injury: technique

A carpal tunnel incision is used and is extended into the forearm via a zigzag extension across the wrist. The transverse carpal ligament then is released to allow adequate exposure of the distal nerve and to remove any compression-related impediment nerve regeneration [36,37]. The median nerve begins to separate into its components within the distal carpal canal. At this level, the fascicles can be identified, and their destination can be presumed according to the lateral to medial order of the fascicles, corresponding to their numbered web spaces. These fascicles then are traced proximally, either by neurolysing them physically from the main nerve or simply by following the segregation visually. The fascicles to the first through third web spaces should be distinct up

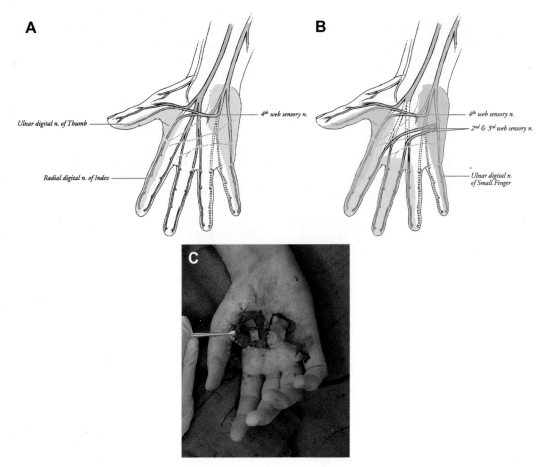

Fig. 12. Sensory transfers for median nerve anesthesia. Nerve transfers within the hand for median nerve sensation. (*A, C*) Fourth to first transfer followed by (*B*) end-to-side strategy for remaining deficits. Yellow = functional nerves or regions of sensation; lighter yellow = lesser quality of sensation; pink = nonfunctional nerves. (*Adapted from* Colbert SH, Mackinnon SE. Nerve transfers in the hand and upper extremity. Tech Hand Up Extrem Surg 2008;12:20–33; with permission.)

to 13 mm above the radial styloid and even more proximally in some cases [56]. The recurrent motor branch must be excluded during this dissection and addressed separately, as discussed previously. Within the wrist, the fascicles to the first and third web spaces are neurolysed from the rest of the nerve, and a loop is placed on each fascicle. The authors recommend the inclusion of the fascicles to the radial border of the thumb with the first web space fascicle to provide sensory coverage to the thumb (Fig. 15).

In the authors' experience, sensory nerve transfers to the first web space have provided moderate sensation, around 4 to 8 out of 10 as measured by the Ten Test [58]. Although the authors have presented their preferred transfers for this deficit, other successfully implemented transfers have included the superficial radial nerve (either at the

web space or the wrist) or the dorsal cutaneous branch of the ulnar nerve [54,55]. These transfers are less ideal because the donor nerve innervates a larger territory, and pain related to recruiting the radial nerve can be a concern [55,57]. As a result, these donor nerves are rarely used.

For sensory transfers, it is important to consider the newly transected proximal ends of the nerves to which the transfers are being made. If there is potential for future axon outgrowth from these severed nerves, they must be directed either into a distal target or into the deep tissues of the forearm to prevent future formation of a painful neuroma [57].

Flexion and pronation

In proximal nerve injuries, once the reconstructive strategies for restoration of opposition

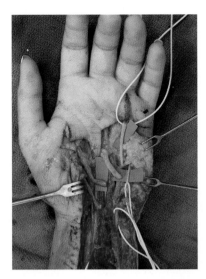

Fig. 13. Exposure for sensory nerve transfers in the hand. Bruner zigzag extensions of the carpal tunnel incision provide exposure of all digital nerves within the palm for transfer.

and sensation have been established, attention can be directed to the restoration of finger flexion and forearm pronation. With an appropriately timed proximal nerve repair or graft, extrinsic muscle function often can be restored [59]. If this restoration is not possible, finger flexion can be reconstructed with side-to-side suturing of the FDP tendons of the index and long finger to the conjoint tendons of the ulnar-innervated ring and small fingers in addition to a transfer of the extensor carpi radialis longus to the index FDP tendon [45]. The authors have found that flexion can be restored effectively to the index finger and thumb by using the corresponding nerve transfers. The ECRB branch of the radial nerve (with or without its contribution to the supinator) can be used to reinnervate the AIN directly without a graft in a tension-free manner [7].

Nerve transfer for restoration of anterior interosseous nerve function: technique

By using the volar forearm exposure described for the median to radial nerve transfer, the tendon of the superficial head of the pronator teres is lengthened, and this muscle is retracted to expose the median nerve. The AIN is identified as it deviates from the radial side of the main trunk of the median nerve. If the AIN is not readily discernable as a discrete fascicle, then a longitudinally oriented prominent vessel commonly marks

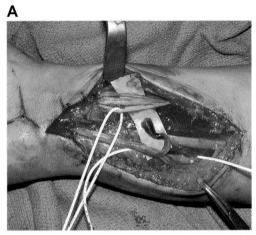

A

B

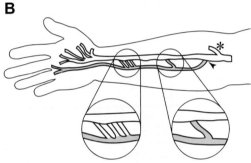

Fig. 14. Anatomy of the median third webspace sensory fascicle. (*A*) The anatomy of the median third webspace sensory contribution has been elucidated carefully. (*B*) Understanding of its reliable location and plexus formation enables its use in several transfers at the level of the wrist. (*Adapted from* Ross D. Intraneural anatomy of the median nerve provides "third web space" donor nerve graft. J Reconstr Microsurg 1992;8(3):231; with permission.)

the cleavage plane between the AIN and the remainder of the median nerve. Gently tapping with the tips of the micro-pickups across the transverse diameter of the median nerve often demonstrates this cleavage as it dips into this interval (Fig. 16). Once the AIN is identified, separated, and looped, attention is turned to the radial nerve exposure.

As described previously, the radial sensory nerve is identified under the brachioradialis and is followed a few centimeters proximally toward the antecubital fossa until the PIN and branch to the ERCB are visualized. These nerves then are followed distally until the PIN enters the arcade of Frohse. The branch to the ERCB continues past the supinator muscle, parallel to but separate from the radial sensory branch. This branch

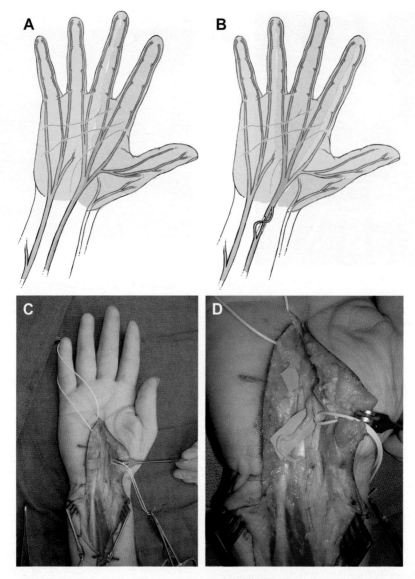

Fig. 15. Sensory transfers for upper plexus injury. (*A*) Anesthesia of the first two webspaces (*pink*) frequently follows an upper plexus injury. (*C*) After internal neurolysis, the medial to lateral positions of the fascicle indicate their ultimate webspace destination. (*B, D*) Cutting and transposing the proximal third webspace fascicle to the first webspace fascicle can rerout quality sensation to this more critical region of the hand.

should be followed as far distally as possible. Several centimeters of the nerve usually are obtainable. If possible, the nerve is transected at the interface with the ERCB muscle belly. If the size discrepancy between this nerve and the AIN is significant, the authors recommend also including the supinator branch of the PIN. To allow some mobilization of the PIN for neurolysis of the supinator branch, the PIN is released at the arcade of Frohse. With retraction of the PIN,

the supinator branch is transected as it enters into the supinator muscle. The AIN then is neurolysed further from the median nerve several centimeters proximally and, if possible, as far as the ante-cubital fossa. If only the branch to the ECRB is used, this proximal dissection will be less imper-ative given its length and accessibility. When the branch to the supinator is used, the proximal mobilization of the AIN is more critical, because the length of the supinator branch is much shorter

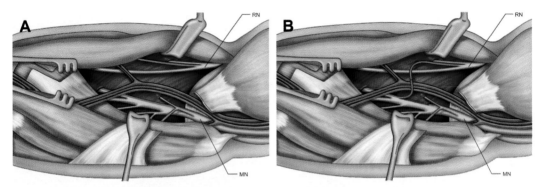

Fig. 16. Radial to median transfers for AIN function. (*A*) As in the median to radial transfer, the respective nerves are exposed, and branches are identified. (*B*) Mobilization of the ECRB branch (*green*) makes for a technically simple transfer to the AIN (*pink*). MN, median nerve; RN, radial nerve.

and less easily mobilized. If it is not possible to obtain sufficient proximal distance, the branch to the palmaris longus is included with the AIN to form the posterior fascicular group, which is separable well into the arm [60]. Once adequate length has been obtained, these groups (ERCB and supinator to AIN) are sutured end-to-end (see Fig. 16).

The authors have encountered an isolated palsy of the AIN in many clinical scenarios. In these cases they often have performed intramedian nerve transfers using branches of the FDS or PL/FCR to restore motor function to this vital median component (Fig. 17).

Once reconstructive strategies for grasp have been addressed, restoration of pronation should be considered. Even with excellent finger function, simple hand functions such as writing, typing, and throwing are difficult without active pronation. The authors have encountered situations in which partial loss of median nerve function has resulted in isolated loss of pronation [15,61]. The pronator teres muscle has less redundancy in the fascicles at the root level, leaving it more susceptible to denervation and loss of function even with proximal pathology. Loss of pronation is found frequently in C6-7 nerve root injuries, lower brachial plexus injuries, and high median nerve injuries. Successful nerve transfers to restore this function have included donors from the FDS, FCR, and FCU [4,5,10,15]. The authors recently have included the ERCB branch as a donor in this nerve transfer when the entire median nerve is involved. Because many actions, such as turning a doorknob, require the simultaneous use of wrist extension and pronation, the retraining

associated with this transfer is relatively intuitive.

Nerve transfer for restoration of pronator teres function: technique

As the median nerve enters the forearm, it gives off three distinct groups of branches. The first group innervates the pronator teres, the second group innervates the PL and FCR, and the third group innervates the FDS. The branches to the PL, FCR, and FDS usually branch from the ulnar side of the nerve, whereas the pronator teres branch exits from the volar aspect of the nerve proximal to the elbow crease and usually runs along its volar surface before dividing to reach the superficial and deep head of the pronator muscle. To facilitate the exposure of this branch, the incision described previously is extended proximal to the antecubital fossa. The tendon of the pronator teres is released, and the muscle is retracted as described previously. Retraction of the pronator teres frequently reveals a branch from the median nerve entering its underside. If this branch is not clearly discernable, the median nerve is followed proximally. The branch can be found exiting from the volar surface of the nerve 1 to 2 cm proximal to the medial epicondyle. Most commonly seen is a single exiting branch that bifurcates after reaching the forearm. The branch is followed distally to ensure its continuity with the pronator teres muscle. This branch then is looped, and the branch to the ECRB is retrieved as described previously. The pronator branches are transected at their exit from the median nerve. In the rare instance that the length is insufficient, an additional 2 to 3 cm can be neurolysed proximally from the main nerve. An end-to-end coaptation is performed (Fig. 18).

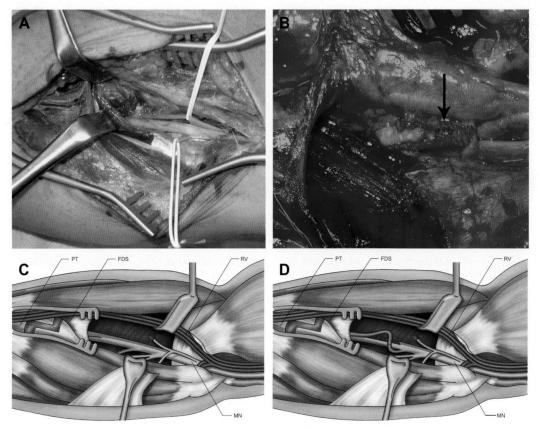

Fig. 17. Intramedian transfers for AIN function. (*A, B*) When the deficit is isolated to a single branch, exposure of the median nerve alone is sufficient. The arrow indicates the nerve tube used to cuff the sutured coaptation. (*C, D*) An expendable branch (in this case, a branch to the flexor digitorum superficialis, *green*) is selected and is transferred directly to the AIN (*pink*). FDS, flexor digitorum superficialis; MN, median nerve; PT, tendon of pronator teres; RV, radial vessels.

In a lower brachial plexus injury with loss of both median and ulnar nerve function, the brachialis branch of the musculocutaneous nerve and branches of the radial nerve may be considered potential donors for nerve transfer. Although the authors sometimes have used the branch to the brachioradialis and have preserved the ECRB branch for pronation, the use of the brachialis branch of the musculocutaneous has gained some popularity recently. The brachialis muscle usually is innervated by a single branch of the musculocutaneous nerve and can be mobilized for a significant length, making it relatively easy to transfer [62]. The brachialis motor branch usually carries more than 2000 axons and, with a normal biceps, loss of this muscle is reported to be inconsequential [63]. The authors argue that reinnervation of both biceps and brachialis is critical in

musculocutaneous palsy because a reinnervated muscle generates less power than its normal counterpart. Therefore this transfer should be considered only in a patient who has a normal biceps muscle.

Nerve transfer for restoration of anterior interosseous nerve function using the brachialis branch of the musculocutaneous nerve: technique

A curvilinear incision is made from the volar forearm 4 to 5 cm distal to the elbow crease that runs along the medial border of the brachioradialis. The incision is curved medially across the antecubital fossa and then is turned proximally again when the interval between the biceps and triceps muscle bellies is reached. This incision then is extended to approximately the midpoint of the arm. The LABC nerve is identified beside the

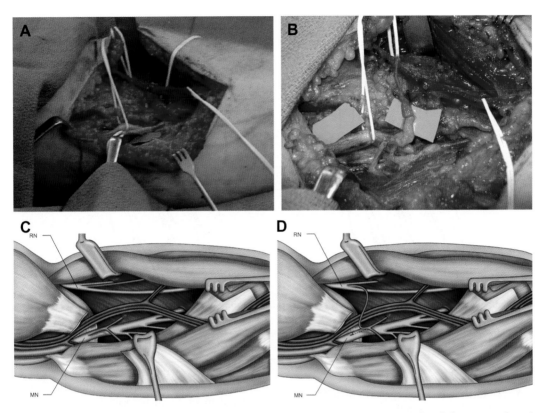

Fig. 18. Transfers for restoration of pronation. (*A, C*) Via the same volar forearm exposure, (*B, D*) the pronator branch (*pink*) is mobilized proximally and the ECRB (*green*) is mobilized distally for a tension-free repair. MN, median nerve, RN, radial nerve.

cephalic or accessory cephalic vein. A loop is placed around the LABC to assist in the identification of the musculocutaneous nerve. After the forearm fascia and lacertus fibrosus is opened, the pronator teres tendon is released, and the median nerve is exposed. The nerve is followed distally until the AIN can be discriminated clearly from the rest of the median nerve. A loop is placed on the nerve at this level. In the proximal region of the incision, the brachial fascia is opened widely and is extended to meet the opening in the lacertus fibrosus. As the dissection proceeds into the arm, the median nerve is identified and, just volar to this structure, the interval between the biceps and brachialis muscles is explored. The surgeon can identify the nerve easily by placing a finger into this interval and tugging on the looped LABC. Because the branch to the biceps muscle usually is in the more proximal portion of this incision in the mid-point of the arm, it should not be within the dissection. Therefore identification of the LABC and neurolysis of this branch from the

rest of the nerve should leave only the branch to the brachialis muscle, which can be followed into the muscle belly. These fascicles may be separated for several centimeters to allow easy mobilization of this nerve branch. The branch is marked with a loop, and attention is redirected to the distal aspect of the incision.

The AIN is dissected from the median nerve. This branch usually can be neurolysed from the main nerve for a significant distance proximally. If this length is insufficient, the branch to the palmaris longus muscle should be included with the AIN fascicle. The AIN and the branch to the palmaris longus form the posterior fascicular group, which can be neurolysed further proximally [64]. The two nerves usually can meet end-to-end in the distal third of the arm for a direct, tension-free coaptation [64]. If the palmaris longus is included in this nerve transfer, the authors recommend cutting this branch distally to avoid diverting axons from the more crucial deep flexors (Fig. 19).

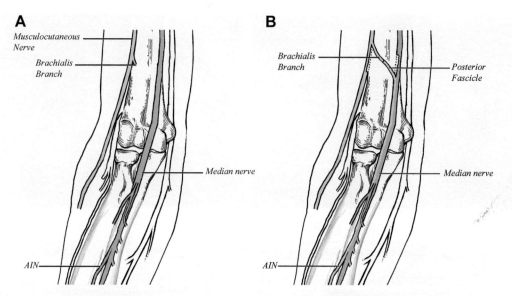

Fig. 19. Brachialis branch to AIN transfer. (*A, B*) Proximal mobilization of the AIN or the posterior fascicular group of the median nerve can allow direct coaptation to the brachialis branch of the musculocutaneous nerve. Yellow = a functional nerve or portion thereof; pink = a denervated or dysfunctional nerve or fascicular group. (*Adapted from* Colbert SH, Mackinnon SE. Nerve transfers in the hand and upper extremity. Tech Hand Up Extrem Surg 2008;12:20–33; with permission.)

Ulnar nerve deficits

Injury to the ulnar nerve results in significant pinch and grip weakness and clawing of the fourth and fifth digits [65]. In a proximal ulnar nerve injury, anatomic suture repair usually can restore protective sensation to the digits, but recovery of useful intrinsic motor function is uncommon even with early intervention [11,59,66]. Some hand surgeons have recommended distal tendon transfers be done at the time of proximal nerve repair [65], but tendon transfers have been found to give only limited results and are considered secondary salvage procedures in this situation [48,67].

When the injury does not involve the median nerve, the preferred nerve transfer to restore intrinsic function uses the distal AIN. The recipient motor branch of the ulnar nerve can be neurolysed up to 14 cm proximal to the radial styloid, providing sufficient length to perform a tension-free direct coaptation within the distal forearm (Fig. 20).

Transfer of the distal anterior interosseous nerve to the ulnar deep motor branch: technique

A carpal tunnel incision in line with the radial border of the fourth digit is used and is extended in a zigzag fashion across the wrist crease and continued about 14 cm into the forearm. Guyon's canal is opened, and the neurovascular bundle is

retracted to reveal the ulnar nerve. The origin of the flexor digiti minimi is noted adjacent to the hook of the hamate, which can be located by palpation. The deep motor branch of the ulnar nerve is found descending beneath the proximal border of this muscle and beneath the ulnar vessels. This leading fascial edge is released to remove any impediment to regeneration. Once identified and released at this level, the nerve is neurolysed from the sensory branch or simply is followed visually into the forearm. The fascicles remain distinct for a long distance, but the relation of the fascicles should be noted. The motor branch shifts from medial to lateral in relation to the sensory branch as it passes from the hand to the forearm. It then is joined by the dorsal cutaneous branch that lies most medial, moving it to the center of the bundle. These branches are separated carefully at the most distal site at which they can be discerned visually, and the motor fascicle is marked with a vessel loop. This location should correspond to the proximal border of the pronator quadratus muscle.

The neurovascular bundle of the pronator quadratus is readily apparent and enters the muscle proximally and centrally. An additional couple of centimeters of nerve can be obtained by separating the nerve from this bundle and following it into the muscle. The nerve is transected here as it begins to arborize. After an adequate length for direct coaptation has been ensured, the motor

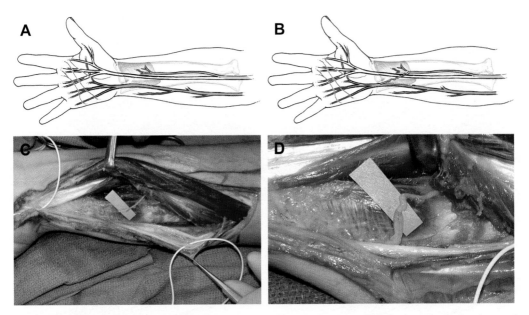

Fig. 20. AIN to ulnar deep motor transfer. (*A, C*) As in the AIN to median recurrent motor branch transfer, the anterior interosseous nerve (*yellow*) is followed into the pronator quadratus, but the need for a graft can be eliminated. (*B, D*) Proximal neurolysis of the ulnar motor fascicle (*pink*) often can allow a direct repair.

branch of the ulnar nerve is transected, and an end-to-end coaptation is performed. Occasionally the motor branch begins to plexify with the other ulnar fascicles at this level. In this case the authors identify and cut small tributaries to obtain sufficient length and avoid a graft.

The disadvantages of this transfer include the lack of a synergistic axon source and the mismatch in donor and recipient size. As noted earlier, the pronator quadratus branch of the AIN contains approximately 900 axons, some being afferents from the joint. The ulnar nerve to the intrinsics contains more than 1200 motor axons, resulting in an axon count discrepancy. When there are very few good reconstructive options, however, one can expect to prevent clawing, improve pinch strength, and avoid tendon transfers [5,26]. In younger patients, the results have been even more substantial [67]. In the authors' experience, this nerve transfer results in a good outcome, and in rare cases it may be necessary to correct Wartenberg's syndrome with a transfer of the extensor digiti quinti to the extensor digiti communis tendon. The authors always would recommend this nerve transfer in a timely presentation of a high ulnar nerve injury in patients without a Martin-Gruber anastomosis [5]. If the median nerve is not available, radial nerve function via the extensor carpi ulnaris and

extensor digiti quinti branches can be used for this transfer via an interposition graft [7].

The next priority for neurologic reconstruction of an ulnar nerve deficit is to provide sensation to the medial border of the hand [68]. Based on the priorities of sensory innervation of the hand, transfer of the third web space of the median nerve to the ulnar sensory fascicle at the wrist has been a useful approach. Restoration of protective sensation to the dorsal ulnar nerve distribution and distal remnant of the third web space then can be addressed with an end-to-side coaptation to the main median sensory trunk. Because of the benefits of the end-to-side strategy, which, as discussed previously, preserves the sensory distribution of the donor nerve while providing that rudimentary level of sensation, the authors have adopted this strategy for residual sensory deficits in the hand after the priorities have been addressed (Fig. 21). Other strategies have included direct end-to-end transfer of the palmar cutaneous branch of the median nerve at the wrist or of the LABC nerve in the forearm to the dorsal ulnar nerve (Fig. 22) [67,69].

Nerve transfers to restore ulnar sensation: technique

Nerve transfers to restore some protective sensation to the medial border of the hand usually

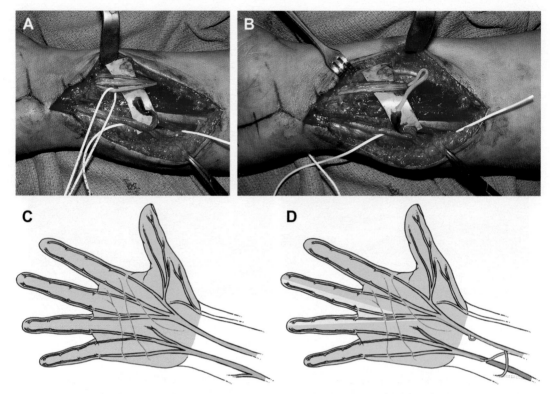

Fig. 21. Nerve transfers for restoration of ulnar sensation. (*C*) Anesthesia secondary to ulnar nerve injury involves a sig-nificant region of the palm (*pink*). (*A*) Mobilization of the median sensory contribution to the third web space allows for a quality sensory donor. (*B*) Direct repair of the end-to-end to the proximally cut end of the ulnar palmar sensory com-ponent moves trades ulnar anesthesia for the less critical third web space numbness. (*D*) Following accomplishment of this primary goal, lesser quality sensation can be restored to the third web space and dorsal ulnar cutaneous distributions by way of the use of an end-to-side strategy with the remaining median sensory trunk.

are performed in conjunction with the AIN to ulnar deep motor nerve transfer described pre-viously. After the deep motor branch has been neurolysed from the ulnar nerve, the remaining fascicles include the dorsal cutaneous and ulnar sensory nerves. The fascicles are separated from each other and then are identified with a loop. The median nerve fascicles then are separated within the distal carpal tunnel and are identified based on their medial to lateral position. The most medial fascicle, which represents the third web space innervation, is identified with a loop and then is neurolysed several centimeters proximally. Once adequate length for the transfer is obtained, the ulnar sensory branch to the palm is cut proxi-mally, and the third web space component of the median nerve is cut distally. The proximal cut end of the third web space then is sutured to the distal end of the ulnar sensory component to the palm.

The remaining branch of the ulnar nerve, which should represent the dorsal ulnar branch, then is cut

quite proximally and transposed to a relaxed posi-tion where it meets the median nerve. The remain-ing distal portion of the nerve to the third web space is neurolysed further distally and also is mobilized to meet the adjacent remaining median nerve. Epineurial windows are cut at the positions on the median nerve where these nerves approximate easily without tension, and the underlying perineu-rium is incised longitudinally. These nerves then are coapted to these perineurial windows.

Flexion of the fourth and fifth digits usually is managed via a side-to-side suture of the FDP tendons to those of the second and third digits [11]. Nerve transfers for the restoration of wrist flexion are not required unless there is accompa-nying median nerve injury as discussed previously.

Postoperative care

In all the nerve transfers described, unless a concomitant tendon transfer has been

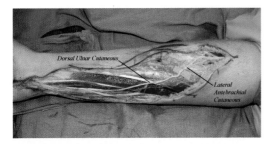

Fig. 22. LABC to dorsal ulnar sensory transfer is one example of alternative strategies for restoring sensation to this territory.

performed, the wounds are closed without the need for a Marcaine infusion pump for pain. The bulky dressing includes an Ortho-Glass splint to hold the forearm in neutral and the elbow flexed at 90°. This bulky dressing is removed 2 to 3 days

---

Box 1. Potential donors

Motor
Median nerve branches
 Flexor digitorum superficialis (if flexor
  digitorum profundus is intact)
 Flexor carpi radialis (if the FCU is
  intact)
 Palmaris longus
 Distal anterior interosseous nerve
Ulnar nerve branches
 FCU (if flexor carpi
  radialis is intact)
Radial nerve branches
 Supinator (if biceps is intact)
 Extensor carpi radialis brevis (when
  other extensors are intact)
 Brachioradialis (when other extensors
  are intact)
Musculocutaneous branches
 Brachialis branch (if biceps is intact)
Sensory
Median nerve branches
 Main sensory trunk (as an end-to-side
  donor only)
 Third webspace
Ulnar nerve branches
 Fourth webspace
Radial nerve branches
 Radial sensory branch
Musculocutaneous branches
 Lateral antebrachial cutaneous

Box 2. Potential recipients

Motor
Median nerve branches
 Anterior interosseous nerve
 Pronator teres branch
Ulnar nerve branches
 Deep motor branch
Radial nerve branches
 Extensor carpi radialis brevis
 Posterior interosseous nerve
Sensory
Median nerve branches
 First webspace and branch to radial
  aspect of thumb
Ulnar nerve branches
 Ulnar sensory branch
 Dorsal ulnar sensory nerve
Radial nerve branches
 Radial sensory branch

---

after surgery, and a splint is used to hold the wrist in neutral position for 2 to 3 weeks. Occasionally, a sling may be used for comfort for the first few days. The sutures are removed 2 to 3 weeks postoperatively, and therapy is instituted at this time to regain passive range of motion. Patients are educated regarding the nerve transfer so that they understand what actions will activate their reinnervated muscles. These actions are practiced daily until there is evidence of reinnervation. Once there is evidence of reinnervation, the tasks are to improve strength and to learn to discriminate the new function from that of the original function of the transferred nerve. Therapy is an extremely important part of all nerve transfers and cannot be overemphasized.

Summary

Nerve transfers within the forearm and hand have been used to restore function successfully in numerous combinations of extremity neurologic deficit. In addition to the more widely recognized solutions of nerve grafting and tendon transfers, the nerve transfer has clearly found a place in the restoration of function to the upper extremity. The authors believe that the peripheral nerve surgeon must understand the indications, timing, and expected results of anatomic nerve repair, local nerve transfer, and functional tendon transfer to select the best reconstruction for the given clinical scenario.

The forearm presents a unique anatomic substrate in which intimate understanding of the microneuroanatomy can allow creative reconstitutions of function. Multiple nerve contributions in relatively close proximity allow numerous donor–recipient combinations to improve function following nerve injury (Boxes 1 and 2). The understanding of the fascicular structure of nerves, the number and location of contributions to each muscle group, and the consequences of discrete denervations has grown rapidly. The addition of innovative concepts such as fascicular transfers and end-to-side coaptation for sensory recovery has reduced donor deficits, and results have been realized in a much more timely fashion. Solutions are rapidly accruing to a problem whose previous solutions often were technically more difficult and yielded results that often were more morbid and less functionally successful.

References

[1] Kline DG, Hudson AR. Mechanisms and pathology of injury. In: Kline DG, Hudson AR, editors. Nerve injuries. 1st edition. Philadelphia: W.B. Saunders Company; 1995. p. 29.

[2] van Alfen N, van Engelen BG. The clinical spectrum of neuralgic amyotrophy in 246 cases. Brain 2006; 129:438–50.

[3] Mackinnon SE, Nakao Y. Repair and reconstruction of peripheral nerve injuries. J Orthop Sci 1997;7: 357–65.

[4] Humphreys DB, Mackinnon SE. Nerve transfers. Operative Techniques in Plastic and Reconstructive Surgery 2003;9:89, 7–11.

[5] Tung TH, Weber RV, Mackinnon SE. Nerve transfers for the upper and lower extremities. Operative Techniques in Orthopaedics 2004;14:213–22.

[6] Chuang DC. Nerve transfers in adult brachial plexus injuries: my methods. Hand Clin 2005;21:71–82.

[7] Colbert SH, Mackinnon SE. Nerve transfers in the hand and upper extremity. Tech Hand Up Extrem Surg 2008;20–33.

[8] Shin AY, Spinner RJ, Bishop AT. Nerve transfers for brachial plexus injuries. Operative Techniques in Orthopaedics 2004;14:199–212.

[9] Tomaino MM. Nonobstetrical brachial plexus injuries. Journal of the American Society for Surgery of the Hand 2001;1:135–53.

[10] Weber RV, Mackinnon SE. Nerve transfers in the upper extremity. Journal of the American Society for Surgery of the Hand 2004;4:200–13.

[11] Weber RV, Mackinnon SE. Upper extremity nerve transfers. In: Slutsky DJ, Hentz VR, editors. Peripheral nerve surgery: practical applications in the upper extremity. Philadelphia: Churchill Livingstone Elsevier; 2006. p. 89.

[12] Lewis RC Jr, Tenny J, Irvine D. The restoration of sensibility by nerve translocation. Bull Hosp Jt Dis Orthop Inst 1984;44:288–96.

[13] Nath RK, Mackinnon SE, Shenaq SM. New nerve transfers following peripheral nerve injuries. Operative Techniques in Plastic and Reconstructive Surgery 1997;4:2–11.

[14] Stocks GW, Cobb T, Lewis RC Jr. Transfer of sensibility in the hand: a new method to restore sensibility in ulnar nerve palsy with use of microsurgical digital nerve translocation. J Hand Surg [Am] 1991; 16:219–26.

[15] Tung TH, Mackinnon SE. Flexor digitorum superficialis nerve transfer to restore pronation: two case reports and anatomic study. J Hand Surg [Am] 2001;26: 1065–72.

[16] Hovius SE. Musculo-tendinous transfers of the hand and forearm. Clin Neurol Neurosurg 1993; 95(Suppl):S92–4.

[17] Omer GE Jr. Reconstructive procedures for extremities with peripheral nerve defects. Clin Orthop Relat Res 1982;80–91.

[18] Omer GE Jr. Tendon transfers in combined nerve lesions. Orthop Clin North Am 1974;5:377–87.

[19] Babiloni C, Vecchio F, Babiloni F, et al. Coupling between "hand" primary sensorimotor cortex and lower limb muscles after ulnar nerve surgical transfer in paraplegia. Behav Neurosci 2004;118:214–22.

[20] Beaulieu JY, Blustajn J, Teboul F, et al. Cerebral plasticity in crossed C7 grafts of the brachial plexus: an fMRI study. Microsurgery 2006;26:303–10.

[21] Malessy MJ, Bakker D, Dekker AJ, et al. Functional magnetic resonance imaging and control over the biceps muscle after intercostal-musculocutaneous nerve transfer. J Neurosurg 2003;98:261–8.

[22] Midha R. Nerve transfers for severe brachial plexus injuries: a review. Neurosurg Focus 2004;16:E5.

[23] Terzis JK, Kostopoulos VK. The surgical treatment of brachial plexus injuries in adults. Plast Reconstr Surg 2007;119:73e–92e.

[24] Tung TH, Mackinnon SE. Brachial plexus injuries. Clin Plast Surg 2003;30:269–87.

[25] Guelinckx PJ, Faulkner JA, Essig DA. Neurovascular-anastomosed muscle grafts in rabbits: functional deficits result from tendon repair. Muscle Nerve 1988;11:745–57.

[26] Mackinnon SE, Novak CB. Nerve transfers. New options for reconstruction following nerve injury. Hand Clin 1999;15:643–66.

[27] Green DP. Radial nerve palsy. In: Green DP, Hotchkiss RN, Pederson WC, et al, editors. Green's operative hand surgery, vol 2. Philadelphia: Elsevier; 2005. p. 1113.

[28] Kim DH, Kam AC, Chandika P, et al. Surgical management and outcome in patients with radial nerve lesions. J Neurosurg 2001;95:573–834.

[29] Lowe JB 3rd, Tung TR, Mackinnon SE. New surgical option for radial nerve paralysis. Plast Reconstr Surg 2002;110:836–43.

[30] Shergill G, Bonney G, Munshi P, et al. The radial and posterior interosseous nerves. Results of 260 repairs. J Bone Joint Surg Br 2001;83:646–9.

[31] Bowden RE, Napier EJ. The assessment of hand function after peripheral nerve injury. J Bone Joint Surg Br 1961;43:481–92.

[32] Lowe JB 3rd, Sen SK, Mackinnon SE. Current approach to radial nerve paralysis. Plast Reconstr Surg 2002;110:1099–113.

[33] Dunnet WJ, Housden PL, Birch R. Flexor to extensor tendon transfers in the hand. J Hand Surg [Br] 1995;20:26–8.

[34] Mackinnon SE, Roque B, Tung TH. Median to radial nerve transfer for treatment of radial nerve palsy [case report]. J Neurosurg 2007;107:666–71.

[35] Skie MC, Parent TE, Mudge KM, et al. Functional deficit after transfer of the pronator teres for acquired radial nerve palsy. J Hand Surg [Am] 2007;32:526–30.

[36] Johnston RB, Zachary L, Dellon AL, et al. The effect of a distal site of compression on neural regeneration. J Reconstr Microsurg 1993;9:271–4.

[37] Schoeller T, Otto A, Wechselberger G, et al. Distal nerve entrapment following nerve repair. Br J Plast Surg 1998;51:227–9.

[38] Amr SM, Moharram AN. Repair of brachial plexus lesions by end-to-side side-to-side grafting neurorrhaphy: experience based on 11 cases. Microsurgery 2005;25:126–46.

[39] Mennen U. End-to-side nerve suture in clinical practice. Hand Surg 2003;8:33–42.

[40] Pienaar C, Swan MC, De Jager W, et al. Clinical experience with end-to-side nerve transfer. J Hand Surg [Br] 2004;29:438–43.

[41] Brenner MJ, Dvali L, Hunter DA, et al. Motor neuron regeneration through end-to-side repairs is a function of donor nerve axotomy. Plast Reconstr Surg 2007;120:215–23.

[42] Tarasidis G, Watanabe O, Mackinnon SE, et al. End-to-side neurorraphy: a long-term study of neural regeneration in a rat model. Otolaryngol Head Neck Surg 1998;119:337–41.

[43] Tarasidis G, Watanabe O, Mackinnon SE, et al. End-to-side neurorrhaphy resulting in limited sensory axonal regeneration in a rat model. Ann Otol Rhinol Laryngol 1997;106:506–12.

[44] Imbriglia JE, Hagberg WC, Baratz ME. Median nerve reconstruction. In: Peimer CA, editor. Surgery of the hand and upper extremity, vol II. New York: McGraw-Hill; 1996. p. 1381.

[45] Davis TRC. Median nerve palsy. In: Green DP, Hotchkiss RN, Pederson WC, et al, editors. Green's operative hand surgery. 5th edition. Philadelphia: Elsevier; 2005. vol 1. p. 1131.

[46] Mackinnon SE, Dellon AL. Anatomic investigations of nerves at the wrist: I. Orientation of the motor fascicle of the median nerve in the carpal tunnel. Ann Plast Surg 1988;21:32–5.

[47] Vernadakis AJ, Humphreys DB, Mackinnon SE. Distal anterior interosseous nerve in the recurrent motor branch graft for reconstruction of a median nerve neuroma-in-continuity. J Reconstr Microsurg 2004;20:7–11.

[48] Haase SC, Chung KC. Anterior interosseous nerve transfer to the motor branch of the ulnar nerve for high ulnar nerve injuries. Ann Plast Surg 2002;49: 285–90.

[49] Ustun ME, Ogun TC, Karabulut AK, et al. An alternative method for restoring opposition after median nerve injury: an anatomical feasibility study for the use of neurotisation. J Anat 2001; 198:635–8.

[50] Huang G. [Experimental reconstruction on intrinsic hand muscle function by anterior interosseous nerve transference]. Zhonghua Yi Xue Za Zhi 1992;72: 269–72 [in Chinese].

[51] Wang Y, Zhu S. Transfer of a branch of the anterior interosseous nerve to the motor branch of the median nerve and ulnar nerve. Chin Med J (Engl) 1997;110:216–9.

[52] Schultz RJ, Aiache A. An operation to restore opposition of the thumb by nerve transfer. Arch Surg 1972;105:777–9.

[53] Ebied AM, Kemp GJ, Frostick SP. The role of cutaneous sensation in the motor function of the hand. J Orthop Res 2004;22:862–6.

[54] Brunelli GA. Sensory nerves transfers. J Hand Surg [Br] 2004;29:557–62.

[55] Ducic I, Dellon AL, Bogue DP. Radial sensory neurotization of the thumb and index finger for prehension after proximal median and ulnar nerve injuries. J Reconstr Microsurg 2006;22:73–8.

[56] Ross D, Mackinnon SE, Chang YL. Intraneural anatomy of the median nerve provides "third web space" donor nerve graft. J Reconstr Microsurg 1992;8:225–32.

[57] Cheng J. Nerve transfers for digital sensation. In: Slutsky DJ, editor. Master skills in nerve repair: tips and techniques. Rosemont (IL): ASSH; 2008.

[58] Strauch B, Lang A. The ten test revisited. Plast Reconstr Surg 2003;112:593–4.

[59] Kim DH, Han K, Tiel RL, et al. Surgical outcomes of 654 ulnar nerve lesions. J Neurosurg 2003;98: 993–1004.

[60] Zhao X, Lao J, Hung LK, et al. Selective neurotization of the median nerve in the arm to treat brachial plexus palsy. An anatomic study and case report. J Bone Joint Surg Am 2004;86–A:736–42.

[61] Boutros S, Nath RK, Yuksel E, et al. Transfer of flexor carpi ulnaris branch of the ulnar nerve to the pronator teres nerve: histomorphometric analysis. J Reconstr Microsurg 1999;15:119–22.

[62] Gu Y, Wang H, Zhang L, et al. Transfer of brachialis branch of musculocutaneous nerve for finger flexion: anatomic study and case report. Microsurgery 2004;24:358–62.

[63] Palazzi S, Palazzi JL, Caceres JP. Neurotization with the brachialis muscle motor nerve. Microsurgery 2006;26:330–3.

[64] Zhao X, Lao J, Hung LK, et al. Selective neurotization of the median nerve in the arm to treat brachial plexus palsy. Surgical technique. J Bone Joint Surg Am 2005;87(Suppl 1):122–35.

[65] Tse R, Hentz VR, Yao J. Late reconstruction for ulnar nerve palsy. Hand Clin 2007;23:373–92.

[66] Lester RL, Smith PJ, Mott G, et al. Intrinsic reinnervation—myth or reality? J Hand Surg [Br] 1993;18: 454–60.

[67] Battiston B, Lanzetta M. Reconstruction of high ulnar nerve lesions by distal double median to ulnar nerve transfer. J Hand Surg [Am] 1999;24: 1185–91.

[68] Anderson GA. Ulnar nerve palsy. In: Green DP, Hotchkiss RN, Pederson WC, editors. Green's operative hand surgery. 5th edition. Philadelphia: Elsevier; 2005. vol 1. p. 1162.

[69] Oberlin C, Teboul F, Severin S, et al. Transfer of the lateral cutaneous nerve of the forearm to the dorsal branch of the ulnar nerve, for providing sensation on the ulnar aspect of the hand. Plast Reconstr Surg 2003;112:1498–500.

Nerve Transfers for Brachial Plexus Reconstruction

Stephen H. Colbert, MD[a],*, Susan E. Mackinnon, MD[b]

[a]Division of Plastic Surgery, University of Missouri School of Medicine, One Hospital Drive,
M349, Columbia, MO 65212, USA
[b]Division of Plastic and Reconstructive Surgery, Department of Surgery, Washington University School of Medicine,
660 South Euclid, Box 8238, St. Louis, MO 63110, USA

Nerve transfers for brachial plexus reconstruction

Brachial plexus injuries are infrequent but incredibly debilitating injuries. Traditional reconstruction in these cases has led to poor results because of the long distances required for nerve regeneration and muscle atrophy before reinnervation. Modern advancements with a rejuvenation of nerve-to-nerve transfer procedures (nerve transfers) that move the reconstruction closer to the target have created a renaissance in peripheral nerve surgery, particularly with respect to brachial plexus reconstruction, with great potential for much-improved patient outcomes.

Blunt trauma occurs frequently, and brachial plexus injuries occur in 1% of multitrauma patients [1]. Although car and truck crashes account for most of the overall number of brachial plexus injuries, the frequency of these injuries is much greater among motorcycle and snowmobile crashes—approaching 5%. Approximately 60% of brachial plexus injuries are closed traction injuries, which generally lead to poor outcomes when compared with open injuries [2]. Traction injuries are more likely to involve nerve root avulsion, thus contributing to the poor outcome. Likewise, all injuries at the level of the brachial plexus are expected to fare poorly compared with distal injuries because of the distance and time of nerve regeneration required. It is well known that

denervated motor end plates lose their reinnervation potential and denervated muscle atrophies after 12 to 18 months in the adult population [3].

Given our inability—as yet—to increase the rate of nerve regeneration, a logical solution to the problem of a nerve injury much more proximal to its target than the physiologic time clock allows is to convert the high injury to a low injury in an effort to speed motor end plate reinnervation and preserve muscle structure and function. Nerve transfers are a natural and elegant way to accomplish this goal. With this technique, a redundant or expendable intact donor nerve is transferred to the distal end of an injured nerve much closer to its end organ. The senior author has taken a lead role in using this strategy for brachial plexus reconstruction, based on an understanding of nerve anatomy, nerve regeneration, nerve surgery, and the principles of tendon transfers and motor re-education. This issue discusses the more common brachial plexus injuries and strategies for reconstruction, with particular emphasis on nerve transfers.

Anatomy

Achieving a complete understanding of the anatomy of the brachial plexus is a daunting yet vitally important task for the diagnosis and treatment of individuals who have brachial plexus injuries. Our understanding of its intricate pathways and that of the nerves of the brachium and forearm is good thanks to the classic studies and life work of Sir Sydney Sunderland [4–6] and others [7–19]. The reader is referred to the anatomy atlas or text for a thorough review. A basic review is presented here to highlight

The authors have no financial interest, professional or other relationship bearing any conflict of interest with the subject matter of this article.
    * Corresponding author.
    E-mail address: colberts@missouri.edu
(S.H. Colbert).

hand.theclinics.com

important surgical anatomy relevant to the more common brachial plexus injuries (Fig. 1).

The brachial plexus is formed by the fifth through eighth cervical (C5, C6, C7, C8) and first thoracic (T1) nerve roots, with occasional contributions from the fourth cervical (C4) nerve root (pre-fixed) and the second thoracic (T2) nerve root (post-fixed). Root origins at the spinal cord and spinal column represent fixed points along the course of the nerves and a potential site of traction injury. Root avulsion injuries are the most proximal and irreparable of brachial plexus injuries. The nerve roots pass between the anterior and middle scalene muscles and merge into three trunks. The upper trunk is formed by the merging of the fifth and sixth cervical roots, the middle trunk is formed by the continuation of the seventh cervical root, and the lower trunk is formed by the merging of the eighth cervical and the first thoracic root. The trunks each diverge into an anterior and posterior division at the level of the clavicle, and these six divisions merge into three cords at the level of pectoralis minor.

The cords are named relative to their positions around the axillary artery. The posterior cord is formed from all three posterior divisions, the lateral cord is formed from the anterior divisions of the upper and middle trunk, and the medial cord is formed from the anterior division of the lower trunk. The cords then each divide into two divisions that selectively reconstitute into infraclavicular branches that are the named nerves. The musculocutaneous nerve is formed from a division of the lateral cord. The posterior cord divides into the axillary and radial nerves and gives off the thoracodorsal nerve and the subscapular nerve. The ulnar nerve is formed from a continuation of the medial cord. The median nerve is formed from the remaining divisions from the lateral and medial cords receiving sensory input from the lateral cord and motor input from the medial cord. The lateral and medial pectoral nerves originate from the cords of the respective name. Other important terminal branches from the brachial plexus emerge above the clavicle. The long thoracic nerve and the dorsal scapular nerve originate from the upper roots, and the cervical contributions to the sympathetic nerve chain originate from the lower roots. The suprascapular nerve originates from the upper trunk.

It is important to note that the roots that eventually contribute to specific terminal branches do not necessarily include all roots that make up the cord from which the branch originates. This fact is important for recognizing patterns of brachial plexus injury. For example, the radial and axillary nerves originate from the posterior cord; however, the axillary nerve receives contributions from only the upper plexus roots (C5, C6), whereas the radial nerve receives contributions from nearly all roots (C5, C6, C7, C8). This helps explain why axillary function is lost and radial function is often retained in isolated upper plexus injuries. Similarly, the median nerve sensory fibers are formed from the upper roots that eventually give rise to the lateral cord, whereas the median nerve intrinsic hand motor fibers are formed from the lower roots that eventually give rise to the medial cord. Thus, avulsions of the upper roots of the plexus affect median nerve sensation but not median nerve intrinsic hand function. Likewise, knowing the level of origin of named nerves helps determine the proximal-distal level of injury. For example, if suprascapular nerve function to the spinatus muscles is intact and musculocutaneous and axillary nerve function to the elbow flexors and deltoid, respectively, are lost, the level of injury is likely to be at or distal to the clavicle.

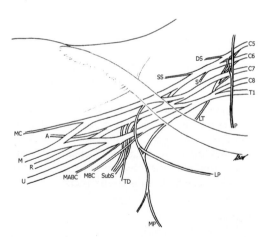

Fig. 1. Brachial plexus anatomy. Note that the roots and trunks of the brachial plexus form the supraclavicular plexus, and the cords and terminal branches form the infraclavicular plexus. C5–8, cervical spine nerve roots; A, axillary nerve; DS, dorsal scapular nerve; LP, lateral pectoral nerve; LT, long thoracic nerve; M, median nerve; MABC, medial antebrachial cutaneous nerve; MBC, medial brachial cutaneous nerve; MC, musculocutaneous nerve; MP, medial pectoral nerves; P, phrenic nerve; R, radial nerve; S, nerve to subclavius; SS, suprascapular nerve; SubS, subscapular nerves; T1, first thoracic nerve root; TD, thoracodorsal nerve; U, ulnar nerve. (*Courtesy of* Stephen H. Colbert, MD, Columbia, MO.)

Diagnosis

With the aforementioned knowledge of anatomy, the diagnosis of brachial plexus injuries generally can be made after a thorough history and physical examination. Imaging studies and electrodiagnostic studies are valuable and occasionally essential tools for accurate diagnosis and operative planning, however.

Physical examination

Proper examination of the brachial plexus requires a thorough, consistent, anatomic approach to the entire forequarter, that is, the upper extremity including the shoulder, chest, back, and neck. An organized, comprehensive approach is not only sage advice for the novice extremity surgeon but also vital to even the most experienced peripheral nerve surgeon in ensuring accurate evaluation of the patient with a brachial plexus injury. Although the following text presents an examination from proximal to distal, the clinician may chose any convention he or she wishes, as long as it ensures an accurate and thorough examination. It is critical to examine the involved and uninvolved extremities for comparison, and although possibly more important in the setting of nerve compression, it is wise to examine sensation before motor function to avoid confounding the sensory examination with the manipulation required by the motor examination.

The quickest and easiest of sensory examinations is testing for the presence of light touch in each dermatome of the brachial plexus roots and terminal branches (Fig. 2). For a more specific test, sensory thresholds may be measured with Semmes-Weinstein filaments and static, and moving two-point discrimination may be measured with a standardized, calibrated Disk-Criminator. In general, threshold testing provides information about neuron conductivity, and discrimination testing provides information about innervation density. Most important for the purpose of examination of a patient with a potential brachial plexus injury, either test can provide information regarding the absolute presence or absence of cutaneous nerve integrity. In this manner, one can gain insight into whether an injury is complete or incomplete and what level is involved.

The motor examination is perhaps more valuable than the sensory examination. It usually can more clearly define the level of injury and is more reflective of functional losses incurred by the patient. To follow changes over time, either preoperatively or postoperatively, it is important to use a standardized motor examination scale, the most common of which is the motor portion of the Medical Research Council scale (Table 1). This scales grades voluntary motor function on a scale from M0, which represents complete flaccidity, to M5, which represents strong function against full resistance. M1 represents a flicker of muscle activity. M2 represents a more full range of motion with gravity eliminated. M3 represents activity against gravity, but not against manual resistance. M4 represents a weakened ability to oppose manual resistance. M4 is often qualified with a (+) or a (−) to indicate whether the function is relatively strong, which is closer to an M5 grade, or relatively weak, which is closer to an M3 grade, respectively.

Following the convention of examining for injuries from a proximal to distal direction, much information can be gained during the observation portion of the examination, even before the sensory examination. The most proximal brachial plexus injury involves avulsion of the spinal roots. When the lower plexus is involved and includes C8 and T1 roots, Horner's syndrome (myosis, ptosis, and anhydrosis) may be noted because of the involvement of the sympathetic nerves. The resting posture of the hand, arm, and shoulder can be revealing, such as assumption of the "waiter's tip" posture in an upper brachial plexus injury, which involves loss of shoulder abduction and external rotation, elbow flexion, and forearm supination, and wrist extension when involvement extends to C7 and affects radial nerve function. Upper plexus injuries may involve the phrenic nerve roots (C3 through C5) and result in hemi-diaphragmatic paralysis, which could be detected by an elevated diaphragm "shadow" on chest percussion or reduced breath sounds on auscultation.

Further evaluation of the nerve roots may be performed by examining the rhomboids and the serratus anterior function, which relate to the integrity of the dorsal scapular (C4, C5) and long thoracic (C5 through C7) nerves, respectively. The rhomboids are tested by having the patient "stand at attention" in a military-style posture and assessing for palpable rhomboid muscles. The serratus anterior is examined by having the standing patient fully flex the arms forward, with elbows extended, and slowly return the arms to the sides while the clinician observes and palpates the scapulae. In the setting of an upper brachial plexus injury with no deltoid or

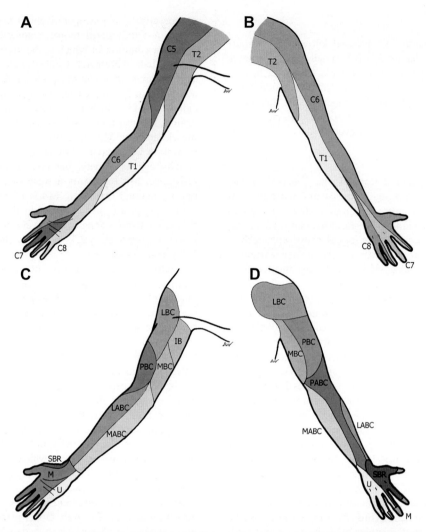

Fig. 2. Dermatomes of roots and terminal branches. (*A*) Volar surface nerve root distributions. (*B*) Dorsal surface nerve root distribution. (*C*) Volar surface terminal branch distribution. (*D*) Dorsal surface terminal branch distribution. C5–8, cervical spine nerve roots; IB, intercostobrachial nerve; LABC, lateral antebrachial cutaneous nerve; LBC, lateral brachial cutaneous nerve; M, median nerve; MABC, medial antebrachial cutaneous nerve; MBC, medial brachial cutaneous nerve; PABC, posterior antebrachial cutaneous nerve; PBC, posterior brachial cutaneous nerve; SBR, superficial branch of radial nerve; T1, first thoracic nerve root; T2, second thoracic nerve root; U, ulnar nerve. (*Courtesy of* Stephen H. Colbert, MD, Columbia, MO.)

spinatus muscle function, this examination is not possible, however. In this situation, the arms may be passively flexed forward with the patient leaning against a wall with elbows extended and the scapulae observed for winging. It is strongly advised that the patient remove his or shirt for accurate examination.

In addition to these functions related to nerves of the brachial plexus, it is imperative that certain muscles not supplied by the brachial plexus be examined to gain information necessary to define potential treatment options. These muscles are, in a sense, more "proximal" than the roots of the plexus and are described here. The most important of these muscles are the trapezius, supplied by C11, the spinal accessory nerve, and the intercostal muscles, supplied by ventral rami of their respective spinal roots. These nerves may be used as donor nerves in specific situations.

Beyond the nerve roots are the trunks of the brachial plexus. Only two branches originate from the level of the trunks, only one of which is

Table 1
Medical Research Council motor grading scale

Grade	Muscle status
0	No contraction
1	Flicker of contraction
2	Active motion, gravity eliminated
3	Active motion against gravitys
4	Active motion against resistance
5	Normal strength

Data from Medical Research Council. Aids to the investigation of peripheral nerve injuries. 2nd edition. London: Her Majesty's Stationery Office; 1943.

amenable to examination. The nerve to subclavius supplies the subclavius muscle, and the suprascapular nerve (C5, C6) supplies the supraspinatus and infraspinatus muscles. The supraspinatus muscle helps initiate lateral abduction of the shoulder and supports the head of the humerus in the glenoid fossa. The infraspinatus muscle is the primary external rotator of the shoulder. Both of these nerves originate from the upper trunk of the brachial plexus; without any branches originating from the middle and lower trunks, no specific information about injury to them can be gained at this point. Likewise, no branches originate from the anterior and posterior divisions of the plexus, just distal to the trunks.

The roots, trunks, and divisions are often considered to comprise the supraclavicular portion of the brachial plexus because of their anatomic location and common injury patterns. The cords and terminal branches are often referred to as the infraclavicular plexus. The three cords of the plexus each have branches that supply muscles that can provide information on examination. From the lateral cord, the lateral pectoral nerve (C5 through C7) provides the only innervation to the clavicular head of the pectoralis major, although it also innervates the sternal and costal heads. Injury to the lateral cord may be suggested by loss of pectoralis tone appreciated by palpation of the clavicular head on attempted forward arm adduction. The posterior cord gives rise to the muscles of the posterior axilla via the thoracodorsal nerve (C6 through C8) to latissimus dorsi and the subscapular nerve (C5, C6) to subscapularis and teres major. Latissimus dorsi may be examined by palpating the muscle as the patient voluntarily coughs, which should elicit muscle flexion. Subscapularis and teres major muscles may be examined by having the patient adduct the

humerus and internally rotate the shoulder. The medial cord is the origin of the medial pectoral nerve (C8, T1), which innervates pectoralis minor and the sternal and costal heads of pectoralis major. Injury to the medial cord would result in more significant loss of pectoral muscle function, and it is worth noting that complete loss of pectoral muscle function requires either injury to the lateral and medial cords or nearly all roots of the brachial plexus.

Finally, the terminal branches of the brachial plexus should be examined individually. The axillary nerve (C5, C6) innervates the deltoid and teres minor muscles. The deltoid allows for lateral abduction of the shoulder beyond 90°. If initiation of abduction exists but does not extend to 90° or beyond, in the absence of a musculoskeletal injury, it implies preservation of the upper trunk of the plexus and suprascapular nerve function with loss of axillary nerve function, suggesting an infraclavicular injury pattern. The radial nerve (C5 through T1) accompanies the axillary nerve as a terminal branch of the posterior cord and controls extension of the wrist and fingers. It is important to remember the susceptibility of the radial nerve to injury at the level of its course along the spiral grove of the humerus. In the absence of such a distal injury or a posterior cord injury, loss of radial nerve function implies relative extensive brachial plexus injury, as the nerve receives contributions from all roots.

Traditionally, the more proximal radial nerve musculature innervation originates from the upper plexus roots, whereas the more distal musculature innervation originates from the lower plexus roots, which may be borne out on physical examination. Nerves to the triceps muscles largely originate from the radial nerve, although there is some evidence that the nerve to the long head of the triceps more commonly originates from the axillary nerve or directly from the posterior cord. The musculocutaneous (C5 through C7) nerve arises from the lateral cord and innervates the coracobrachialis, brachialis, and biceps muscles, which control elbow flexion. The median nerve (C5 through T1) is formed by contributions from the lateral and medial cords; its sensory components come largely from the former and its motor components come largely from the latter. Motor evaluation of median nerve functions, such as flexion of the proximal interphalangeal joints and thumb opposition, reflect function of the lower plexus roots through the lower trunk and medial cord. The ulnar nerve (C8, T1) is comprised of the remaining elements of the medial cord, and its motor function is examined via finger abduction and adduction, lateral thumb-to-index pinch, ulnar wrist flexion, and flexion of the distal interphalangeal joints of the ring and small fingers.

To summarize, examination of the upper extremity from the shoulder through the elbow, forearm, and hand tends to parallel a proximal to distal evaluation of the brachial plexus and provides an orderly and thorough convention. Both sides should be examined for comparison, and palpating for muscle tone is helpful and often necessary, particularly when function seems to be absent or is in question.

Objective studies

The complex and intricate anatomy of the region of the brachial plexus presents a challenge for current imaging techniques. CT myelography remains the gold standard for imaging of the traumatic brachial plexus injury, largely because of its ability to identify nerve root avulsions [20,21]. MRI has become the preferred method for imaging nontraumatic brachial plexus injuries because of its ability to identify and locate associated structures, such as tumors. Other imaging techniques have limited value in the evaluation of the brachial plexus.

Electrodiagnostic studies are generally much more valuable in the evaluation of brachial plexus injury. These studies commonly consist of nerve conduction studies (NCSs) and electromyography, which are helpful in determining the location and severity of injury. These studies are operator and setting dependent. The peripheral nerve surgeon should have good knowledge of the setting and reliability of electrodiagnostic studies that may present with patients, and a good working relationship with a local professional electrodiagnostician is invaluable.

NCSs test motor and sensory nerves. The amplitude of action potentials recorded after supramaximum stimulation correlates to the number of functioning axons. The conduction velocity of action potentials recorded along the course of the nerve tends to correlate to the integrity of the myelin sheath and the degree of compression or injury. NCSs can be particularly valuable in determining a preganglionic root lesion from a postganglionic root lesion. The peripheral sensory neuron is unique in that its cell body is contained in the dorsal root ganglion outside the spinal cord. If it is disrupted distal to the dorsal root ganglion, then Wallerian degeneration (degeneration of the distal axon segment) occurs just as with peripheral motor neurons, and no response is recorded on NCSs. If it is disrupted proximal to the dorsal root ganglion, however, then distal degeneration does not occur and responses can be recorded on NCSs, although function is lost. If sensory responses are recorded on NCSs and motor responses are not and the patient has a functional sensory and motor deficit, it identifies the location of the lesion to a preganglionic level.

As helpful as these findings may be, electromyography tends to provide much more valuable information in the setting of a brachial plexus injury than do NCSs. Immediately after a peripheral motor nerve injury, electrodiagnostic studies may show few, if any, abnormalities because of the retained electrochemical elements in the transected segment and intact motor end plate. After 2 to 3 days, those chemicals dissipate and the axons and myelin sheaths break down; after 5 to 7 days, the muscle shows fewer motor unit potentials (MUPs), which tend to fire at higher frequency, seemingly to try to regain lost force. This pattern represents one of the hallmarks of peripheral motor neuron injury and is called reduced recruitment. After 4 to 6 weeks, muscle fibers tend to exhibit firing of their internal pacemakers, which is displayed as fibrillation potentials on electromyography. If some axons are intact, MUPs show higher amplitudes and longer durations. If an injury is complete, then no MUPs are recorded. Fibrillation potentials and reduced recruitment tend to be early signs of peripheral motor nerve injury, and lack of MUPs at a later date indicates more significant injury.

Electrodiagnostic studies are generally first recommended in the setting of a brachial plexus injury 6 weeks after injury to establish baseline information. At 12 weeks, if recovery is occurring, then MUPs should be present and representative of recovery of uninjured axons or nerves suffering low-grade injury. Nascent units represent actual regeneration of injured axons or nerves suffering high-grade injury. Both MUPs and nascent units almost always are predictors of spontaneous recovery. These studies, combined with thorough sequential physical examinations, are generally more than adequate to identify the location and severity of a brachial plexus lesion and allow for appropriate operative planning.

In the preoperative period, electrodiagnostic studies can help classify peripheral nerve injuries, which in turn aids in operative planning. The most common classification schemes for peripheral nerve injuries are presented in Table 2. Seddon [22] described three degrees of injury: neurapraxia, axonotmesis, and neurotmesis. Neurapraxia represents a mild injury leading to a conduction block. Demyelination may occur, typically affecting large fibers more than small fibers, resulting in reduced conduction velocities and increased conduction latencies. No significant axonal injury occurs and there is no Wallerian degeneration; thus, innervation density and action potential amplitude remain normal. Neurapraxic lesions alone do not result in fibrillation potentials on electromyography, but conduction block does block motor action potentials and leads to changes in recruitment. These injuries recover spontaneously, often within days or weeks, and assuming that no persistent injuries occur, recovery is complete at 3 to 4 months.

Axonotmesis represents injury to the myelin sheath and the axon, with varying degrees of injury to the endoneurium and perineurium. Wallerian degeneration does occur, and the degree and speed of recovery depend on the integrity of the endoneurial sheath. Axon regeneration must occur, necessitating a more prolonged recovery time than with neurapraxia.

Neurotmesis represents a complete nerve injury that affects all structures from the axon out, including the epineurial sheath. Axonal regeneration leading to reinnervation of distal segments

does not occur, and the prognosis is poor. Sunderland [23] added to the classification of nerve injuries by further breaking down axonotmetic injuries to create a more clinically useful system. A first-degree injury corresponds to neurapraxia. A second-degree injury corresponds to an axonotmetic injury without disruption of the basal lamina or endoneurium. These injuries recovery spontaneously, only much slower than neurapraxia, at a rate approximating 1 mm/day because of the need for axonal regeneration. A third-degree injury involves disruption of the basal lamina with subsequent development of some scar tissue. It inhibits spontaneous recovery to a variable degree, and surgery may be warranted in only rare circumstances. A fourth-degree injury involves injury to the endoneurium and perineurium and results in complete scar blockage of regeneration, the so-called "neuroma-in-continuity." Surgery is necessary for any hope of recovery. A fifth-degree injury corresponds to neurotmesis and necessitates surgical repair. In 1988, Mackinnon and Dellon [24] introduced another clinically important category of nerve injury, the sixth-degree injury, which describes a combination of varying degrees of nerve injury intermixed, potentially with normal fascicles. The importance of this type of injury rests in the difficulty in treating the portions of the nerve having fourth- and fifth-degree injury without disrupting the portions having lesser degrees of injury that recover spontaneously.

Indications

The poor prognosis associated with peripheral nerve injuries generally is related to motor nerve injuries because of the time-dependent nature of motor end plate survival after denervation. In an adult, the motor end plates and muscle undergo irreversible fibrosis and atrophy approximately 12 to 18 months after denervation. On the other hand, the potential for sensory recovery is under no apparent time constraint, because the sensory end organs tend to remain capable of responding to reinnervation [25]. The long distance of regeneration in high nerve injuries or the lack of a viable proximal nerve for repair are the situations that stand to gain the most from nerve reconstruction with nerve transfer. Another scenario might involve an injury that is at a level expected to reinnervate the muscle before atrophy if repaired shortly after injury but has required delay of repair such that recovery would no longer be

Table 2
Classification of nerve injury

Degree	Injury
I	Conduction block; resolves spontaneously
II	Axonal rupture with intact basal lamina
III	Axonal and basal lamina rupture; some scar; perineurium intact
IV	Complete scar; perineurium ruptured; epineurium intact; "neuroma in-continuity"
V	Complete transaction
VI	Combination of normal nerve and type I-V injuries

Data from Sunderland S. A classification of peripheral nerve injuries producing loss of function. Brain 195;74(4):491–516; and Mackinnon SE, Dellon AL. Surgery of the peripheral nerve. New York: Thieme Medical Publishers, Inc; 1988.

expected. Another example may be an extremity injury that involves inadequate tissue bed homeostasis to allow nerve regeneration or successful nerve grafting. The basic indications for nerve transfer are injuries in which direct repair is not possible or functional recovery with direct repair or nerve grafting is not expected.

Traditionally, before the use of nerve transfers, poor outcomes were treated with tendon transfers where possible. That is, expendable musculotendinous units were transferred to perform the lost functions of the denervated musculotendinous units. Those donor musculotendinous units naturally required intact nerves. Nerve transfers may be viewed as an alternate means of achieving the same goal as tendon transfers, only via the transfer of the intact nerve rather than the musculotendinous unit. Many of the principles of nerve transfers parallel those of tendon transfers. First and foremost, the donor nerve must be functioning and expendable. The donor nerve must be of the same type—motor or sensory—as the recipient and must be near the recipient nerve end organ. The donor nerve should have an adequate number of donor axons. Synergy of donor and recipient function is preferable, although not always necessary, because re-education is possible for functional recovery. Understanding these principles, presented in Table 3, is requisite for appreciating appropriate indications for nerve transfers, and the peripheral nerve surgeon who keeps them in mind will avoid costly errors.

Nerve transfers have one significant advantage over tendon transfers: they allow for maintenance of the original musculotendinous dynamics [26]. Line of pull and excursion should remain unchanged. In general, they should have the potential to provide better functional recovery than tendon transfers. A disadvantage of nerve transfers, however, is that they cannot be delayed indefinitely, as tendon transfers can. Situations may exist, however, in which the expected power of recovery from an available nerve transfer may be inferior to that of a tendon transfer. All of these factors should be considered when weighing the option of nerve transfer.

Upper brachial plexus injury

Injury to the upper trunk of the brachial plexus is one of the most common injury patterns, particularly in the adult trauma population. A diagram of a representative injury is presented in Fig. 3. The major functions affected include those of the suprascapular nerve, the axillary nerve, and the musculocutaneous nerve, which results in dysfunction of elbow flexion, shoulder abduction, shoulder internal rotation, and glenohumeral stability. Because elbow flexion is generally considered the most important upper extremity function and shoulder function is considered next most important, these injuries are

Table 3
Principles of nerve transfer

Principles of motor nerve transfers	Principles of sensory nerve transfers
Donor nerve near target motor end plates	Donor nerve near target sensory receptors
Expendable donor nerve	Expendable, noncritical donor nerve
Pure motor donor nerve	Pure sensory donor nerve
Donor–recipient size match	Donor–recipient size match
Donor function synergy with recipient function	Side-to-end (terminolateral) repair if necessary; end-to-end repair is preferable
Motor re-education improves function	Sensory re-education improves function

Data from Mackinnon SE, Novak CB. Nerve transfers: new options for reconstruction following nerve injury. Hand Clin 1999;15:643–66.

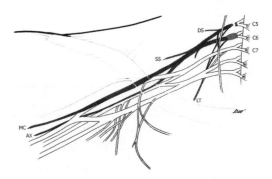

Fig. 3. Upper brachial plexus injury. In this injury, the fifth cervical root has been completely avulsed and the sixth root exhibits an incomplete avulsion injury (grade VII). C7 sometimes may be involved in these injuries. The most commonly affected terminal branches are highlighted and labeled. C5–7, cervical spine nerve roots; Ax, axillary nerve; DS, dorsal scapular nerve; LT, long thoracic nerve; MC, musculocutaneous nerve; SS, suprascapular nerve. (*Courtesy of* Stephen H. Colbert, MD, Columbia, MO.)

devastating. An extended upper brachial plexus injury involves C7 and may affect radial nerve function. The following sections describe the specific nerve transfers used to restore these lost functions.

Double nerve transfer for shoulder function

The suprascapular nerve and the axillary nerve are both formed from the C5 and C6 roots through the upper trunk of the brachial plexus. If the level of injury is distal to the clavicle, which is distal to the origin of the suprascapular nerve, then suprascapular nerve function may be spared. If the level of injury is at the upper trunk or cervical root level, however, then the function of both nerves is generally affected. Because more proximal injuries tend to be more common, the reconstructive procedures for both of these nerves are presented together. Each reconstructive technique may be used individually.

In 1948, Lurje [27] reported the first nerve transfer for reconstruction of shoulder function. Lurje promoted use of the phrenic nerve for transfers but also described a case in which a nerve to the triceps was used to reconstruct the axillary nerve. Subsequently, many other donor nerves have been promoted, including intercostal nerves [28–30], thoracodorsal nerve [28], medial pectoral nerve [28,31], long thoracic nerve [28], distal accessory nerve [28,29], ipsilateral C7 root [32], contralateral C7 root [33], suprascapular nerve [28], and hypoglossal nerve [34]. The selection of the most appropriate donor nerves and the techniques by which they are transferred has been refined as our experience increases. Early transfers used more proximal approaches. More distal approaches take greater advantage of the nerve transfer maxim of being closer to the target muscle and have shown excellent results, such as an axillary approach for reconstruction of the axillary nerve by transfer of a triceps fascicle reported by Nath and Mackinnon in 2000 [35]. Others have shown similar results using a posterior approach to reconstruct the axillary nerve with various components of the radial nerve [36–39] and reconstruct the suprascapular nerve with the distal spinal accessory nerve [40,41]. These approaches provide excellent and rather direct access to the most distal portions of the donor and recipient nerves. The following sections represent the authors' preferred techniques for suprascapular nerve and axillary nerve reconstruction for upper brachial plexus deficits [42].

Distal spinal accessory to suprascapular nerve transfer

The standard locations of the donor and recipient nerves are marked at the posterior shoulder preoperatively. Accuracy with this step substantially facilitates operative identification of the nerves. The distal spinal accessory nerve is marked at a point 40% of the distance from the midline of the cervicothoracic spine to the acromion. The suprascapular nerve is marked at its course through the suprascapular notch, which is located at a point 50% of the distance from the superior angle of the medial border of the scapula to the acromion (Fig. 4). The surgical incision is planned and marked as a transverse line encompassing these two points. The patient is under general anesthesia and placed prone with the arm adducted but prepped into the field. It is critically important that either short-acting paralytic agents or, preferably, no paralytic medications are used to allow for proper intraoperative assessment of neuromuscular function. No local anesthesia should be used before assessment of the donor and recipient nerve status, although infiltration of the incision with a plain epinephrine solution facilitates hemostasis.

Loupe magnification is used for the initial dissection. The incision is made and dissection begun toward the suprascapular nerve. The trapezius muscle is split along the course of its fibers, and the suprascapular notch is approached above the supraspinatus muscle. Identification of the notch is facilitated by palpating the superior transverse scapular ligament, which is appreciated as firm, thin, and fibrous, distinct from the more rounded and smooth superior border of the scapula bone. Just inferior to the ligament, the depression of the foramen is identified by palpation. This is a "tactile" approach, and the notch is located just at the "turn" of the free border of the scapula, where it takes a superior angle, not on the "flat" aspect of the border. Care should be taken to avoid injury to the suprascapular artery during this dissection, because it generally runs over the superior border of the scapula outside of the notch lateral to the nerve (the senior author remembers this by the pneumonic "NM" for "nerve medial" or Neiman Marcus). The suprascapular nerve is identified by blunt dissection of its surrounding adipose within the notch after division of the ligament and is stimulated with a portable nerve stimulator to ensure lack of function. The nerve is dissected as far proximally (anteriorly) as possible.

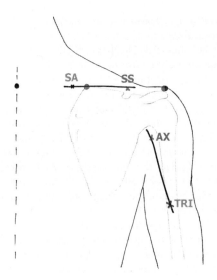

Fig. 4. Markings for posterior shoulder transfers. The midline spinous process is marked (*dark dot*), as is the acromion (*light/dark dot*). The location of the spinal accessory nerve is marked (SA) at a distance 40% from the dorsal midline to the acromion parallel to a line along the superior border of the scapula. The superior angle of the scapula is marked (*light dot*), and the location of the suprascapular notch containing the suprascapular nerve is identified and marked (SS) at the midpoint between the superior angle of the scapula and the acromion along the superior border of the scapula. The surgical incision is planned in a transverse fashion to expose both nerves. The posterior approach to the quadrangular space containing the axillary nerve (AX) is marked at the posterior border of the deltoid muscle just inferior to the scapular neck and infraglenoid tubercle. The surgical incision is planned from this point distally along the posterior border of the arm in line with the interval between the long and lateral heads of the triceps muscle, approximately 10 to 12 cm in length. At the distal aspect of this approach, the nerve branch to the medial head of the triceps muscle (TRI) is located. (*From* Colbert SH, Mackinnon SE. Posterior approach for double nerve transfer for restoration of shoulder function in upper brachial plexus palsy. Hand 2006;1(2):72; with permission.)

The medial portion of the wound is then dissected just deep to the trapezius muscle, where the distal spinal accessory nerve is found running in a superior-to-inferior direction. Its localization is often facilitated by use of the nerve stimulator, because this nerve is also generally surrounded by adipose tissue and at this level rests deep to—not within—the muscle. Its function is confirmed via stimulation, and then it is dissected as far distally as possible into the trapezius muscle, divided, and

transposed laterally toward the suprascapular nerve. The suprascapular nerve is divided as far proximally as possible, and the distal segment is withdrawn from the suprascapular notch and transposed medially. We emphasize the mantra "donor-distal and recipient-proximal." This advice is necessary to avoid tension or the need for a nerve graft. With this technique, the proximal branches of the spinal accessory nerve to the upper trapezius muscle do not need to be divided, and enough length is provided for a tension-free nerve coaptation without the need for a graft. The proximal segment of the distal spinal accessory nerve is sutured to the distal segment of the suprascapular nerve with microsurgical technique (Fig. 5). When this transfer is performed in combination with reconstruction of the axillary nerve, the nerve coaptation suturing is performed after preparation of the triceps and axillary nerves to allow efficient use of time spent with the operating microscope.

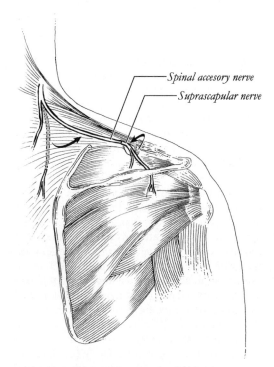

Fig. 5. Distal spinal accessory to suprascapular nerve transfer. The distal spinal accessory nerve has been transected distally and transferred to the suprascapular nerve, which has been transected proximally to the suprascapular notch. (*From* Mackinnon SE, Colbert SH. Nerve transfers in the hand and upper extremity surgery. Tech Hand Up Extrem Surg 2008;12(1):24; with permission.)

Medial triceps nerve to axillary nerve transfer

The location of the axillary nerve at the quadrangular space and the triceps nerve branches are identified at the posterior shoulder and upper brachium. The quadrangular space often can be palpated in thinner patients between the thumb and fingers by gently clasping the posterior apex of the axilla. The triceps branches run along with the radial nerve along the posterior surface of the humerus. A line encompassing these two locations is marked beginning proximally along the posterior border of the deltoid muscle and running distally along the interval between the lateral and long heads of the triceps (see Fig. 4). This line identifies the surgical incision. The preparation of the patient is the same as that previously described for the spinal accessory to suprascapular nerve transfer. It is important to avoid paralytic medications and local anesthesia to allow for proper assessment of nerve function after dissection. Loupe magnification is used for the initial dissection.

Although dissection of the recipient nerve is preferentially performed first, it is occasionally easier to identify the radial nerve and triceps branches on the posterior surface of the humerus first and then trace them proximally to the inferior border of the teres major. The teres major forms the inferior boundary of the quadrangular space and is the key landmark for this dissection. Its white musculotendinous fascia running in a transverse direction toward the neck of the humerus generally identifies it. The axillary nerve is comprised of motor components to the teres minor and deltoid muscles and a sensory component to the lateral upper arm, namely the lateral brachial cutaneous nerve. Identification of the axillary nerve at the quadrangular space may be facilitated by preliminary identification of the lateral brachial cutaneous nerve coursing through or around the posterior border of the deltoid muscle and tracing it proximally to its origin. The axillary nerve is dissected as proximally as possible from within the quadrangular space, taking care not to injure the accompanying posterior circumflex humeral artery. In some situations there may be significant scarring in the quadrangular space, and it is important to remember that the axillary nerve is superior to the vessels to avoid vessel injury and subsequent bleeding that can obscure the dissection.

By dissecting proximally, the axillary nerve branch to the teres minor is always included in the reconstruction. Inclusion of the teres minor is critical for an excellent result. The lateral brachial cutaneous nerve may be excluded when possible, although no heroic effort is made because it is not felt to be absolutely necessary at the risk of damage to the recipient motor fibers. The axillary nerve is confirmed as nonfunctional with a portable nerve stimulator. The dissection is then performed distally between the long and lateral triceps head interval to identify the radial nerve and branches to each of the three heads of the triceps. Function of these nerves is confirmed with the nerve stimulator, and the nerve to the medial head is singled out and dissected as distally as possible. The reader is reminded that extended upper brachial plexus injuries may affect radial nerve function. Function is generally determined preoperatively, but maintaining a healthy awareness at the time of operation can prevent surprises.

The axillary nerve is divided as proximally as possible and reflected inferiorly. Our preference for the medial triceps branch is that it is already "pre-dissected" lying adjacent to the radial nerve and has a long length. It is quickly dissected and more easily transferred to the axillary nerve than either the branch to the long or lateral head. The nerve to the medial triceps nerve is divided as distally as possible, dissected free of surrounding tissue, and transposed proximally, which allows adequate length for a tension-free repair. The medial triceps nerve is sutured to the axillary nerve using microsurgical technique (Fig. 6).

After completion of one or both of these transfers, the wounds are irrigated and hemostasis achieved using bipolar electrocautery. The wounds are closed in layers over drains and indwelling anesthetic catheters as needed. A soft dressing is applied and a shoulder immobilizer is used for 1 to 2 weeks, taking care to allow intermittent range of motion to prevent stiffness. Full range of motion is resumed 2 weeks after surgery.

These specific techniques that incorporate posterior approaches provide distinct advantages over other techniques that we feel are worth re-emphasizing. Taking the spinal accessory nerve at its most distal point where it branches within the trapezius muscle allows for preservation of the more proximal branches to the upper portions of the muscle, which preserves shoulder shrug. Releasing the suprascapular nerve from the suprascapular notch removes the notch as a potential point of compression that could block nerve regeneration. For axillary nerve reconstruction,

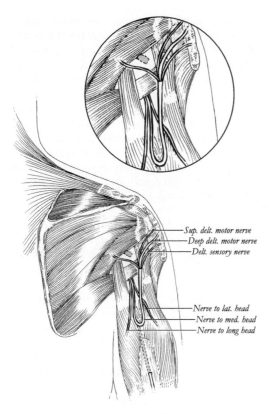

Fig. 6. Medial triceps to axillary nerve transfer. The branch to the medial head of the triceps has been transected distally and transferred to the axillary nerve. The axillary nerve has been transected as proximally as possible in the quadrangular space. The nerve to teres major is included as a recipient in the transfer. (*From* Mackinnon SE, Colbert SH. Nerve transfers in the hand and upper extremity surgery. Tech Hand Up Extrem Surg 2008;12(1):26; with permission.)

Sup. delt. motor nerve
Deep delt. motor nerve
Delt. sensory nerve

Nerve to lat. head
Nerve to med. head
Nerve to long head

other described techniques are performed at the level of the axilla or more proximally, use the long triceps nerve as the donor, or exclude the branch to teres minor from the reconstruction. Using the medial triceps nerve provides a longer donor nerve that obviates the need for a nerve graft, intramuscular dissection, or sectioning of the teres major to achieve a tension-free repair. The medial head of the triceps tends to be a purer elbow extender, similar to the lateral head, whereas the long head acts additionally as an arm adductor, which is contrary to deltoid function and the principle of synergy of donor and recipient function. Incorporating the axillary nerve branch to teres minor allows for return of its function as an external rotator of the shoulder—a principle

goal of shoulder reconstruction—and a stabilizer of the glenohumeral capsule. Finally, the suprascapular nerve and the axillary nerve reconstruction techniques described here take full advantage of the concept of performing the reconstruction as close to the target end organ as possible, which minimizes the distance of nerve regeneration and maximizes the potential for recovery.

Double fascicular transfer for elbow function

The history of musculocutaneous nerve reconstruction reveals an ever-increasing degree of sophistication. Early nerve transfers were performed using intercostal nerves, first with then without interposition nerve grafts, or the spinal accessory nerve, each proximal to the target. In 1993, Brandt and Mackinnon [43] described transfer of the medial pectoral nerves to the musculocutaneous nerve at a more distal point than previous transfers. In 1994, Oberlin and colleagues [44] described an innovative technique for reconstructing the biceps nerve by using donor fascicles from the ulnar nerve at the level of the brachium. This approach allowed for reconstruction at the most distal portion of the recipient nerve, and because a redundant fascicle was used, it preserved donor nerve function [45,46]. More recently, Humphreys and Mackinnon [47] described a technique that incorporated reconstruction of the biceps branch and the brachialis branch of the musculocutaneous nerve with redundant donor fascicles from the ulnar and median nerves (Fig. 7). It recognized the importance of return of brachialis function and maximized functional recovery [48,49].

In this procedure the patient is placed supine under general anesthesia with the arm and hand extended on a hand table. The incision is marked in the mid portion of the medial arm along the bicipital groove. Plain epinephrine may be infiltrated to assist with hemostasis, but no local anesthesia should be applied. Paralytics also are prohibited to ensure accurate assessment of neuromuscular function after dissection. Dissection is carried through the deep fascia, taking care not to injure the medial antebrachial cutaneous nerve. The ulnar nerve, brachial artery, and median nerve are often easiest to first identify, but they are not dissected. The musculocutaneous nerve is identified lateral to these structures deep to the biceps, often first by palpation. With the biceps retracted, the biceps branch originates proximal to the other branches and runs laterally, the brachialis branch originates distal to the biceps

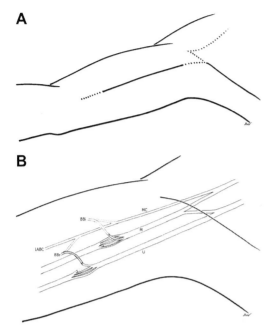

Fig. 7. Double fascicular transfer. (*A*) Marking for incision at the upper medial arm. The dotted lines represent possible extensions of the incision. (*B*) Transfer of a redundant median nerve fascicle to the biceps branch of the musculocutaneous nerve and transfer of a redundant ulnar nerve fascicle to the brachialis branch of the musculocutaneous nerve. BBi, biceps branch of musculocutaneous nerve; BBr, brachialis branch of musculocutaneous nerve; LABC, lateral antebrachial cutaneous nerve; M, median nerve; MC, musculocutaneous nerve; U, ulnar nerve. (*Courtesy of* Stephen H. Colbert, MD, Columbia, MO.)

branch and runs medially, and the lateral antebrachial cutaneous nerve continues straight distally. The biceps and brachialis branches are identified, isolated, and interrogated with a portable nerve stimulator to ensure lack of function. They are transected at their origins and draped toward the median and ulnar nerves.

The donor for the brachialis branch is usually selected first, because the length of the brachialis nerve branch may be more limiting than that of the biceps branch. Either the median or the ulnar nerve may serve as a donor for either recipient nerve branch, and both options for transfer should be assessed before donor selection to find the most appropriate match. The median and ulnar nerves then undergo internal neurolysis to identify the appropriate donor fascicles. The location of fascicle dissection is planned to allow transfer to the recipient nerve without tension,

including during full range of motion of the shoulder and elbow. The ideal donors are redundant fascicles that innervate the wrist flexors, the flexor carpi radialis and flexor carpi ulnaris, or the superficial finger flexors, the flexor digitorum superficialis. Motor components of the median nerve originate from the medial cord and are generally found on the medial side of the nerve, whereas the motor components of the ulnar nerve are generally found in the central and lateral portion of the nerve. The fascicles are separated carefully with microsurgical technique, and potential donor fascicles are identified via nerve stimulation.

It is critically important to confirm function not only of the potential donor fascicle but also of the remaining fascicles to preserve all forearm and hand function. Fascicles that mediate forearm pronation and intrinsic muscles of the hand and long finger flexors—both median and ulnar innervated—should not be sacrificed. The appropriate fascicles are selected, transected distally, transposed toward the respective recipient nerve, and sutured with microsurgical technique (see Fig. 7). The extremity is always moved through range of motion to ensure no tension on the repairs. The wound is irrigated, bipolar electrocautery is used for hemostasis, and the wound in closed in layers over drains and indwelling anesthetic catheter as needed. A soft wrap is applied and a shoulder immobilizer placed for 1 to 2 weeks, taking care to allow intermittent range of motion to prevent stiffness. Full range of motion is allowed 2 weeks after surgery.

Medial pectoral nerve

In 1993, Brandt and Mackinnon [43] reported use of the medial pectoral nerve as an improved alternative over nerve grafting from the root level, which was the standard at the time, for upper brachial plexus injuries. This technique used the medial pectoral nerve in transfer to the musculocutaneous nerve distal to the branch to coracobrachialis with redirection and neurotization (implantation of nerve into muscle) of the lateral antebrachial cutaneous nerve into the biceps muscle, setting the nerve repair site much closer to the end organ and effectively maximizing the channeling of motor fibers to the biceps and brachialis muscles. The success of the more distal transfers of fascicles from the median and ulnar nerves to the muscular branches of the musculocutaneous nerves has limited the need to rely on more proximal donor nerves. Situations may still arise that require the use of more traditional donors. In addition to reconstruction of the musculocutaneous nerve, the medial pectoral nerve has been used for reconstruction of the proximal spinal accessory nerve [50], the long thoracic nerve [51], and the axillary nerve [31] with excellent success.

The pectoral nerve anatomy is such that some pectoral function is preserved in virtually any partial brachial plexus injury. The main root contribution to the lateral pectoral nerve is from C7, followed by C6 and C5, in order. The main root contribution to the medial pectoral nerve is C8, more so than T1 [52]. With pure upper root or upper trunk injuries (C5 and C6), lateral and medial pectoral nerve function may be maintained. In that case, use of the medial pectoral nerve as a donor may not result in complete pectoral dysfunction. Even in cases in which pectoral function is compromised, the resulting dysfunction is well tolerated and more than accounted for by any recovery of elbow or shoulder function supplied in return.

The medial pectoral nerve (or nerves, if multiple) and infraclavicular brachial plexus are accessed via a zigzag incision at the axilla that extends proximally in a curved fashion along the course of the cephalic vein in the deltopectoral groove. Dissection is carried down to the pectoralis major muscle, which is isolated at its insertion onto the humerus. Sectioning of the tendon is planned with the intent of leaving a cuff of tendon at its insertion onto the humerus. Placement of stay sutures along this cuff, before actual release, greatly facilitates reapproximation of the tendon to its insertion at closure. Sutures are then placed in the proximal end of the cut tendon for ease of handling, and the pectoralis major muscle is reflected anteriorly. The pectoralis minor muscle is then isolated and elevated, as the medial pectoral nerve is found entering the deep surface of the pectoralis minor muscle (Fig. 8). The nerve is traced as distally as possible to within the pectoralis major muscle to maximize donor nerve length, stimulated to confirm activity, transected, and transposed toward its previously dissected recipient.

Transfers for serratus anterior function

The serratus anterior muscle is innervated by the long thoracic nerve, which originates from C5 through C7. The muscle originates from the lateral portions of the upper eight ribs and inserts onto the anterior surface of the entire medial

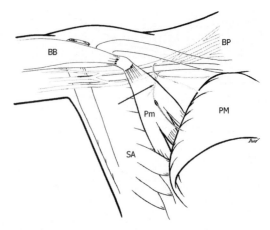

Fig. 8. Medial pectoral donor nerve. The medial pectoral nerves and relevant anatomy are depicted. The medial pectoral nerves (*arrow*) course deep to pectoralis minor and pierce pectoralis minor to innervate the deep surface of pectoralis major. Note that the lateral pectoral nerves do not encounter or innervate pectoralis minor. BB, biceps brachii muscle; BP, brachial plexus roots; PM, pectoralis major muscle; Pm, pectoralis minor muscle; SA, serratus anterior muscle. (*Courtesy of* Stephen H. Colbert, MD, Columbia, MO.)

border of the scapula. It pulls the scapula forward, stabilizes the scapula against the chest wall, and assists with upward rotation of the scapula during forward flexion of the shoulder and forward abduction of the arm. Loss of serratus function generally implies a root avulsion injury at the upper brachial plexus and is commonly associated with the aforementioned nerve injuries involving the suprascapular, axillary, and musculocutaneous nerves. Patients may complain of winging, limitation of shoulder elevation, pain, and weakness. The medial pectoral nerve has been used to restore innervation to the long thoracic nerve [51]. Tomaino [51] described successful return of serratus anterior function after a medial pectoral to long thoracic nerve transfer with an 11-cm interposed sural nerve graft 4 months after nerve injury during axillary node dissection.

Thoracodorsal nerve

Mackinnon and Novak [53,54] described transfer of the thoracodorsal nerve to the long thoracic nerve for reconstruction of serratus anterior function. In this transfer, no interposition nerve graft is needed. The patient' s chest and arm are prepped into the operative field, and an incision is made in the mid-axillary line, anterior to the free border of the latissimus muscle. The thoracodorsal and long thoracic nerves are identified, and the long thoracic nerve is stimulated to confirm lack of function. The thoracodorsal nerve is dissected to identify its branching points deep to the latissimus muscle, and it is likewise stimulated to confirm function of its branches. The transfer is planned at a point as proximal as possible along the long thoracic nerve to allow maximum reinnervation of the serratus anterior muscle, particularly the upper portion of the muscle. An appropriate posterior branch of the thoracodorsal nerve is selected so that the transfer may be performed without tension and without a nerve graft as the arm moves through full shoulder range of motion. The long thoracic nerve is transected proximally and reflected toward the thoracodorsal nerve; the thoracodorsal branch is transected distally and reflected toward the long thoracic nerve. The two are sutured in an epineurial fashion with microsurgical technique (Fig. 9).

Intercostal nerves

The intercostal nerves have been well used for nerve transfers and may be one of the only available options for donor nerves. Different techniques for intercostal nerve harvest exist, some of which have been well described [55]. Harvest of these nerves does not seem to have any effect on respiratory function, although ipsilateral rib fractures and phrenic nerve palsy are contraindications to their use as donor nerves [56]. Intercostal nerves may be used in transfer to reconstruct the long thoracic nerve (Fig. 10). Generally, a single curved incision along the course of the fourth rib centered about the anterior axillary line is sufficient for intercostal nerve harvest and can be hidden in the bra line and along the inframammary fold in women for better cosmesis.

Multiple incisions may be required for harvest of more than two or three intercostal nerves, and a longitudinal incision at the anterior axillary line can be extended in a zigzag fashion across the anterior axillary fold to the infraclavicular area or to the brachium to allow further dissection as needed. Intercostal nerves from T3 and T4 are most commonly used; however, T5 and T6 and—rarely—T2 are available options. The lateral border of the pectoralis major muscle is elevated and the origins of pectoralis minor serve as a landmark for the third through fifth ribs. The superficial periosteum of the ribs is incised, and a subperiosteal dissection is performed around the inferior costal border to avoid injury to the

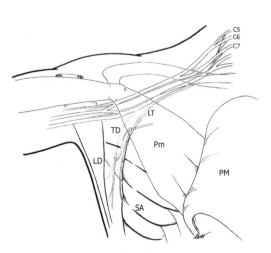

Fig. 9. Thoracodorsal to long thoracic nerve transfer. The thoracodorsal donor nerve (solid arrow) is transected as distally as possible and the long thoracic recipient nerve (open arrow) is transected as proximally as possible. C5–C7, cervical spine nerve roots. LT, long thoracic nerve. TD, thoracodorsal nerve. LD, latissimus dorsi muscle. Pm, pectoralis minor muscle. PM, pectoralis major muscle. SA, serratus anterior muscle. (*Courtesy of* Stephen H. Colbert, MD, Columbia, MO.)

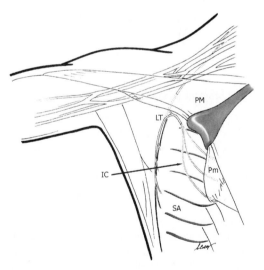

Fig. 10. Intercostal nerves to long thoracic nerve transfer. The third, fourth, and fifth intercostal nerves (*arrow*) are dissected posterior to the origin of pectoralis minor for added length and transferred to the long thoracic nerve, which has been transected as proximally as possible. Pectoralis major and pectoralis minor are being retracted. IC, intercostal nerves; LT, long thoracic nerve; PM, pectoralis major muscle; Pm, pectoralis minor muscle; SA, serratus anterior muscle. (*Courtesy of* Stephen H. Colbert, MD, Columbia, MO.)

nerves, blood vessels, and pleura. The deep periosteum of each rib is opened to identify the nerve and vessels, with the nerve situated inferior to the artery and the artery inferior to the vein. The nerve is dissected distally, or anteriorly, to a point at which motor function, as assessed by interrogation with a portable nerve stimulator, is lost. It is then freed proximally, or posteriorly, as far as necessary for tension-free transfer, generally to the anterior axillary line or the serratus anterior origins. These nerves are delicate and should not receive direct handling with forceps during the dissection. Hemostasis is performed with bipolar electrocautery only after the entire lengths of the nerves have been freed. We would re-emphasize that the long thoracic nerve should be dissected as proximally as possible to allow return of function to as much of the muscle as possible, including the important upper slips of serratus anterior. It is transected proximally and reflected toward the two to three donor nerves, which are grouped and sutured to the long thoracic nerve using micro-surgical technique.

After nerve transfer to the long thoracic nerve, the patient is kept in a shoulder immobilizer to prevent abduction for 2 weeks. Gentle intermittent limited active range-of-motion exercises are performed to prevent undue shoulder stiffness, but abduction beyond 90° is prevented until 2 to 3 weeks after surgery to avoid tension on the nerve repair.

Total brachial plexus injury

Complete injuries to the brachial plexus naturally affect the lower plexus and the upper plexus, as described previously. The arm is completely flaccid, with loss of shoulder, elbow, wrist, and hand function. Unlike isolated upper brachial plexus injuries, total brachial plexus avulsion injuries leave few donor nerves available for reconstruction, with those remaining being resigned to extraplexal sources. Such donors include the phrenic nerve [57], the spinal accessory nerve [58], motor branches of the cervical plexus [59], and intercostal nerves [60,61]. Gilbert [62] and Gu [63] recognized the availability of the intact contralateral brachial plexus as a source of donor nerves and first reported its use independently. Gilbert used the medial pectoral nerve and Gu used the C7 root. C7 was known to contribute not only to the lateral cord, mainly median nerve sensory fibers, and the posterior cord, mainly radial nerve motor fibers, but also to the pectoral,

musculocutaneous, long thoracic, subscapular, and thoracodorsal nerves [64]. All of the nerves that receive contributions from C7 maintain other nerve roots as their dominant contributors. C7 was felt to be an ideal donor nerve for total brachial plexus injuries. As pointed out by Chuang and colleagues [65], these transfers require long distances of regeneration through nerve grafts, staged operative procedures, intensive biofeedback retraining, and—rarely—achieve independent muscle function. Contralateral C7 transfers were recommended as best reserved for reconstruction of wrist and hand function in select cases.

Doi and colleagues [66] developed a double free muscle transfer for total brachial plexus reconstruction with a focus on achieving grip and finger extension for prehensile function. The procedure involves free gracilis muscle transfer innervated by the spinal accessory nerve to achieve elbow flexion and finger extension and a second free gracilis transfer innervated by intercostal nerves to achieve finger flexion. Other intercostal nerves are transferred to the nerves to the triceps for elbow extension. The shoulder is stabilized by glenohumeral arthrodesis, the thumb is stabilized by basal joint arthrodesis, and tenolysis of the transferred muscles is often required secondarily. Reported results revealed that 96% of patients achieved satisfactory elbow flexion, whereas 65% achieved more than 30° of total active finger motion and 54% were able to use the hand for two-handed activities (eg, lifting a heavy object or opening a bottle) [67].

The same group reported use of the double free muscle transfer in children combined with other techniques using ipsilateral upper plexus nerve roots and contralateral C7 as donor nerves via free vascularized ulnar nerve grafts to reconstruct the upper trunk, suprascapular nerve, posterior cord, and median nerves, selectively [68]. Similar results for free-functioning muscle transfers in adults have been reported by others [69,70], although they are keen to point out that more reliable results are achieved when the transferred muscle is used for a single function rather than for multiple functions [69] and that resulting hand function suggests much room for improvement.

Better functional results are achieved with shorter transfers closer to the target muscles. When available, the spinal accessory to suprascapular nerve and intercostal to musculocutaneous nerve transfers are recommended. When these transfers are successful, ever-important shoulder function and elbow flexion should be regained, and free-functioning muscle techniques may be considered for wrist or finger function reconstruction. When these transfers are unsuccessful or unavailable because of prolonged delay after injury, free-functioning muscle techniques are often the best options for functional recovery. Proper selection of the muscle is determined by desired strength, excursion, tendinous component, overall length and bulk, and vascular supply. Although the gracilis muscle is the preferred muscle of transfer, other muscles have been used, including the pectoralis major, latissimus dorsi, and tensor fascia lata. The arterial and venous donors of choice, such as the subclavian vasculature, the brachial artery, the thoracoacromial trunk and the thoracodorsal vessels, should be uninjured to provide reliable donor blood supply. Finally, the patient must be appropriately healthy to undergo prolonged administration of anesthesia.

Elbow flexion is the single most valuable upper extremity function, and free-functioning muscle transfers for reconstruction of elbow flexion tend to provide the most reliable results. Our recommendation is to give priority to restoration of elbow flexion with a free-functioning gracilis muscle powered by intercostal nerves (Fig. 11). The same technique may be used in patients with incomplete brachial plexus injuries that have undergone time-dependent atrophy of biceps and brachialis muscles. In these cases, other donor nerves, such as a redundant flexor carpi ulnaris fascicle from the ulnar nerve, would be preferred over the intercostal nerves.

The surgical technique for free-functioning muscle transfer involves careful planning and timing. The patient should be well positioned and padded to expose all operative sites. The recipient site is dissected first to ensure an adequate bed for the transferred muscle, and the donor vasculature and nerve supply are prepared. Although evidence indicates that spinal accessory nerve provides better results as a donor nerve than intercostal nerves [71], the intercostal nerves may be the best available option. When the intercostal nerves are used, two or three nerves—generally T3, T4, and possibly T5—are dissected via one or multiple incisions along the course of the ribs. The superficial surfaces of the ribs are identified and a subperiosteal dissection is performed around the inferior costal border to avoid injury to the nerves, blood vessels, and pleura. The deep periosteum of each rib is opened to identify the nerve and vessels. The nerve is dissected

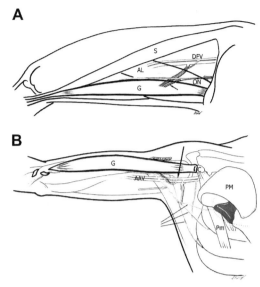

Fig. 11. Free-functioning gracilis muscle for total brachial plexus injury. (*A*) The gracilis muscle is shown at the posteromedial aspect of the right thigh with relevant anatomy. The nerve to gracilis (*arrow*) arises from the obturator nerve, and its vascular supply arises from the deep femoral system. AL, adductor longus; DFV, deep femoral vessels; G, gracilis muscle; ON, obturator nerve; S, sartorius muscle. (*B*) The gracilis muscle has been inset in the relative position of the biceps brachii muscle. The origin is fixated rapidly and vascular anastomoses completed promptly to available nearby vessels. In this case, vascular supply comes from the axillary vessels (*single solid arrow*) and nerve supply to the gracilis nerve (*open arrow*) comes from intercostal donor nerves (*multiple solid arrows*). Tension is set and the muscle insertion is secured. AAV, axillary artery and vein; C, coracoid process; G, gracilis muscle; PM, pectoralis major muscle; Pm, pectoralis minor muscle. (*Courtesy of* Stephen H. Colbert, MD, Columbia, MO.)

distally, or anteriorly, to a point at which motor function, as assessed by interrogation with a portable nerve stimulator, is lost. It is freed proximally, or posteriorly, as far as necessary for tension-free transfer, generally to the anterior axillary line.

The gracilis muscle may be approached via a longitudinal incision directly over the muscle at the medial thigh or via endoscopic technique. The nerve to the gracilis enters the muscle from superiorly and laterally at an oblique angle from its origin from the obturator nerve. The vascular pedicle originates from the profunda femoris. As much length as possible should be obtained from the vessel and nerve pedicles to ensure a tension-free transfer without the need for interposition grafts. If nerve grafts are felt to be necessary, they can be placed at the time of initial dissection of the donor nerves as the first of a staged procedure, with the muscle being transferred as a second stage at a later date. Once adequate length has been determined, the gracilis muscle is marked at regular length intervals along its course with suture to facilitate restoration of normal resting length at the time of inset, as described by Manktelow and colleagues [72]. The muscle is harvested, with a skin paddle—if necessary—for monitoring, transferred to its recipient bed, and immediately definitively secured to its origin and tentatively secured to its insertion. The microvascular repair is performed first to minimize ischemia time, followed by nerve repair. The nerve repair is performed as close to the muscle as possible to minimize time to reinnervation. Appropriate muscle tension is set using the previously placed marking sutures and the insertion definitively secured. Closure is completed and the tissue is monitored appropriately postoperatively.

Rehabilitation

Rehabilitation for patients undergoing brachial plexus reconstruction begins before surgery. Supple joints and a healthy tissue bed are critical for a successful outcome, and preoperative therapy may be required to prepare the patient adequately. Preparation may include splints at the hand and wrist to prevent joint contraction in an undesired position, slings or other supports at the shoulder to maintain capsular integrity, range-of-motion exercises to maintain joint motion, and potentially direct muscular stimulation of the denervated muscle.

The appropriate therapy is crucial to re-educate and retrain neuromuscular function after surgical reconstruction has been performed. Nerve repairs are always performed in a tension-free manner through full joint range of motion. These microsurgical repairs are delicate, however. We recommend 1 to 2 weeks in a shoulder immobilizer after surgery at the shoulder, axilla, or upper arm level, with intermittent gentle range-of-motion exercises three to four times daily to prevent stiffness. Motion of the wrist and hand is not restricted during this time. Full range-of-motion exercises four to six times daily are begun 2 weeks after surgery, and all restrictions are lifted 6 weeks after surgery. A notable exception to this rule applies to patients who have undergone a free-functioning muscle transfer. In those cases, shoulder and elbow immobilization is maintained strictly for 2 to 3 weeks, with the shoulder abducted and the elbow flexed at or beyond 30°. Thereafter, the elbow is not extended beyond 30° of flexion, because a small degree of flexion contracture generally improves function. For all postoperative patients, edema and scar management measures are instituted, and electrical stimulation may be beneficial.

Neuromuscular re-education is a critical element of successful nerve transfer. Without the potential of re-education and retraining, nerve transfers would not provide any useful return of function. This issue emphasizes the importance of a good working relationship between therapist and surgeon. The therapist must have a clear understanding of the surgical procedure, including the specific donor and recipient nerves. Patients are educated preoperatively about what exercises are needed for re-education in the postoperative period. Re-education in earnest is begun when reconstructed muscle contraction is observed or voluntary MUPs are identified on electromyography. The concept behind re-education involves cognitive recognition of the previous donor function as the initiator of the reconstructed function followed by relearning for subconscious control. Biofeedback is the most powerful tool for this type of re-education. Because muscle function is weak upon return, exercises are performed with gravity eliminated. As strength increases, motion against gravity is introduced, as are specific strengthening exercises. Patients are taught to contract the donor muscle to achieve function of the reconstructed muscle, which is often facilitated by simultaneous co-contraction of the muscle groups on the affected extremity and the contralateral unaffected extremity. With training, the new function is learned independently. Sensory re-education is performed, generally some time later than motor re-education, depending on the length of sensory nerve regeneration required. Motor and sensory re-education allows the central nervous system to be "remapped" to provide this independent function.

Summary

Brachial plexus injuries are functionally devastating and present incredibly difficult problems for peripheral nerve surgeons. Typical injuries tend to be from blunt trauma and involve significant components of root avulsions or other proximal injuries. Functional recovery after reconstruction traditionally has been far from optimal. The rejuvenation of the concept of nerve transfers has added new options for brachial plexus reconstruction, however, many of which have produced superior results to traditional nerve grafting procedures and quickly have become the gold standards of treatment. These procedures effectively reduce a high nerve injury to a low injury, hasten muscle reinnervation, and preserve muscle integrity and function. In total brachial plexus injuries, free-functioning muscle transfers are being refined to provide better elbow function and occasional return of useful active hand function. The potential of nerve transfers for brachial plexus reconstruction is only just being realized, and although there is still substantial room for improvement, nerve transfers have provided the ability to achieve functional results for patients, the likes of which we have never seen before.

References

[1] Midha R. Epidemiology of brachial plexus injuries in a multitrauma population. Neurosurgery 1997; 40(6):1182–8 [discussion: 1188–9].

[2] Dubuisson AS, Kline DG. Brachial plexus injury: a survey of 100 consecutive cases from a single service. Neurosurgery 2002;51(3):673–82 [discussion: 682–3].

[3] Gorio A, Carmignoto G. Reformation, maturation and stabilization of neuromuscular junctions in peripheral nerve regeneration. In: Gorio A, Millesi H, Mingrino S, editors. Posttraumatic peripheral nerve regeneration. New York: Raven Press; 1981. p. 481–92.

[4] Sunderland S. Nerves and nerve injuries. Baltimore (MD): Williams and Wilkins Company; 1968.

[5] Sunderland S. Nerves and nerve injuries. Edinburgh (NY): Churchill Livingstone; 1978.

[6] Sunderland S. Nerve injuries and their repair: a critical appraisal. Edinburgh (NY): Churchill Livingstone; 1991.

[7] Williams HB, Jabaley ME. The importance of internal anatomy of the peripheral nerves to nerve repair in the forearm and hand. Hand Clin 1986;2(4): 689–707.

[8] Millesi H. Healing of nerves. Clin Plast Surg 1977; 4(3):459–73.

[9] Millesi H. Peripheral nerve repair: terminology, questions, and facts. J Reconstr Microsurg 1985; 2(1):21–31.

[10] Kline DG, Hudson AR, Hacket ER, et al. Progression of partial experimental injury to peripheral nerve. Part 1. Periodic measurements of muscle contraction strength. J Neurosurg 1975; 42(1):1–14.

[11] Hudson AR, Kline DG. Progression of partial experimental injury to peripheral nerve. Part 2. Light and electron microscopic studies. J Neurosurg 1975;42(1):15–22.

[12] Kline DG, Hayes GJ, Morse AS. A comparative study of response of species to peripheral-nerve injury. I. Severance. J Neurosurg 1964;21:968–79.

[13] Kline DG, Hayes GJ, Morse AS. A comparative study of response of species to peripheral-nerve injury. II. Crush and severance with primary suture. J Neurosurg 1964;21:980–8.

[14] Terzis JK. Sensory mapping. Clin Plast Surg 1976; 3(1):59–64.

[15] Breidenback WC, Terzis JK. The blood supply of vascularized nerve grafts. J Reconstr Microsurg 1986;3(1):43–58.

[16] Narakas AO. Brachial plexus surgery. Orthop Clin North Am 1981;12(2):303–23.

[17] Herzberg G, Narakas A, Comtet JJ, et al. Microsurgical relations of the roots of the brachial plexus: practical applications. Ann Chir Main 1985;4(2): 120–33.

[18] Narakas A. My early experiences in microsurgery. J Reconstr Microsurg 1994;10(2):97–9.

[19] Kline DG, Hudson AR. Stretch injuries to the brachial plexus. In: Kline DG, Hudson AR, editors. Nerve injuries: operative results for major nerve injuries, entrapments, and tumors, Philadelphia: WB Saunders; 1995; 135. p. 415–6.

[20] Yoshikawa T, Hayashi N, Yamamoto S, et al. Brachial plexus injury: clinical manifestations, conventional imaging findings, and the latest imaging techniques. Radiographics 2006;26(Suppl 1): S133–43.

[21] Amrami KK, Port JD. Imaging the brachial plexus. Hand Clin 2005;21(1):25–38.

[22] Seddon HJ. Three types of nerve injury. Brain 1943; 66(4):238–88.

[23] Sunderland S. A classification of peripheral nerve injuries producing loss of function. Brain 1951;74(4): 491–516.

[24] Mackinnon SE, Dellon AL. Surgery of the peripheral nerve. New York: Thieme Medical Publishers, Inc; 1988.

[25] Novak CB, Kelly L, Mackinnon SE. Sensory recovery following median nerve grafting. J Hand Surg 1992;17A(1):59–68.

[26] Guelinckx PJ, Carlson BM, Faulkner JA. Morphologic characteristics of muscles grafted in rabbits with neurovascular repair. J Reconstr Microsurg 1992;8(6):481–9.

[27] Lurje A. Concerning surgical treatment of traumatic injury of the upper division of the brachial plexus (Erb' s-type). Ann Surg 1948;127:317–26.

[28] Samardzic M, Grujicic D, Antunovic V. Nerve transfer in brachial plexus traction injuries. J Neurosurg 1992;76(2):191–7.

[29] Chuang DC, Lee GW, Hashem F, et al. Restoration of shoulder abduction by nerve transfer in avulsion brachial plexus injury: evaluation of 99 patients with various nerve transfers. Plast Reconstr Surg 1995;96:122–8.

[30] Celli L, Rovesta C, Balli A. Neurotization of brachial plexus avulsion with intercostal nerves (personal techniques). In: Brunelli G, editor. Textbook of microsurgery. Milano (Italy): Masson; 1988. p. 789–95.

[31] Samardzic M, Grujicic D, Rasulic L, et al. Transfer of the medial pectoral nerve: myth or reality? Neurosurgery 2002;50(6):1277–82.

[32] Gu YD, Cai PQ, Xu F, et al. Clinical application of ipsilateral C7 nerve root transfer for treatment of C5 and C6 avulsion of brachial plexus. Microsurgery 2003;23(2):105–8.

[33] Gu YD, Zhang GM, Chen DS, et al. Cervical nerve root transfer from contralateral normal side for treatment of brachial plexus root avulsions. Chin Med J 1991;104:208–11.

[34] Malessy MJ, Hoffmann CF, Thomeer RT. Initial report on the limited value of hypoglossal nerve transfer to treat brachial plexus root avulsions. J Neurosurg 1999;91:601–4.

[35] Nath RK, Mackinnon SE. Nerve transfers in the upper extremity. Hand Clin 2000;16:131–9.

[36] Witoonchart K, Leechavengvongs S, Uerpairojkit C, et al. Nerve transfer to deltoid muscle using the nerve to the long head of the triceps. Part I. An anatomic feasibility study. J Hand Surg 2003;28A: 628–32.

[37] Leechavengvongs S, Witoonchart K, Uerpairojkit C, et al. Nerve transfer to deltoid muscle using the nerve to the long head of the triceps. Part II. A report of 7 cases. J Hand Surg 2003;28A:633–8.

[38] Bertelli JA, Ghizoni MF. Reconstruction of C5 and C6 brachial plexus avulsion injury by multiple nerve transfers: spinal accessory to suprascapular, ulnar fascicles to biceps branch, and triceps long or lateral head branch to axillary nerve. J Hand Surg 2004; 29A:131–9.

[39] Kawai H, Akita S. Shoulder muscle reconstruction in the upper type of the brachial plexus injury by partial radial nerve transfer to the axillary nerve. Tech Hand Up Extrem Surg 2004;8:51–5.

[40] Bahm J, Naoman H, Becker M. The dorsal approach to the suprascapular nerve in neuromuscular reanimation for obstetric brachial plexus lesions. Plast Reconstr Surg 2005;115:240–4.

[41] Bertelli JA, Ghizoni MF. Improved technique for harvesting the accessory nerve for transfer in brachial plexus injuries. Neurosurgery 2006;58(4 Suppl 2) ONS-366-70; discussion ONS-370.

[42] Colbert SH, Mackinnon SE. Posterior approach for double nerve transfer for restoration of shoulder function in upper brachial plexus palsy. Hand 2006;1(2):71–7.

[43] Brandt KE, Mackinnon SE. A technique for maximizing biceps recovery in brachial plexus reconstruction. J Hand Surg 1993;18A:726–33.

[44] Oberlin C, Beal D, Leechavengvongs S, et al. Nerve transfer to biceps muscle using a part of ulnar nerve for C5-C6 avulsion of the brachial plexus: anatomical study and report of four cases. J Hand Surg. 1994;19A(2):232–7.

[45] Leechavengvongs S, Witoonchart K, Uerpairojkit C, et al. Nerve transfer to biceps muscle using a part of the ulnar nerve in brachial plexus injury (upper arm type): a report of 32 cases. J Hand Surg 1998;23A:711–6.

[46] Sungpet A, Suphachatwong C, Kawinwonggowit V, et al. Transfer of a single fascicle from the ulnar nerve to the biceps muscle after avulsions of upper roots of the brachial plexus. J Hand Surg 2000; 25B:325–8.

[47] Humphreys DB, Mackinnon SE. Nerve transfers. Operative Techniques in Plastic and Reconstructive Surgery 2002;9:89–99.

[48] Tung TH, Novak CB, Mackinnon SE. Nerve transfers to the biceps and brachialis branches to improve elbow flexion strength after brachial plexus injuries. J Neurosurg 2003;98:313–8.

[49] Mackinnon SE, Novak CB, Myckatyn TM, et al. Results of reinnervation of the biceps and brachialis muscles with a double fascicular transfer for elbow flexion. J Hand Surg 2005;30A:978–85.

[50] Novak CB, Mackinnon SE. Treatment of a proximal accessory nerve injury with nerve transfer. Laryngoscope 2004;114(8):1482–4.

[51] Tomaino MM. Neurophysiologic and clinical outcome following medial pectoral to long thoracic nerve transfer for scapular winging: a case report. Microsurgery 2002;22(6):254–7.

[52] Lee KS. Anatomic variation of the spinal origins of lateral and medial pectoral nerves. Clin Anat 2007; 20(8):915–8.

[53] Mackinnon SE, Novak CB. Nerve transfers: new options for reconstruction following nerve injury. Hand Clin 1999;15(4):643–66 [review].

[54] Novak CB, Mackinnon SE. Surgical treatment of a long thoracic nerve palsy. Ann Thorac Surg 2002;73(5):1643–5.

[55] Wahegaonkar AL, Doi K, Hattori Y, et al. Technique of intercostal nerve harvest and transfer for various neurotization procedures in brachial plexus injuries. Tech Hand Up Extrem Surg 2007;11(3):184–94.

[56] Giddins GE, Kakkar N, Alltree J, et al. The effect of unilateral intercostal nerve transfer upon lung function. J Hand Surg 1995;20B(5):675–6.

[57] Gu YD, Wu MM, Zhen YL, et al. Phrenic nerve transfer for brachial plexus motor neurotization. Microsurgery 1989;10(4):287–9.

[58] Allieu Y, Cenac P. Neurotization via the spinal accessory nerve in complete paralysis due to multiple avulsion injuries of the brachial plexus. Clin Orthop Relat Res 1988;(237):67–74.

[59] Brunelli G, Monini L. Neurotization of avulsed roots of brachial plexus by means of anterior nerves of cervical plexus. Clin Plast Surg 1984;11(1): 149–52.

[60] Minami M, Ishii S. Satisfactory elbow flexion in complete (preganglionic) brachial plexus injuries: produced by suture of third and fourth intercostal nerves to musculocutaneous nerve. J Hand Surg 1987;12A(6):1114–8.

[61] Nagano A, Tsuyama N, Ochiai N, et al. Direct nerve crossing with the intercostal nerve to treat avulsion injuries of the brachial plexus. J Hand Surg 1989; 14A(6):980–5.

[62] Gilbert A. Neurotization by contralateral pectoral nerve. Presented at the 10th Symposium on the Brachial Plexus. Lausanne, Switzerland, January 19–22, 1992.

[63] Gu YD. Neurotization by contralateral C7. Presented at the 9th Symposium on the Brachial Plexus. Villars, Switzerland, March 30–31, 1989.

[64] Slingluff CL, Terzis JK, Edgerton MT. The quantitative microanatomy of the brachial plexus in man: reconstructive relevance. In: Terzis JK, editor. Microreconstruction of nerve injuries. Philadelphia: WB Saunders; 1987. p. 285–324.

[65] Chuang DC, Wei FC, Noordhoff MS. Cross-chest C7 nerve grafting followed by free muscle transplantations for the treatment of total avulsed brachial plexus injuries: a preliminary report. Plast Reconstr Surg 1993;92(4):717–25 [discussion: 726–7].

[66] Doi D, Sakai K, Duwata N, et al. Double free-muscle transfer to restore prehension following complete brachial plexus avulsion. J Hand Surg 1995;20A: 408–14.

[67] Doi K, Muramatsu K, Hattori Y, et al. Restoration of prehension with the double free muscle technique following complete avulsion of the brachial plexus: indications and long-term results. J Bone Joint Surg Am 2000;82(5):652–66.

[68] Hattori Y, Doi K, Ikeda K, et al. Restoration of prehension using double free muscle technique after complete avulsion of brachial plexus in children: a report of three cases. J Hand Surg 2005;30A(4): 812–9.

[69] Barrie KA, Steinmann SP, Shin AY, et al. Gracilis free muscle transfer for restoration of function after complete brachial plexus avulsion. Neurosurg Focus 2004;16(5):E8.

[70] Songcharoen P, Wongtrakul S, Spinner RJ. Brachial plexus injuries in the adult: nerve transfers. The Siriraj Hospital experience. Hand Clin 2005; 21(1):83–9.

[71] Hattori Y, Doi K, Ikedu K, et al. Ultrasonographic evaluation of functioning free muscle transfer: comparison between spinal accessory and intercostal nerve reinnervation. J Reconstr Microsurg 2006; 22(6):423–7.

[72] Manktelow RT, Zuker RM, McKee NH. Functioning free muscle transplantation. J Hand Surg 1984; 9A:32–9.

Nerve Transfers in Brachial Plexus Birth Palsies: Indications, Techniques, and Outcomes

Scott H. Kozin, MD[a,b,*]

[a]*Department of Orthopaedic Surgery, Temple University, 3401 Broad Street, Philadelphia, PA 19140, USA*
[b]*Upper Extremity Center of Excellence, Shriners Hospitals for Children,*
3551 North Broad Street, Philadelphia, PA 19140, USA

Brachial plexus birth palsies occur in approximately 0.87 to 2.5 per 1000 live births [1–4]. Most lesions involve the upper trunk (C5 and C6), with or without additional injury to C7. Total plexus involvement (C5 through T1) occurs less frequently. Isolated lower trunk injury is rare and may not even exist in birth palsies (Table 1).

Infants who have upper trunk birth palsies who demonstrate considerable recovery within the first 2 months usually recover normal function [5,6]. Biceps activity is the best indicator of upper trunk function. Lack of elbow flexion against gravity is the primary indication for microsurgery. The timing of surgery for upper trunk lesions remains controversial and varies between 3 and 8 months [7–12]. In contrast, infants who have global lesions should undergo early microsurgery by 3 months of age [7–9]. This early intervention allows lower trunk reconstruction and the potential for hand function [9]. Delayed surgery allows end plate degradation and lessens the chances of hand reinnervation.

Neurolysis has little benefit in brachial plexus palsy [10,11]. Nerve grafting and nerve transfers are the mainstay of treatment. The use of nerve transfers in brachial plexus birth palsies is evolving; however, their precise role is still not clearly defined. The decision to perform nerve transfers versus nerve grafting is even more controversial. Many factors influence the decision-making

process, including injury pattern, age of the child, and physical examination. In addition, surgeon's preference appears to play a dominant role. This article provides an overview of nerve transfers for infants who have brachial plexus birth palsies. Indications, technique, and outcome will be discussed. The author's personal preference will be highlighted with a disclaimer that he will likely amend his indications and contraindications in the future as scientific evidence provides more concrete support for specific surgical techniques.

Evaluation

The author's center advocates early referral to a qualified center for infants who have brachial plexus palsy. For upper ± middle trunk injuries, lack of full recovery by 2 months necessitates evaluation. For global lesions, immediate referral is encouraged. This early evaluation allows us to obtain accurate baseline data, to educate the family, to empower the family to participate in the decision-making process, and to develop a relationship with the family before any surgical intervention.

The initial evaluation uses a brachial plexus intake form to obtain all relevant information (Fig. 1). This form ensures completeness and facilitates the development of a database. Many inexperienced physicians feel overwhelmed when trying to examine an infant who has a brachial plexus palsy; however, a concise preliminary examination can be accomplished, keeping in mind several key concepts. The goal is to assess upper, middle, and lower trunk function and to

---

* Upper Extremity Center of Excellence, Shriners Hospitals for Children, 3551 North Broad Street, Philadelphia, PA 19140.

E-mail address: skozin@shrinenet.org

Table 1
Types of brachial plexus injuries and associated findings

Pattern	Nerve roots involved	Primary deficiency
Erb-Duchenne lesion Upper brachial plexus (50%)	C5 and C6	Shoulder abduction and external rotation Elbow flexion
Extended Erb palsy Upper & middle plexus (30%)	C5 through C7	As above plus elbow and finger MP joint extension
Dejerine-Klumpke paralysis Lower brachial plexus	C8 and T1	Hand intrinsic muscles Finger flexors
Total or global lesion Entire brachial plexus (20%)	C5 through T1	Entire extremity

Abbreviation: MP, metacarpophalangeal.

determine the type of injury. For the upper trunk, the assessment involves shoulder motion, elbow flexion, and wrist extension (extensor carpi radialis longus). For the middle trunk, the evaluation consists of elbow extension, wrist extension (extensor carpi radialis brevis), and digital metacarpophalangeal joint extension. For the lower trunk, the assess examination focuses on extrinsic finger and thumb flexion by way of grasp. Certainly, other functions can be examined, such as supination (upper trunk), pronation (middle trunk), and intrinsic function (lower trunk). However, these movements are a challenge to elicit in uncooperative infants. In the author's clinic, the therapists play an integral role in the examination process and family education. Their examination focuses on specific movement patterns using the active movement scale (see Fig. 1) [13]. This scale is designed for infants and provides reliable data before and after surgical intervention [14].

Once the type of injury is determined, the extent of injury is defined. Transient neurapraxias resolve spontaneously within the first 2 months and are a distinct entity. Axonotmesis and neurotmesis are more extensive injuries and are more difficult to discriminate from one another. Furthermore, all components of each trunk may not have sustained a similar degree of injury. For example, an upper trunk injury may have a portion that has undergone complete separation (neurotmesis) and an adjacent part where the nerve fiber integrity has been disrupted with preservation of the axonal sheath and framework (axonotmesis). In the neurotmetic portion, no recovery can occur without surgical intervention. In the axonotmesis position, wallerian degeneration and nerve fiber regeneration can occur for recovery. Therefore, the differentiation of a neurotmesis and an axonotmesis is not initially

discernable, because within the same trunk, different degrees of nerve injuries can coexist (Fig. 2).

Consideration factors for nerve transfers

Various factors must be considered when developing a surgical plan. First and foremost is the injury pattern. For global lesions, axonal inflow is always a problem because avulsions are likely (Fig. 3). Nerve transfers can increase the inflow and allow additional reconstruction, compared with nerve grafting alone. In addition, available axons from any available root are often biased toward the avulsed lower trunk, which leaves little axonal inflow for shoulder and elbow motion [15–19]. Typical donors that can provide inflow axons are the spinal accessory for shoulder motion and the intercostal nerves for elbow motion. Contralateral C7 transfer has been reported in birth palsy, although the author has not performed this transfer in infants [20].

For upper ± middle trunk lesions, the number of available nerve transfers increases considerably. In addition, the indications become more controversial.

When considering nerve transfers for upper ± middle trunk lesions, additional factors must be considered. Nerve transfers are especially useful for infants who present late, often older than 1 year of age [21]. In these cases, nerve transfers would reach the targeted muscle before nerve grafting and diminish ongoing motor end plate demise. Nerve transfers are also useful when neuroma resection would create too great a loss of function. For example, some infants regain good shoulder function but still lack elbow flexion. Adequate is hard to define, but the author usually defines 90 degrees against gravity as sufficient,

Patient's Age: ______ **Visit Type:** routine follow up ___ post-op follow up (___ months)
History of Condition:

______

PROM: **ER (scapula stabilized, shoulder add)** ________ **IR (scapula stabilized, shoulder add)** ________
Scapulo-Humeral Abduction Contracture: ________ **Elbow Extension:** ________

Active Movement Scale (AMS)

Shoulder Abduction	_______		
Shoulder Adduction	_______	Gravity Eliminated	Score
Shoulder Flexion	_______	No contraction	0
Shoulder External Rotation	_______	Contraction, no motion	1
Shoulder Internal Rotation	_______	<50% motion	2
Elbow Flexion	_______	>50% motion	3
Elbow Extension	_______	Full Motion	4
Forearm Supination	_______	Against Gravity	
Forearm Pronation	_______	<50% motion	5
Wrist Flexion	_______	>50% motion	6
Wrist Extension	_______	Full Motion	7
Finger Flexion	_______		
Finger Extension	_______		
Thumb Flexion	_______		
Thumb Extension	_______		
Total	_______		

Toronto Score

Elbow Flexion (0-2)	_____
Elbow Extension (0-2)	_____
Wrist Extension (0-2)	_____
Finger Extension (0-2)	_____
Thumb Extension (0-2)	_____
Total	_____

Table for Scoring Toronto
(all movement scored against gravity)

	Grade	Weight
No Joint Mov't	0	0.0
Flicker	0+	0.3
<50%ROM	1-	0.6
=50%	1	1.0
>50% ROM	1+	1.3
Good but not full	2-	1.6
Full ROM	2	2.0

Modified Mallet Classification (grade I = no function, Grade V = normal function)

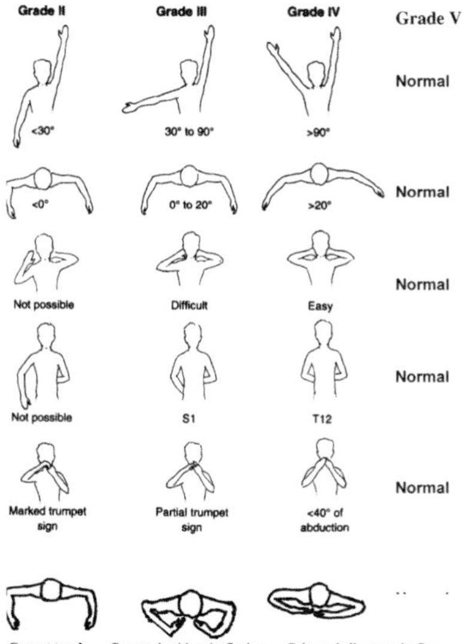

	Not Testable	Grade I	Grade II	Grade III	Grade IV	Grade V
Global Abduction	Not Testable	No function	<30°	30° to 90°	>90°	Normal
Global External Rotation	Not Testable	No function	<0°	0° to 20°	>20°	Normal
Hand to neck	Not Testable	No function	Not possible	Difficult	Easy	Normal
Hand on spine	Not Testable	No function	Not possible	S1	T12	Normal
Hand to mouth	Not Testable	No function	Marked trumpet sign	Partial trumpet sign	<40° of abduction	Normal
Internal Rotation	Not Testable	No Function	Cannot touch	Can touch with wrist flexion	Palm on belly, no wrist flex	.. .

Strength (MMT/AROM)

Shoulder ABD
MMT ___/5
AROM ___

Shoulder IR (at belly)
MMT ___/5
AROM ___

Pronation
MMT ___/5
AROM ___

Digit ext
MMT ___/5
AROM ___

Wrist ext
MMT ___/5
AROM ___

Elbow Flex
MMT ___/5
AROM ___

Supination
MMT ___/5
AROM ___

Assessment: ______

______

Intervention: ______
Plan: ______

Today's Date: ______ Therapist's Signature: ______

Fig. 1. Upper Extremity Brachial Plexus Clinic Form. ABD, abduction; AROM, active range of motion; ER, external rotation; IR, internal rotation; MMT, manual muscle testing; PROM, passive range of motion; ROM, range of motion.

especially considering the positive outcomes associated with secondary tendon transfers. Figs. 4–6 show an example of a 7-month-old child who had forward flexion and abduction to 90 degrees with, however, no evident biceps activity. In this case, isolated nerve transfer for elbow flexion could preserve shoulder motion and was performed. Nerve transfers are also performed in

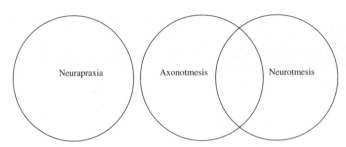

Fig. 2. Neurapraxia is a distinct entity, but axonotmesis and neurotmesis can overlap.

upper ± middle trunk lesions when intraoperative assessment reveals poor root quality or avulsions at the time of surgery.

The choice of nerve transfers versus nerve grafting also appears to be surgeon biased. Some surgeons prefer one technique over the other option, based on their experience, results, and familiarity. This lack of consensus is confusing to families trying to decide what is best for their child and seeking multiple opinions (Table 2).

Principles of nerve transfer

The principles of nerve transfer are remarkably similar to those of tendon transfer [22]. The proper selection of a donor and recipient nerve requires a clear understanding of the principles. In general, a motor donor should have many motor fibers and a sensory donor should have many sensory fibers. In addition, the donor and recipient nerves should be in close proximity.

Selection of the donor nerve

The donor nerve has to be available and expendable. Available implies a functioning, normal nerve that can sustain a loss of a portion of its axons. Fortunately, many nerves have built-in redundancy in their proximal aspect. As the nerve travels in a distal direction, less overlap is found. Expendable means that if the donor harvest causes some loss of function, the effect is minimal. For example, harvesting the intercostal nerves has a negligible effect on pulmonary function, as long as the phrenic nerve is working [15,23]. Similarly, selection of a radial nerve to a single head of the triceps has a miniscule effect on elbow extension, as long as the other two heads are preserved. An additional consideration during nerve transfer is synergism. Logically, using a donor nerve that provides synergistic function with the intended action would facilitate relearning after reinnervation. For example, when selecting an ulnar nerve fascicle for elbow flexion, selecting the fascicle

Table 2
Indications and considerations for nerve transfers

Indication/consideration	Rationale	Common transfers
Global injury	To increase axonal inflow	Spinal accessory Intercostal ± Contralateral C7
Upper ± middle with late presentation	For quicker motor reinnervation to preserve end plates	Spinal accessory Ulnar Median Thoracodorsal
Upper ± middle with mixed recovery, but persistent deficit	To avoid iatrogenic loss of function associated with neuroma resection	Spinal accessory Ulnar Median
Upper ± middle with poor root quality or avulsions	For additional axonal inflow	Spinal accessory Ulnar Median Thoracodorsal

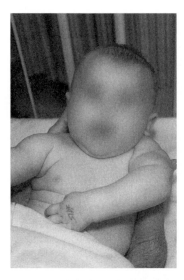

Fig. 3. A 4-month-old child who has left global brachial plexus palsy and Horner's syndrome. Surgical reconstruction usually involves nerve grafting and nerve transfers, depending on intraoperative findings.

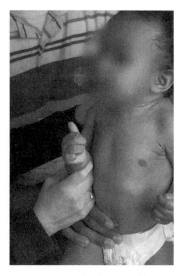

Fig. 5. A 7-month-old child who has right upper trunk brachial plexus palsy and 90 degrees of forward flexion, no external rotation, and no elbow flexion.

that innervates the flexor carpi ulnaris would enhance firing.

Selection of the recipient nerve

The recipient nerve should be chosen selectively to achieve the desired function. A motor donor should be directed into a motor recipient and a sensory donor placed into a sensory recipient. In addition, the motor nerve recipient should be close to the end plate to minimize reinnervation time. When selecting recipient motor nerves, the trend is to provide dual reinnervation to achieve a desired function. For example, nerve transfers for elbow flexion attempt to

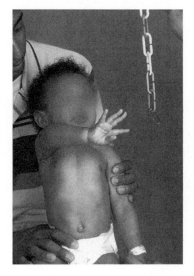

Fig. 4. A 7-month-old child who has right upper trunk brachial plexus palsy and 90 degrees of forward flexion, no external rotation, and no elbow flexion.

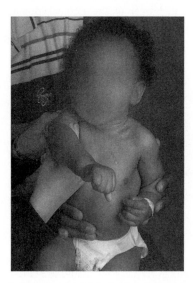

Fig. 6. A 7-month-old child who has right upper trunk brachial plexus palsy and 90 degrees of forward flexion, no external rotation, and no elbow flexion.

reinnervate both the biceps and brachialis muscles. Similarly, nerve transfers for shoulder motion try to reinnervate both deltoid and rotator cuff function.

Nerve transfers for shoulder motion

Shoulder movement is a complex interaction between the rotator cuff and the deltoid. Nerve transfers can be directed toward the suprascapular nerve or the axillary nerve [17,18,22,24–33]. In the flail shoulder, the author prefers to perform both nerve transfers to maximize shoulder motion. In selected cases that have adequate deltoid function but no external rotation, isolated nerve transfer to the suprascapular nerve is an alternative technique.

Suprascapular nerve transfer

Suprascapular nerve transfer requires attention to detail [32,34,35]. The infant is placed supine on the operating room table. After general anesthesia is induced, a rolled towel is placed along the child's back between the scapulae, and the head is turned to the opposite side (Fig. 7). This towel elevates the shoulder and neck from the table and provides access to the spinal accessory nerve. On occasion, a second towel is used to make a T-shape to elevate the trapezius muscle from the table better.

Initial attention is directed to the supraclavicular approach. A transverse incision is made from the lateral border of the sternocleidomastoid to the trapezius muscle (Fig. 8). Hemostasis is obtained with electrocautery. Loupe magnification

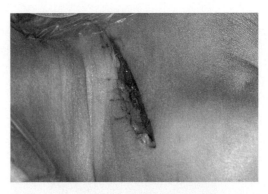

Fig. 8. A transverse incision from the lateral border of the sternocleidomastoid to the trapezius muscle.

is used throughout the procedure. Deeper dissection identifies the omohyoid, which is retracted carefully. Deep to the omohyoid, the upper trunk is palpated and retracted. The suprascapular nerve is found exiting the upper trunk and a vessel loop is placed around the nerve (Fig. 9).

The lateral border of the trapezius muscle is then released from the clavicle and acromioclavicular joint using electrocautery (Fig. 10). Dissection is then performed on the anterior surface of the trapezius muscle, looking for the spinal accessory nerve. The landmark for detection of the spinal accessory nerve is the transverse cervical artery and vein. These vessels enter the muscle at the base of the neck and then descend vertically midway between the vertebral column and the medial border of the scapula and accompany the spinal accessory nerve. Identification of these vessels facilitates isolation of the spinal accessory nerve. An electric stimulator can be used around the vessels to identify the distal part of the spinal

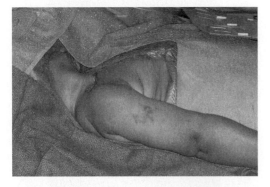

Fig. 7. The child depicted in Fig. 4 was carefully positioned on the operating room table with a rolled towel between the scapulas and the head turned to the opposite side to provide access to the spinal accessory and suprascapular nerves.

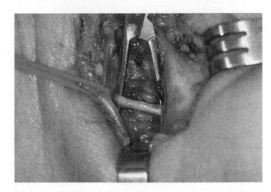

Fig. 9. The omohyoid is retracted with a vessel loop and the suprascapular nerve is identified exiting the upper trunk.

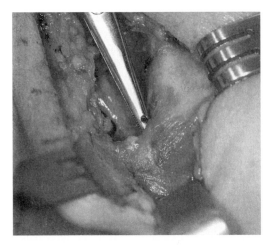

Fig. 10. The lateral border of the trapezius muscle is identified at its insertion into the clavicle before release with an electrocautery.

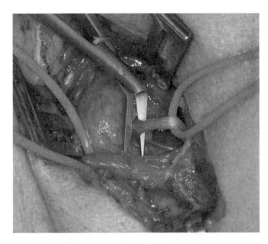

Fig. 12. The suprascapular nerve is cut from the upper trunk.

accessory nerve. A vessel loop is placed around the spinal accessory nerve. Small branches from the cervical plexus in the vicinity can be confused with the spinal accessory nerve. However, these branches are small and will not elicit any muscle response when stimulated. The terminal division of the nerve is dissected as far distal as possible, divided, and transferred to the supraclavicular fossa for transfer (Fig. 11). Proximal dissection is not necessary and not warranted because the proximal innervation of the trapezius muscle is preserved.

The suprascapular nerve is traced as proximal as possible and cut from the upper trunk (Fig. 12). The operating microscope is then brought into the field (Fig. 13). Nerve coaptation is performed with

a combination of 9-0 nylon suture and fibrin glue. The supraclavicular fat is then placed over the nerve repair to enhance vascular ingrowth. The wound is closed in a layered fashion with absorbable suture.

Radial nerve transfer

A longitudinal incision is made from the posterior border of the deltoid muscle along a line between the long and lateral heads of the triceps muscles (Fig. 14) [17,18,26,27,36]. Deep dissection exposes the long and lateral heads of the triceps and the quadrangular space above the teres major muscle. The axillary nerve is identified as it emanates from this space (Fig. 15). The

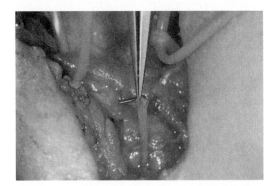

Fig. 11. The terminal division of the spinal accessory nerve has been dissected as far distal as possible, divided, and transferred toward the supraclavicular nerve (ligaclip on spinal accessory nerve, vessel loops around omohyoid and suprascapular nerve).

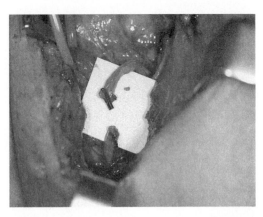

Fig. 13. The suprascapular and spinal accessory nerves are placed adjacent to each other before nerve coaptation with suture and fibrin glue.

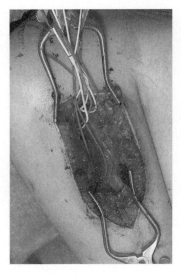

Fig. 14. The posterior aspect of left arm in a child who has avulsions of C5 and C6. Exposure for radial to axillary nerve transfers.

braches to the lateral, long, and medial heads of the triceps are isolated. Electric stimulation is useful to verify the motor branches.

As recommended by Colbert and Mackinnon [36], the author prefers to use the nerve branch to the medial head as the donor nerve (Fig. 16). This nerve has tremendous length and easily reaches the axillary nerve. The lateral and long head branches, however, are other options for nerve transfer. The medial branch is found closely adjacent to the radial nerve in the central aspect of the triangular space. The nerve is traced in a distal direction to gain adequate length for tension-free transfer to the recipient axillary nerve. It is cut sharply and reflected toward the axillary nerve, which has been cut proximal to the teres minor branch (Fig. 17). The operating microscope is then brought into the field. Nerve coaptation is performed with a combination of 9-0 nylon suture and fibrin glue (Fig. 18). The wound is closed in a layered fashion with absorbable suture.

sensory branch is usually encountered first and is traced in a proximal direction to its main portion. The nerve is dissected in a retrograde direction until the axillary nerve is isolated proximal to the motor branch to the teres minor. The radial nerve is isolated as it exits the triangular space below the teres major muscle and between the long and lateral heads of the triceps. The specific nerve

Other donors

Alternative donors for shoulder reinnervation have been used, including the intercostal nerves, thoracodorsal nerve, medial pectoral nerve, long thoracic nerve, phrenic nerve, ipsilateral C7 root,

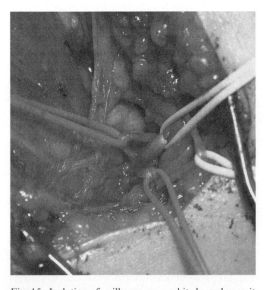

Fig. 15. Isolation of axillary nerve and its branches as it exits the quadrangular space.

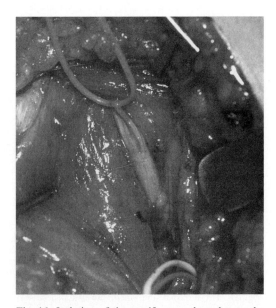

Fig. 16. Isolation of the specific nerve branches to the lateral, long, and medial heads of the triceps. The nerve branch to the medial head is usually selected as the donor nerve.

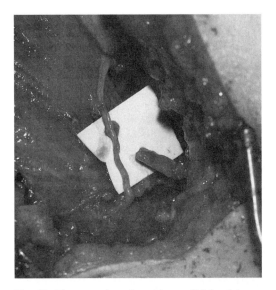

Fig. 17. The nerve branch to the medial head is cut sharply and reflected toward the axillary nerve, which has been cut proximal to the teres minor branch.

contralateral C7 root, and hypoglossal nerve (see Refs. [20,23,25,29,31]).

Nerve transfers for elbow motion

Elbow motion is critical to upper extremity function and has a high priority during nerve

reconstruction (see Refs. [17–19,21–23,25,37–42]). Nerve transfers can be directed to the biceps muscle or the brachialis muscle. The brachialis muscle is the primary elbow flexor; the biceps muscle is a primary forearm supinator and secondarily provides elbow flexion. Therefore, reinnervation of the brachialis muscle and the biceps muscle makes sense, with an additional advantage of improving elbow flexion strength [22,38].

The decision-making process usually involves careful consideration of the injury pattern, an assessment of available donors, and the preference of the surgeon. In infants who have upper ± middle trunk lesions, local ulnar ± median nerve transfers are preferable because median and ulnar motor function is predominantly from C8 and T1 root contribution. In global lesions, local transfers are unavailable and intercostal transfers may be necessary.

Ulnar nerve transfer

An incision is performed over the midline of the arm, beginning distal to the pectoralis major tendon (Fig. 19) [38–41]. The anterior fascia over the biceps muscle is divided and the muscle is dissected from the coracobrachialis muscle. The musculocutaneous nerve is identified between the biceps and the brachialis. The nerve is carefully followed in a distal direction, looking for the motor branch of the biceps muscle, which is identified on the undersurface of the muscle (Fig. 20). The

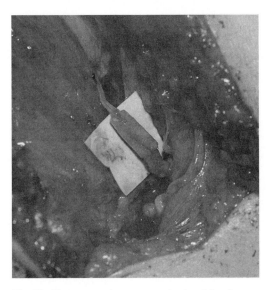

Fig. 18. The nerve ends are coapted using 9-0 nylon suture and fibrin glue. In this case, a nerve tube was placed around the repair site for augmentation.

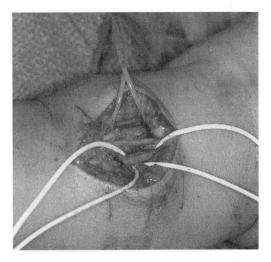

Fig. 19. The child's right arm depicted in Fig. 4 with medial incision. Red vessel loop is around biceps motor branch from musculocutaneous nerve, yellow vessel loops are around ulnar nerve.

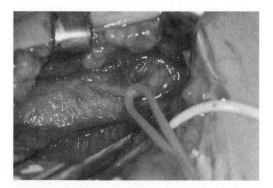

Fig. 20. The motor branch from musculocutaneous nerve to biceps muscle.

motor branch exits the musculocutaneous nerve in the proximal third to midportion of the arm. Distal to the biceps motor branch, the division into the lateral antebrachial cutaneous nerve and the brachialis branch is seen. The brachialis branch is more medial and the lateral antebrachial cutaneous nerve continues into the forearm. Stimulation can facilitate identification as long as some innervation is still present. The motor nerve is dissected in a proximal direction and divided from the musculocutaneous nerve in preparation for transfer.

A second fascia incision is performed posterior to the intermuscular septum, and the ulnar nerve is isolated 1 cm distal to the motor branch of the biceps muscle. Using loupe magnification, a longitudinal epineurotomy is made along the ulnar nerve and the individual group fascicles are separated (Fig. 21). Usually, three sizeable group fascicles are present. From a topographic

standpoint, the expendable motor component of the ulnar nerve is usually located on the lateral or central portion of the nerve [38]. Electric stimulation is used to confirm those group fascicles that contain motor fibers to the extrinsic hand muscles. The selected donor fascicle is mobilized for 1 to 3 cm as permitted by the fascicular anatomy. This group fascicle is divided and transferred to the biceps motor branch (Fig. 22). The donor fascicle is divided as distal as possible and the recipient nerve as proximal as achievable to facilitate a direct repair without tension. The operating microscope is then brought into the field. Nerve coaptation is performed with a combination of 9-0 or 10-0 nylon suture and fibrin glue (Fig. 23). The nerve coaptation is performed with the elbow in extension and the elbow immobilized in flexion to relieve any tension across the nerve repair.

Median nerve transfer

A incision and approach are used similar to those for ulnar nerve transfer [22,38]. The anterior fascia over the biceps muscle is divided and the muscle is dissected from the coracobrachialis muscle. The musculocutaneous nerve is identified between the biceps and the brachialis (Fig. 24). The nerve is carefully followed in a distal direction looking for the motor branch of the biceps muscle, which is identified on the undersurface of the muscle (Fig. 25). The motor branch exits the musculocutaneous nerve in the proximal third to midportion of the arm. Distal to the biceps motor branch, the division into the lateral antebrachial cutaneous nerve and the brachialis branch is seen. The brachialis branch is more medial and

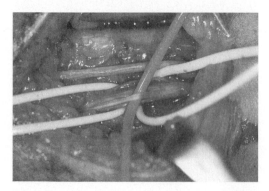

Fig. 21. A longitudinal epineurotomy along the ulnar nerve to identify the individual group fascicles and to isolate an expendable motor component. The adjacent parallel nerve is medial antebrachial cutaneous.

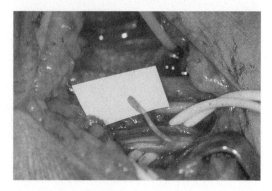

Fig. 22. The group fascicle of ulnar nerve to extrinsic muscles is divided and transferred toward the biceps motor branch.

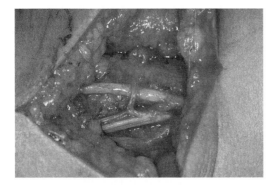

Fig. 23. The group fascicle of the ulnar nerve is coapted to the biceps motor branch using 9-0 nylon suture and fibrin glue. In this case, a nerve tube was placed around the repair site for augmentation.

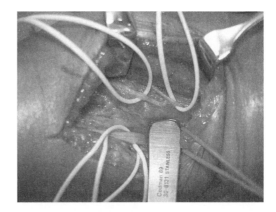

Fig. 25. This case had a common motor branch to the biceps and brachialis muscles.

the lateral antebrachial cutaneous nerve continues into the forearm. Stimulation can facilitate identification as long as some innervation is still present. The motor nerve is dissected in a proximal direction and divided from the musculocutaneous nerve in preparation of transfer.

The median nerve is identified adjacent to the musculocutaneous nerve within the neurovascular sheath. From a topographic standpoint, the motor fascicles in the median nerve are found on the medial side of the median nerve and the sensory component on the lateral side of the median nerve [38]. Using loupe magnification, a longitudinal epineurotomy is made along the median nerve and the individual group fascicles are separated. Electric stimulation is used to confirm those group fascicles that contain motor fibers to the extrinsic hand muscles (flexor carpi

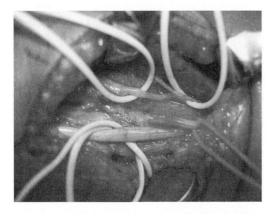

Fig. 24. A medial approach to the arm with identification of the musculocutaneous nerve (red vessel loop) and median nerve (double yellow loop).

radialis, flexor digitorum superficialis, or palmaris longus). The selected donor fascicle is mobilized for 1 to 3 cm as permitted by the fascicular anatomy. This group fascicle is divided and transferred to the brachialis motor branch. The donor fascicle is divided as distal as possible and the recipient nerve as proximal as achievable, to facilitate a direct repair without tension. The operating microscope is then brought into the field. Nerve coaptation is performed with a combination of 9-0 or 10-0 nylon suture and fibrin glue. The nerve coaptation is performed with the elbow in extension and the elbow immobilized in flexion to relieve any tension across the nerve repair.

Intercostal nerve transfer

The intercostal transfer is performed through a transverse thoracic incision in the interspace between the third and fourth ribs, from the midaxillary line to the costochondral junction (Fig. 26) [15,16,23]. The anterior surfaces of the ribs are exposed by separation of the pectoralis major and minor muscles. The ribs are mobilized by subperiosteal dissection, with protection of the underlying pleura. An umbilical tape is placed around the nerve for traction. The rib is retracted in a cephalad direction and the upper portion of the intercostal muscle spread to identify the motor portion of the intercostal nerve. The nerve is dissected from the costochondral junction to the midaxillary line. This length of dissection will avoid the need for an intervening nerve graft. The third, fourth, and fifth intercostal nerves are harvested in similar fashion (Fig. 27). Through a linear incision in the arm, the musculocutaneous nerve is exposed on the undersurface of the biceps

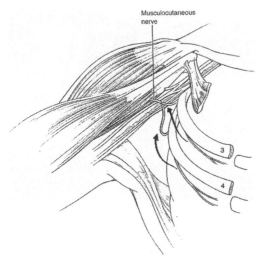

Fig. 26. An intercostal nerve transfer to the musculocutaneous nerve for elbow flexion. (*Reprinted from* Kozin SH. Injuries of the brachial plexus. In: Iannotti JP, Williams GR, editors. Disorders of the shoulder: diagnosis and management. 2nd edition. Philadelphia: Lippincott, Williams & White; 2007. p. 1087–134; with permission.)

brachii muscle. A subcutaneous tunnel is developed between the biceps, axilla, and thoracic incision. The intercostal nerves are then passed to the biceps motor nerve and coapted with epineural sutures or fibrin glue.

Other donors

Alternative donors for elbow flexion have been used, including thoracodorsal, hypoglossal, and pectoral nerves [29,31,37]. These nerve transfers can be coapted to the musculocutaneous nerve.

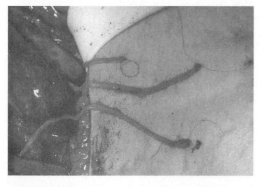

Fig. 27. Three intercostal nerves harvested from left chest wall for transfer to the musculocutaneous nerve for elbow flexion.

Outcomes of nerve transfers

Reports of nerve transfers for brachial plexus birth palsies are limited. In addition, many series include variable injury patterns, concomitant nerve grafting, and secondary procedures [7,8,12,24].

Most of the nerve transfer results in children have addressed shoulder motion [32,33,43]. Kawabata and colleagues [32] reported on 13 spinal accessory nerve transfers to various targets. Sixty-seven percent regained M4 strength in the deltoid muscle and 88% in the infraspinatus muscle. No functional compromise of the trapezius muscle was noted. In contrast, Malessy and colleagues [43] rigorously assessed the results following nerve grafting of C5 to the suprascapular nerve (n = 65) or nerve transfer of the accessory nerve to the suprascapular nerve (n = 21) in a retrospective analysis 3 years after surgery. Outcome was expressed in degrees of true glenohumeral external rotation, which can be executed only by infraspinatus muscle contraction. Only 17 (20%) of the 86 patients reached more than 20 degrees of external rotation, whereas 35 (41%) were unable to perform true external rotation. The difference between nerve grafting from C5 and nerve transfer using the accessory nerve was not statistically significant. Functional scores were better, with 88% of children able to reach their mouths and 75% able to touch their heads. The investigators concluded that restoration of true glenohumeral external rotation after neurotization of the suprascapular nerve in infants who have brachial plexus birth palsies, whether by nerve grafting from C5 or by nerve transfer of the spinal accessory nerve, is disappointingly low. However, compensatory techniques allow a considerable range of motion.

van Ouwerkerk and colleagues [33] reported on late suprascapular nerve transfer performed as a separate procedure at a mean age of 21.7 months in 54 children. Preoperative MRI scans showed only minor wasting of spinatus muscles, intraoperative stimulation of suprascapular nerves elicited spinatus muscle reaction in 44 out of 48 patients, and histology of suprascapular nerves was normal. External rotation and abduction substantially improved in 53 and 27 patients, respectively. The investigators conclude that spinal accessory to suprascapular nerve transfer is effective in restoring active external rotation when performed as a primary procedure or a separate secondary procedure in children older than 10 months. They hypothesized that the lack of MRI wasting and the normal histology imply central nervous changes or a developmental apraxia that may be the main cause for lack of external rotation. The results of this study need additional assessment and repeat analysis.

Most nerve transfers for elbow flexion have been reported in adults, with few results in children. A few cases of nerve transfers for elbow flexion in children using various donors have been reported [21]. Noaman and colleagues [21] reported a series of 7 children who underwent ulnar nerve transfer to the biceps at an average age of 16 months. Five children recovered M3 or greater elbow flexion, whereas 2 children recovered less than M3 strength. Blaauw and Slooff [37] published a large series of 25 children who underwent transfer of the pectoral nerves to the musculocutaneous nerve as part of an extended brachial plexus reconstruction. Results were considered excellent in 17 cases and fair in 5, with 2 failures. An additional Steindler flexorplasty was necessary in 3 patients.

Transfer of the hypoglossal nerve to various targets has been disappointing. Sacrifice of the hypoglossal nerve is associated with early and late oral problems. In addition, volitional control has been inconsistent and associated movement in the arm during tongue activity is an ongoing problem [29,31]. Regarding the phrenic nerve, this transfer is avoided in infants because the diaphragm is not yet firmly fixed to the vertebral bodies and severe respiratory problems can occur [44].

Summary

The advent of nerve transfers has greatly increased surgical options for children who have brachial plexus birth palsies. Nerve transfers have considerable advantages, including easier surgical techniques, avoidance of neuroma resection, and direct motor and sensory reinnervation. Therefore, any functioning nerve fibers within the neuroma are preserved. Furthermore, a carefully selected donor nerve results in little or no clinical deficit. However, some disadvantages and unanswered questions remain. Because of a lack of head-to-head comparison between nerve transfers and nerve grafting, the window of opportunity for nerve grafting may be missed, which may degrade the ultimate outcome. Time will tell the ultimate role of nerve transfer or nerve grafting in brachial plexus birth palsies. The optimal strategy for different types of lesions remains to be determined. A randomized study is necessary to solve these ongoing questions, which will oblige the author to reconsider the opinions expressed in this article.

References

[1] Gilbert A, Whitaker I. Obstetrical brachial plexus lesions. J Hand Surg [Br] 1991;16:489–91.

[2] Greenwald AG, Schute PC, Shiveley JL. Brachial plexus birth palsy: a 10-year report on the incidence and prognosis. J Pediatr Orthop 1984;4:689–92.

[3] Hardy AE. Birth injuries of the brachial plexus: incidence and prognosis. J Bone Joint Surg Br 1981;63:98–101.

[4] Jackson ST, Hoffer MM, Parrish N. Brachial-plexus palsy in the newborn. J Bone Joint Surg Am 1988;70:1217–20.

[5] Hoeksma AF, ter Steeg AM, Nelissen RG, et al. Neurological recovery in obstetric brachial plexus injuries: an historical cohort study. Dev Med Child Neurol 2004;46(2):76–83.

[6] Pondaag W, Malessy MJ, van Dijk JG, et al. Natural history of obstetric brachial plexus palsy: a systematic review. Dev Med Child Neurol 2004;46:138–44.

[7] Antoniadis G, Konig RW, Mohr K, et al. Management bei geburtstraumatischen Lasionen des Plexus brachialis - Eigene Erfahrungen mit der primaren operativen Behandlung [Management of obstetrical brachial plexus palsy–own experience with the primary operative technique]. Handchir Mikrochir Plast Chir 2003;352:98–105 [in German].

[8] Grossman JA, Price AE, Tidwell MA, et al. Outcome after later combined brachial plexus and shoulder surgery after birth trauma. J Bone Joint Surg Br 2003;85:1166–8.

[9] Pondaag W, Malessy MJ. Recovery of hand function following nerve grafting and transfer in obstetric brachial plexus lesions. J Neurosurg 2006;105(Suppl):33–40.

[10] Capek L, Clarke HM, Curtis CG. Neuroma-in-continuity resection: early outcome in obstetrical brachial plexus palsy. Plast Reconstr Surg 1998;102:1555–62.

[11] Clarke HM, Al-Qattan MM, Curtis CG, et al. Obstetrical brachial plexus palsy: results following neurolysis of conducting neuromas-in-continuity. Plast Reconstr Surg 1996;97:974–82.

[12] Chen QH, Chen DS, Fang YS. [Early microsurgical treatment of upper obstetrical brachial plexus injury]. Zhongguo Xiu Fu Chong Jian Wai Ke Za Zhi 2003;17:400–2 [in Chinese].

[13] Clarke HM, Curtis CG. An approach to obstetrical brachial plexus injuries. Hand Clin 1995;11:563–80.

[14] Bae DS, Waters PM, Zurakowski D. Reliability of three classification systems measuring active motion in brachial plexus birth palsy. J Bone Joint Surg Am 2003;85:1733–8.

[15] Krakauer JD, Wood MB. Intercostal nerve transfer for brachial plexopathy. J Hand Surg [Am] 1994;19:829–35.

[16] Minami M, Ishii S. Satisfactory elbow flexion in complete (preganglionic) brachial plexus injuries: produced

by suture of the third and fourth intercostal nerves to the musculocutaneous nerve. J Hand Surg [Am] 1987;12:1285–301.

[17] Leechavengvongs S, Witoonchart K, Uerpairojkit C, et al. Combined nerve transfers for C5 and C6 brachial plexus avulsion injury. J Hand Surg [Am] 2006;31:183–9.

[18] Bertelli JA, Ghizoni MF. Reconstruction of C5 and C6 brachial plexus avulsion injury by multiple nerve transfers: spinal accessory to suprascapular, ulnar fascicles to biceps branch, and triceps long or lateral head branch to axillary nerve. J Hand Surg [Am] 2004;29:131–9.

[19] Samardzic M, Grujicic D, Antunovic V. Nerve transfer in brachial plexus traction injuries. J Neurosurg 1992;76:191–7.

[20] Chen L, Gu YD, Hu SN, et al. Contralateral C7 transfer for the treatment of brachial plexus root avulsions in children - a report of 12 cases. J Hand Surg [Am] 2007;32:96–103.

[21] Noaman HH, Shiha AE, Bahm J. Oberlin's ulnar nerve transfer to the biceps motor nerve in obstetric brachial plexus palsy: indications, and good and bad results. Microsurgery 2004;24:182–7.

[22] Tung TH, Novak CB, Mackinnon SE. Nerve transfers to the biceps and brachialis branches to improve elbow flexion strength after brachial plexus injuries. J Neurosurg 2003;98:313–8.

[23] Malessy MJ, Thomeer RT. Evaluation of intercostal to musculocutaneous nerve transfer in reconstructive brachial plexus surgery. J Neurosurg 1998;88:266–71.

[24] Aydin A, Mersa B, Erer M, et al. Dogumsal brakiyal pleksus yaralanmalarinda sinir cerrahisinin erken sonuclari [Early results of nerve surgery in obstetrical brachial plexus palsy]. Acta Orthop Traumatol Turc 2004;38:170–7 [in Turkish].

[25] Samardzic MM, Grujicic DM, Rasulic LG, et al. The use of thoracodorsal nerve transfer in restoration of irreparable C5 and C6 spinal nerve lesions. Br J Plast Surg 2005;58:541–6.

[26] Leechavengvongs S, Witoonchart K, Uerpairojkit C, et al. Nerve transfer to deltoid muscle using the nerve to the long head of the triceps, part II: a report of 7 cases. J Hand Surg [Am] 2003;28(4):633–8.

[27] Witoonchart K, Leechavengvongs S, Uerpairojkit C, et al. Nerve transfer to deltoid muscle using the nerve to the long head of the triceps, part I: an anatomic feasibility study. J Hand Surg [Am] 2003;28:628–32.

[28] Malessy MJ, de Ruiter GC, de Boer KS, et al. Evaluation of suprascapular nerve neurotization after nerve graft or transfer in the treatment of brachial plexus traction lesions. J Neurosurg 2004;101:377–89.

[29] Malessy MJ, Hoffmann CF, Thomeer RT. Initial report on the limited value of hypoglossal nerve transfer to treat brachial plexus root avulsions. J Neurosurg 1999;91:601–4.

[30] Grossman JA, Di Taranto P, Alfonso D, et al. Shoulder function following partial spinal accessory nerve transfer for brachial plexus birth injury. J Plast Reconstr Aesthet Surg 2006;59:373–5.

[31] Blaauw G, Sauter Y, Lacroix CL, et al. Hypoglossal nerve transfer in obstetric brachial plexus palsy. J Plast Reconstr Aesthet Surg 2006;59:474–8.

[32] Kawabata H, Kawai H, Masatomi T, et al. Accessory nerve neurotization in infants with brachial plexus birth palsy. Microsurgery 1994;15:768–72.

[33] van Ouwerkerk WJ, Uitdehaag BM, Strijers RL, et al. Accessory nerve to suprascapular nerve transfer to restore shoulder exorotation in otherwise spontaneously recovered obstetric brachial plexus lesions. Neurosurgery 2006;59:858–67.

[34] Hattori Y, Doi K, Toh S, et al. Surgical approach to the spinal accessory nerve for brachial plexus reconstruction. J Hand Surg [Am] 2001;26:1073–6.

[35] Bertelli JA, Ghizoni MF. Improved technique for harvesting the accessory nerve for transfer in brachial plexus injuries. Neurosurgery 2006;58(Suppl 2):366–70.

[36] Colbert SH, Mackinnon S. Posterior approach for double nerve transfer for restoration of shoulder function in upper brachial plexus palsy. Hand 2006;1:71–7.

[37] Blaauw G, Slooff AC. Transfer of pectoral nerves to the musculocutaneous nerve in obstetric upper brachial plexus palsy. Neurosurgery 2003;53:338–41.

[38] Mackinnon SE, Novak CB, Myckatyn TM, et al. Results of reinnervation of the biceps and brachialis muscles with a double fascicular transfer for elbow flexion. J Hand Surg [Am] 2005;30:978–85.

[39] Teboul F, Kakkar R, Ameur N, et al. Transfer of fascicles from the ulnar nerve to the nerve to the biceps in the treatment of upper brachial plexus palsy. J Bone Joint Surg Am 2004;86:1485–90.

[40] Shigematsu K, Yajima H, Kobata Y, et al. Oberlin partial ulnar nerve transfer for restoration in obstetric brachial plexus palsy of a newborn: case report. J Brachial Plex Peripher Nerve Inj 2006;1:1–5.

[41] Leechavengvongs S, Witoonchart K, Uerpairojkit C, et al. Nerve transfer to biceps muscle using a part of the ulnar nerve in brachial plexus injury (upper arm type): a report of 32 cases. J Hand Surg [Am] 1998;23:711–6.

[42] Novak CB, Mackinnon SE, Tung TH. Patient outcome following a thoracodorsal to musculocutaneous nerve transfer for reconstruction of elbow flexion. Br J Plast Surg 2002;55:416–9.

[43] Pondaag W, de Boer R, van Wijlen-Hempel MS, et al. External rotation as a result of suprascapular nerve neurotization in obstetric brachial plexus lesions. Neurosurgery 2005;57:530–7.

[44] Chuang DCC. Neurotization procedures for brachial plexus injuries. Hand Clin 1995;11:633–45.

Nerve Transfer with Functioning Free Muscle Transplantation

David Chwei-Chin Chuang, MD

Department of Plastic Surgery, Chang Gung Memorial Hospital, Chang Gung University, Taipei-Linkou, 5, Fu-Hsing Street, Kuei-Shan, Taoyuan 33305, Taiwan

Nerve graft and nerve transfer are the two major methods of nerve reconstruction [1,2]. Nerve transfer, neurotization, and nerve crossing are commonly used interchangeably. Nerve transfer in brachial plexus injury is a surgical option involving intentional division of a physiologically active nerve with low morbidity, and transfer of that nerve to a distal, more important, but irreparable denervated nerve within the golden period [3,4]. The term "neurotization" means either a surgical procedure of nerve-to-nerve neurorrhaphy, or a result of a denervated muscle or skin or even nerve reinnervated by direct contact without neurorrhaphy. Narakas [5] described five possible types of neurotization: cutaneocutaneous neurotization (healthy skin reinnervates the neighboring denervated skin), musculomuscular neurotization (healthy muscle reinnervates the neighboring denervated muscle), neuromuscular neurotization (functional nerve implants to a denervated muscle), neurocutaneous neurotization (functional nerve implants to the dermis of the skin), and neuroneural (motor or sensory nerve coaptation) neurotization. Nerve transfer is actually a neuroneural neurotization, a procedure requiring division and coaptation of a healthy donor nerve to a denervated recipient nerve. Some investigators used the term "nerve crossing" [6] synonymously with "nerve transfer." However, after Viterbo [7] reported end-to-side neurorrhaphy with removal of the epineural sheath in 1994, end-to-side neurorrhaphy became an exceptional nerve transfer without division of the healthy donor nerve. Chuang [4] classified the nerve transfer into four

methods in the brachial plexus reconstruction: extraplexus neurotization, intraplexus neurotization, close-target neurotization, and end-to-side neurotization. These four types of neurotization are all of nerve transfer. In this article, the term "nerve transfer" is uniformly applied, instead of the term "neurotization." The term "close-target nerve transfer" from Chuang [4] is equivalent to the term "distal nerve transfer," described by Watchmaker and Mackinnon [8], referring to direct nerve coaptation at a more distal site (muscle or skin) closer to the end organ targets to achieve faster recovery. Various close-target nerve transfer techniques have been reported [3,4], including spinal accessory (XI) nerve transfer to the suprascapular nerve from a posterior trunk approach, medial pectoral nerve transfer to the suprascapular or axillary nerve, or triceps branch of the radial nerve to the axillary nerve for restoration of shoulder abduction, transfer of ulnar nerve fascicle to the branch to biceps, fascicle of median nerve transfer to the branch to brachialis for elbow flexion are all of distal nerve transfer. The advantages of proximal nerve transfer versus close-target nerve transfer are the subject of much debate. Close-target nerve transfer has the advantages of direct nerve coaptation without the need for nerve grafting, a short operating time because dissection in the traumatized scar zone is avoided, and healthy nerve stumps with no scarring. The major disadvantages of the technique are a requirement for brain reeducation, less power than the original mother nerve, and increasing clinical or subclinical deficits from dividing the donor nerve in a more distal region.

Most extraplexus nerve transfer and intraplexus nerve transfer are kinds of proximal nerve

E-mail address: micro@adm.cgmh.org.tw

0749-0712/08/$ - see front matter © 2008 Elsevier Inc. All rights reserved.
doi:10.1016/j.hcl.2008.03.012

transfer. Extraplexus nerve transfer means transfer of a non–brachial plexus component nerve to the avulsed brachial plexus for neurotization of a denervated nerve. The reported donor nerves in common use are mostly for motor reinnervation, and they include the phrenic (Ph) nerve, XI nerve, deep motor branches of the cervical plexus, intercostal (IC) nerve, hypoglossal nerve, and contralateral C7 spinal (CC7) nerve [1–6]. Ph nerve transfer to the distal C5, XI nerve transfer to the suprascapular nerve from an anterior approach, and CC7 nerve transfer to the median nerve are all extraplexus nerve transfers. Intraplexus nerve transfer is used in cases of non–global root avulsion, in which at least one of the spinal nerves is still available for transfer, not to its original pathway but to other, more important, nerves. Examples include ipsilateral C5 nerve grafting to the median nerve, or C5 nerve grafting to the C6.

All nerve transfers in the series described here are for neurotizing a transferred free muscle, either by extraplexus, intraplexus, or close-target nerve transfer. Nerve transfer is now a reliable and popular reconstructive option, indicated in root avulsion injury of brachial plexus within a golden time period of 5 months [4] and in functioning free muscle transplantation (FFMT) with no need for time consideration.

Functioning free muscle transplantation

FFMT is an advanced microneurovascular technique indicated in patients who have an advanced injury with a major functional muscle or muscle group loss or denervation and in whom no locally available or ideal musculotendinous donor unit exists. FFMTs have been successfully applied clinically in cases involving adult brachial plexus injury, obstetric brachial plexus palsy, facial palsy, severe Volkmann's ischemia, severe crushing and traction injuries of the forearm or arm with major muscle loss or major nerve injury, major limb avulsion amputation where replantation was initially performed but without nerve repair, severe spastic hand, and congenital problems (such as arthrogryposis) [9–13]. When applying FFMT for Volkmann's ischemia, traumatized major soft tissue or major nerve injury, or post–major limb replantation, the neurotizer always comes from its original mother motor nerve (eg, musculocutaneous nerve-innervated FFMT for biceps replacement, anterior interosseous nerve-innervated FFMT for finger flexion, and posterior interosseous nerve- or radial nerve-innervated FFMT for finger extension or triceps replacement). In applying FFMT in adult brachial plexus injury, obstetric brachial plexus palsy, arthrogryposis, or severe spastic hand, the original mother motor nerve is denervated because of proximal root avulsion, congenital absence, or cortical disorganization. The neurotizer in these circumstances comes either from a nearby nerve transfer or from the contralateral side nerve transfer. In this article, the author focuses on nerve transfer with FFMT. Any free muscle reinnervated by its original motor nerve, not by nerve transfer, is excluded. FFMT may be the only solution to situations where the original mother motor nerve is absent (trauma or congenital). It can provide not only motor function but also an including overlying skin flap for monitoring and limb contour.

Nerve transfer with functioning free muscle transplantation

"Nerve transfer with FFMT" is a new challenge for the reconstructive microsurgeon. The source of the recipient neurotizer usually comes from the very proximal brachial plexus or from the contralateral brachial plexus. The reconstructive microsurgeon should be familiar with the brachial plexus anatomy, extraplexus and intraplexus. The surgeon should also be familiar with interfascicular neurolysis, which should be performed carefully and delicately under microscopic view because the neurotizer sometimes comes from a nearby intact nerve, such as a fascicle of the ulnar nerve or a fascicle of the median nerve [14–16]. Sometimes, a two-stage procedure is required for proximal nerve elongation, with a nerve graft or grafts in the first stage, followed by FFMT in the second stage [4,9,11,17]. The following only deals with nerve transfer with FFMT, because it is now the author's major reconstructive option for many challenging and complicated cases in adult brachial plexus injury, child obstetric brachial plexus palsy, polio-like brachial plexus neuritis, severe spastic hand, and congenital arthrogryposis. Three hundred and thirty-three patients received FFMT between 1995 and 2005 in the author's hospital, Chang Gung Memorial Hospital, Taipei-Linkou (Table 1). Most reconstructions were for brachial plexus injuries, adult or obstetric (Table 2). The indications for "nerve transfer with FFMT" were mostly for failed nerve

Table 1

Functioning free muscle transplantation for upper limb injuries, 1995–2005

Cause	No. of patients
Adult brachial plexus injury	186
Obstetric brachial plexus palsy	73
Major soft tissue or major nerve injury	24
Volkmann's ischemia	25
Post–major limb replantation	22
Arthrogryposis	2
Spastic hand	1
Total	333

reconstruction or chronic root avulsion (lasting more than 1 year after injury). Some FFMTs were used in the acute brachial plexus injury to enhance outcome function and nerve reconstruction. For example, sometimes five IC nerves were harvested, three for musculocutaneous nerve neurotization and the remaining two for neurotizing an additional FFMT to enhance the elbow flexion results in cases of late brachial plexus injury, 6 to 12 months after injury (Fig. 1). The functions restored included elbow flexion (135 FFMTs); finger extension (extensor digitorum communis [EDC] ± extensor pollicis longus [EPL]) (66 FFMTs); finger flexion (flexor digitorum profundus [FDP] ±

Table 2

Nerve transfer with functioning free muscle transplantation for reconstruction with various procedures (1995–2005)

IC nerve–innervated FFMT for elbow flexion	108
XI nerve–innervated FFMT for finger extension (EDC ± EPL)	64
C7T-innervated FFMT for finger flexion (FDP ± APB)	24
Part ulnar nerve–innervated FFMT for elbow flexion	14
XI nerve–innervated FFMT for elbow flexion	12
XI nerve–innervated FFMT for finger flexion	8
Ph nerve–innervated FFMT for elbow extension	2
XI nerve–innervated FFMT for elbow extension	1
XI nerve–innervated FFMT for deltoid	1
Part median nerve-innervated FFMT for FDP	1
IC nerve–innervated FFMT for finger extension	1
Ph nerve–innervated FFMT for finger extension	1
CC7T–innervated FFMT for elbow flexion. CC7T, contralateral C7 (spinal nerve) transfer	1
Total	238

flexor pollicis longus [FPL]) (33 FFMTs); elbow extension (3 FFMTs); and deltoid replacement (1 FFMT), for a total of 238 FFMTs (see Table 2). The transferred donor nerves used as the muscle neurotizers included the IC nerve (109 FFMTs), XI nerve (86 FFMTs), CC7 nerve (25 FFMTs), fascicle of ulnar nerve (14 FFMTs), fascicle of median nerve (1 FFMT), and Ph nerve (3 FFMTs). The most common transfers in this investigation were IC nerve-innervated FFMT for elbow flexion, XI-innervated FFMT for finger extension (EDC), and CC7-innervated FFMT for finger flexion (see Table 2).

General principles for nerve transfer with functioning free muscle transplantation

1. The principles of FFMT regarding patient selection, muscle selection, muscle inset at optimum tension, motor nerve chosen, and postoperative rehabilitation are all identical to previous descriptions by Manktelow and Zuker [18], Doi and colleagues [19], and Chuang [12].
2. The principles of nerve transfer are identical to those described by Chuang [4].
3. Nerve transfer with FFMT is used primarily for functional restoration, not for wound coverage. It is therefore suitable for elective, well-prepared cases, not for acute injured cases.
4. The indications are stronger in chronic cases (more than 1 year after injury). Sometimes it can be applied with simultaneous nerve reconstruction for enhancement, or for staged reconstruction when the original mother motor nerve is not available (Fig. 2).
5. In neurotization, direct nerve suture without tension is always superior to indirect nerve suture with a nerve graft, the same general principle as that of the regular nerve transfer and regular FFMT. The motor branch to the transferred muscle and the recipient motor nerve should be dissected as distal as possible to make direct nerve coaptation easy. If the proximal nerve transfer is far from the transferred muscle inset region, it is better to switch to a two-stage procedure, with initial nerve elongation from the proximal donor nerve in the first stage, followed by FFMT in the second stage for functional restoration.
6. The health of the neurotizing motor nerve is an important determinant factor for success.
7. Ipsilateral nerve transfer is always superior to contralateral nerve transfer.

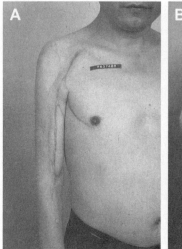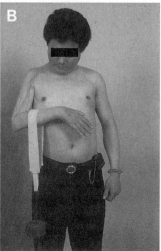

Fig. 1. (*A*) A patient had C5–7 root avulsion of his right brachial plexus for 11 months. He received five IC nerves transfers: three to coapt to the musculocutaneous nerve directly, and two to neurotize a gracilis FFMT for augmentation of the elbow flexion strength. (*B*) One and a half years following FFMT, he achieved M4 elbow flexion.

8. All patients who have received FFMT with nerve transfer require "induction exercise" in the rehabilitation phase after surgery. The patient's motivation and cooperation are therefore important factors for success. Once the muscle has achieved M1 grade, that is, when squeezing the reinnervated muscle or muscles causes chest skin pain in the case of IC nerve transfer, dyspnea in the case of Ph nerve transfer, or contralateral digits tingling in the case of CC7 nerve transfer, induction exercise should start. Several

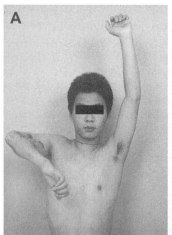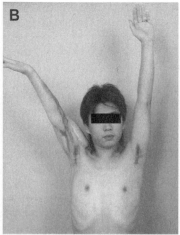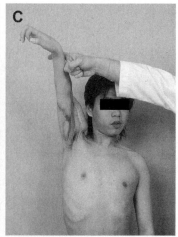

Fig. 2. (*A*) A case of traction avulsion amputation at the lower third arm level after replantation and rehabilitation for 1 year; the patient achieved improved elbow and finger flexion but no extension of elbow and fingers. He received four banking nerve grafts: two (20 cm each) were coapted to the infraclavicular radial nerve, passing through the pectoralis major muscle and biceps muscle, and embedded into the L/3 triceps; and another two (8 cm each) were coapted to the infraclavicular axillary nerve, passing through deltopectoral sulcus, and embedded into the biceps muscle in the first stage. (*B*, *C*) One year later, a rectus femoris FFMT was used for elbow extension, neurotized by an elongated axillary nerve graft. M4 elbow extension was achieved 1 year after the FFMT.

exercises are used to induce the reinnervated muscle to exercise more. After Ph or IC nerve transfer, patients are directed and encouraged to run, walk, or hill climb (2 km a day). After XI nerve transfer, shoulder raising or shoulder bracing backward against resistance should be performed 1000 times per day. After CC7 nerve transfer, contralateral shoulder grasp (adduction) exercises with resistance 1000 times per day are advised. These exercises are all a kind of motor reeducation. The realization of the importance of these exercises is crucial, because good results are commonly achieved by psychologically strong and ambitious patients who cooperate fully in their rehabilitation programs, whereas poor results are often obtained by lazy or uncooperative patients. The following descriptions use FFMTs with different nerve transfer techniques for different purposes:

Extraplexus nerve transfer with functioning free muscle transplantation

The four common uses of nerve transfer with FFMT in the upper extremity for irreparable brachial plexus injury (see Table 2) are

1. FFMT for elbow flexion, using XI or IC nerve transfer
2. FFMT for elbow extension, using Ph nerve with nerve graft in a one-stage, axillary, or radial nerve elongation with nerve graft in a two-stage procedure (see Fig. 2).
3. FFMT for EDC, using XI nerve transfer
4. FFMT for finger flexion, using IC nerve innervation, or CC7 nerve elongation with nerve graft, in a two-stage procedure

Functioning free muscle transplantation for elbow flexion using spinal accessory nerve transfer

The XI nerve is the motor nerve of the sternocleidomastoid and trapezius muscles, lying behind the sternocleidomastoid muscle at a point within one finger breadth above the emergence point of the greater auricular nerve, going laterally and obliquely and posteriorly in front of the trapezius muscle. The XI nerve can be found through the regular C-curved incision for brachial plexus exploration [20], or through a supraclavicular incision parallel and above the clavicle. It can be found on the anterior and deep surface of the

trapezius muscle while detaching the trapezius muscle from the clavicle. Nerve stimulation can confirm the identity of the XI nerve. Dissection should be as distal as possible, below the cervical sensory branch, which comes from the cervical plexus and joins with the XI nerve, until it reaches two or three terminal muscular rami that enter into the muscle, which are divided for transfer. The proximal stump can be transferred to the infraclavicular region over or under the clavicle and prepared for nerve coaptation. In addition to the main distal ramus coapted to the motor branch of the FFMT, the other two or three proximally divided rami can be elongated with a nerve graft (1–2 cm in length) and implanted into the transferred muscle for nerve-to-muscle neurotization with no axon sources wasted. The branches to the sternocleidomastoid muscle and the first branch to the upper trapezius are generally spared. The XI nerve is thought to be more powerful than the IC nerve. Sources of donor vessels include the thoracodorsal artery, superior ulnar collateral artery, circumflex humeral artery, and lateral thoracic artery (Table 3). The recipient veins may come from the cephalic or basilar vein in the axilla. The contralateral gracilis muscle or musculocutaneous flap is the ideal choice for elbow flexion. The gracilis muscle, including 5 cm tendon distal to the tenomuscular junction, is harvested. The motor branch of the gracilis muscle should be dissected to a length as long as possible, up to the obturator foramen. The vessels should be dissected proximally to the bifurcation of the femoral profunda artery. The proximal end of the gracilis muscle is fixed at the lateral clavicle, instead of at the coracoid process of the scapula, and the distal end is sutured to the distal biceps tendon under tension, with the elbow in flexion. The nerve is coapted to the transferred XI nerve directly, where it is over the deltoid muscle. The vessel anastomoses are performed in the axilla, and the nerve coaptation is on the other side of the gracilis muscle.

Functioning free muscle transplantation for elbow flexion using intercostal nerve transfer

The IC nerves are located beneath the periosteum of the ribs after dissection through the external and internal IC muscles. Each IC nerve has two main branches: the deep central and superficial lateral branches. The deep central branch, predominantly motor and commonly used for transfer, passes along the rib; in T1 to

Table 3

Recommendation of nerve transfer with functioning free muscle transplantation for different functions of the upper limb

Purpose	Donor muscle	Proximal attachment	Distal attachment	Nerve transfer	Recipient artery
Elbow flexion	Gracilis with 5 cm tendon	Lateral third of clavicle Coracoid process of the scapula	Distal biceps tendon	XI or IC	Thoracodorsal Superior ulnar collateral Circumflex humeral Lateral thoracic
Elbow extension	RF LD	Humeral head	Distal triceps tendon	Ph (1 stage) More proximal nerve (2 stage)	Thoracodorsal
FDP	Gracilis with longer tendon	Second rib	FDP with elbow pulley	IC or CC7 (2 stage)	Thoracodorsal Circumflex humeral Lateral thoracic
EDC	Gracilis with longest tendon	Lateral third of the clavicle	EDC with elbow pulley	XI	Thoracodorsal Superior ulnar collateral Circumflex humeral

Abbreviations: LD, latissimus dorsi; RF, rectus femoris.

T3, it lies on the upper margin of the rib, in T4 to T6, it is located at the lower margin of the rib, and in T7 and below, it is found in the IC and rectus abdominis muscles inferior to the rib. The T3–5 three deep central branches are usually transected at the costochondral junction and transferred to neurotize the FFMT. IC nerve transfer is effective in children more than in adult patients. The gracilis from the opposite thigh is harvested for FFMT. It is unnecessary to dissect a long obturator nerve for nerve coaptation directly. The proximal end of the muscle is fixed at the coracoid process of the scapula. Thoracodorsal vessels, or even lateral thoracic vessels, are often used for vessel anastomoses.

Functioning free muscle transplantation for elbow extension using phrenic nerve transfer in one stage, or using proximal nerve transfer in a two-stage procedure

The Ph nerve is the motor nerve to the diaphragm, originating from C3 to C5, but chiefly from C4. In most cases, it lies on the ventral and medial surface of the scalene anterior muscle but sometimes it is found on the lateral surface of the muscle, and descends obliquely toward the medial clavicle. It is always the first nerve encountered after cleavage of the adipofascial tissue, localized below the transverse cervical vessels.

Nerve stimulation is required to identify it. The Ph nerve is such a powerful nerve that it has become an important donor nerve for transfer, although its transect can cause palsy of the diaphragm and a decrease in pulmonary capacity. Ph nerve transect can cause severe respiratory distress in children younger than 2 years old but in most adults, it causes no significant respiratory problem, except for one-night dyspnea in a few cases. The Ph nerve is superior to the XI or IC nerve for transfer because of its characteristic of spontaneous rhythmic impulse discharge, which simulates a continuous internal nerve stimulator (termed autophysiotherapy). The Ph nerve can be dissected as distal as possible, down to the medial clavicle, by direct visualization with loupe magnification, or longer, by endoscopic-assisted technique. The Ph nerve can be elongated with a sural nerve graft, passing under the clavicle and out from the Chuang's triangle [20], and left in the biceps muscle for nerve coaptation. The rectus femoris myocutaneous flap is an ideal muscle for elbow extension. The femoral nerve branch to the rectus femoris should be dissected as long as possible. The nutrient vessels should also be dissected as long as possible. The proximal end of the muscle is fixed at the lateral clavicle or humeral head, and the distal rectus femoris tendon is sutured to the distal triceps tendon at olecranon insertion in a sandwich fashion. The thoracodorsal vessel and axillary vein are the vessels for anastomoses (see Table 3).

Functioning free muscle transplantation for finger flexion using intercostal nerve transfer, or contralateral C7 spinal nerve transfer in a two-stage procedure

The author prefers to use the three T3–5 IC nerves for FFMT reinnervation to restore FDP ± FPL function. The IC nerve has a deep central branch and a superficial lateral branch. Only the deep central branch is used for reinnervation. The gracilis myocutaneous FFMT is usually fixed proximally at the second rib. The muscle passes through a subcutaneous tunnel to the medial elbow, where the pronator teres and long wrist flexor muscle origins are elevated to produce a below-elbow pulley. The muscle passes under the pulley and is sutured to the FDP by weaving under tension while the elbow is kept in 30 to 90 degrees of flexion, depending on the power of the elbow flexion recovery. The thoracodorsal artery, lateral thoracic artery, or circumflex humeral artery, and axillary veins are used for the vessel anastomoses (see Table 3).

Functioning free muscle transplantation for finger extension using spinal accessory nerve transfer

This procedure is the most common in the author's series, first described by Doi [21]. The gracilis should be harvested as long as possible, including part of the periosteum of the tibial attachment. The muscle origin is fixed at the lateral clavicle. The gracilis muscle is passed through a subcutaneous tunnel to the elbow, where the origins of the brachioradialis and EDC are elevated to form a pulley, which also aids in the efficiency of elbow flexion. If the muscle is passed through the distal insertion of the triceps, it may also help elbow extension. The gracilis muscle and tendon pass under the pulley and are sutured to the EDC under tension. The thoracodorsal artery, circumflex humeral artery, and nearby veins are used for vascular anastomoses. The obturator nerve is easily coapted to the XI nerve over the deltoid muscle.

Contralateral C7 spinal nerve elongation with nerve graft as the first stage, followed by functioning free muscle transplantation for elbow or finger function as the second stage

This concept is similar to the staged cross-chest nerve graft procedure [22]. Following a 1-year nerve regeneration, detected by advance of the Tinel sign, the FFMT technique can be applied using the elongated nerve graft for motor reinnervation. CC7 nerve elongation may be performed either by two sural nerve grafts (if C8 and T1 are still in function) or by vascularized ulnar nerve graft (if C8 and T1 are both avulsed). CC7 nerve dorsal division elongation with cable nerve grafts are commonly used for single function of elbow extension. A nerve passer is used to pass the nerve graft subcutaneously, and the cable nerve grafts are embedded into the biceps muscle for the second-stage FFMT. The whole C7 can also be used, transferring to the median nerve by using a vascularized ulnar nerve graft in the acute stage [22]. If the forearm flexor muscles do not achieve function by nerve transfer because of the motor nerve plate degeneration, then a new FFMT can be applied for enhancement of the outcome [9]. The CC7 nerve transect has been proved to produce little significant loss of any specific muscle function.

Intraplexus nerve transfer with functioning free muscle transplantation

Proximal nerve elongation with sural nerve graft or grafts as a first stage in preparation for a subsequent FFMT is actually not a new technique. It has often been applied by the author in the upper limb since 1995 [9], and also in lower limb reconstruction. It is mostly applied for elbow extension and finger flexion. The motor nerve source may come from the supraclavicular or infraclavicular higher proximal nerve or nerves. A 6-month to 1-year waiting period for second-stage reconstruction is required.

Close-target nerve transfer with functioning free muscle transplantation

To nerve transfer with FFMT, the recipient motor nerve should be not only close to the neuromuscular junction of the transferred muscle for motor reinnervation, but also functional and long enough for nerve coaptation. Nerve graft elongation from a proximal donor nerve transfer, from either the ipsilateral side or the contralateral side, requires a two-stage procedure. Fascicle of the ulnar nerve (mostly for flexor carpi ulnaris), or fascicle of the median nerve (mostly for flexor carpi radialis) is selected in the arm level to innervate an FFMT for elbow or finger flexion. Branches of the anterior interosseous nerve or

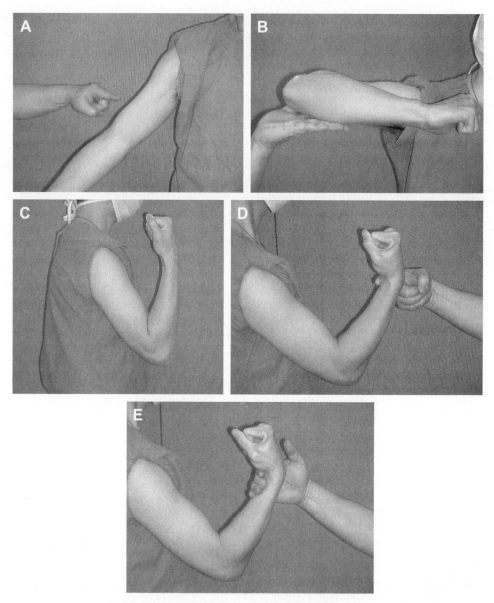

Fig. 3. Motor reevaluation of the elbow flexion strength. (*A*) M0–1, biceps (or brachialis) no movement (M0), or muscle contraction without elbow joint movement (M1); (*B*) M2, with examiner's hand support (no gravity), patient can flex the elbow; (*C*) M3, elbow flexion against gravity; (*D*) M4, elbow flexion against examiner's one finger resistance (about 1 kg weight); (*E*) M5, elbow flexion against examiner's four fingers resistance (at least 5 kg weight).

branches of the posterior interosseous nerve can also be chosen as a neurotizer for an FFMT for finger flexion or extension while the median or radial nerve has been neurotized or is functional.

End-to-side neurorrhaphy nerve transfer

End-to-side neurorrhaphy nerve transfer with FFMT was first proposed by Frey and Giovanoli [23] to enhance the results from major nerve repair. He repaired the ruptured median nerve in the elbow. In addition, he used a free muscle transplantation for finger flexion, coapting the free end of the motor nerve to the transferred muscle, to the proximal median nerve by an end-to-side neurorrhaphy technique. The author has not yet experienced this technique.

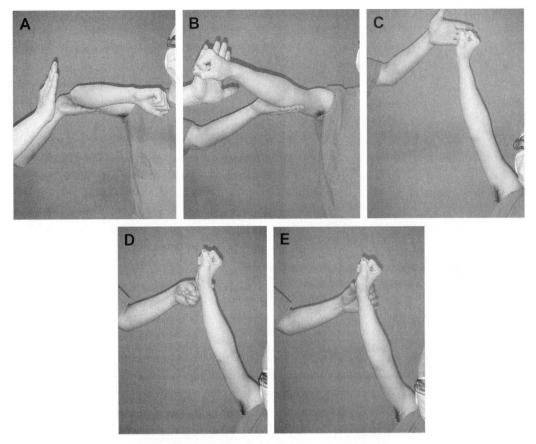

Fig. 4. Motor evaluation of the elbow extension strength. (*A*) M0–1, triceps no movement (M0), or muscle contraction without elbow joint movement (M1), while examiner asks patient to do elbow extension with examiner's hand to support the patient's elbow; (*B*) M2, with examiner's hand support (no gravity), patient can extend the elbow; (*C*) M3, elbow extension against gravity; (*D*) M4, elbow extension against examiner's one finger resistance; (*E*) M5, elbow extension against examiner's four fingers resistance.

The role of nerve transfer with functioning free muscle transplantation in acute brachial plexus injury

Before 1995, the author performed about 10 cases a year of FFMT, but subsequent to 2000, this number has increased up to 50 or more cases a year. The author had performed more than 800 cases of FFMT up to the end of 2006 for a number of different purposes, nearly one half of which were for brachial plexus injury. Most FFMT for BPI were indicated in chronic BPI, enhancement of results following nerve reconstruction, or stage reconstruction for functional improvements. Only a few FFMT were applied in acute BPI (ie, in cases within 1 year of injury). An across-elbow FFMT with a below elbow pulley, as described by Doi

[21], in the acute case of proved brachial plexus avulsion, represents a kind of "distal to proximal" reconstruction priority, which is different from the traditional "proximal to distal" reconstruction. FFMT in the author's series is predominantly an adjuvant palliative reconstruction to enhance the results in the late stage. FFMT applied in the acute stage is only for uncooperative patients or for those who do not understand the importance of following the necessary postoperative rehabilitation.

Postoperative management and rehabilitation

Postoperative splinting is applied immediately and maintained for 3 weeks for the coapted nerve, and for 6 weeks for the sutured tendon. Nerve

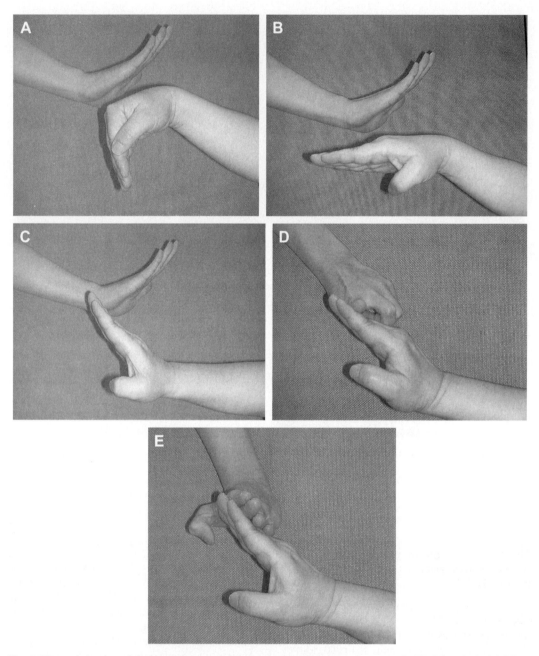

Fig. 5. Motor evaluation of the finger metacarpophalangeal joint (MPJ) extension strength (EDC function). (*A*) M0–1, MPJ no movement (M0), or muscle contraction without MPJ movement (M1), while wrist is kept in maximal flexion; (*B*) M2, positive finger MPJ extension while wrist is kept in neutral position; (*C*) M3, positive finger MPI extension while wrist is kept in full extension; (*D*) M4, positive finger MPJ extension against examiner's one finger resistance; (*E*) M5, positive finger MPJ extension against examiner's four fingers resistance.

stimulation can be started earlier, at 3 weeks postoperatively. Passive exercise of the muscle under supervision starts 4 weeks after surgery. Patients are encouraged to use electric muscle stimulation at home twice a day. In cases of XI nerve transfer, immediate neck splintage is additionally required for at least 3 weeks postoperatively. In cases of IC nerve transfer, passive

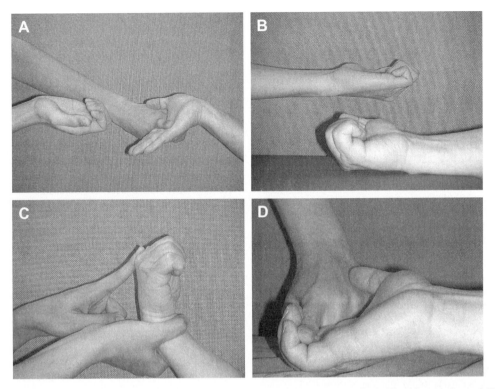

Fig. 6. Motor evaluation of the finger flexion strength (FDP function): (*A*) M0–1, finger distal interphalangeal (DIP) joint no movement (M0), or muscle contraction without DIP movement (M1), while wrist is kept in maximal extension; (*B*) M2, positive finger DIP flexion while wrist is kept in neutral position; (*C*) M3, positive finger DIP flexion while wrist is kept in full flexion; (*D*) M4, positive finger DIP flexion against examiner's one finger resistance.

shoulder elevation remains restricted to less than 90° for 6 months, until the transferred muscle has muscle-squeezing chest pain, which becomes a warning sign for limitation of shoulder elevation. "Induction exercise" is an important muscle exercise for patients with nerve transfer for an FFMT. Patients should be followed periodically, every 3 to 4 months.

Outcome evaluation

A successful FFMT implies that the transferred muscle has the power to function against resistance (ie, M4 muscle strength in the Medical Research Council scale system, in which the muscle can resist at least one examiner's finger of resistance, or at least 1 kg of resistance [10]). M5 describes movement against four-finger resistance. A successful, or good, result of an FFMT is defined as M4. In actuality, M4 describes useful function, in which the patient can use the achieved function for daily activity. Although the British Medical Research Council scale provides the possibility of homogeneity and consensus in motor evaluation, a considerable degree of heterogeneity exists in outcome evaluation of shoulder, elbow, and finger and/or thumb. In the author's opinion, establishing an international consensus on motor evaluations of different movements is vital and imperative for the advance of our understanding and mutual comparison. The schemata represent the author's opinion on precisely evaluating motor recovery of the transferred muscle on different movements: elbow flexion (Fig. 3), elbow extension (Fig. 4), finger extension (EDC function) (Fig. 5), and finger flexion (FDP function) (Fig. 6).

Acknowledgment

The author would like to thank Mr. C.P. O'Boyle, MD, MRCS (England), microreconstructive fellow, Chang Gung Memorial Hospital, for his expert assistance, including English and grammar correction.

References

[1] Terzis JK, Papakonstantinou KC. The surgical treatment of brachial plexus injuries in adults. Plast Reconstr Surg 2000;106(5):1097–122.

[2] Millesi H. Update on the treatment of adult brachial plexus injuries. In: Gilbert A, editor. Brachial plexus injuries. London: Martin Dunitz Ltd; 2001. p. 77–90.

[3] Dvali L, Mackinnon SE. The role of microsurgery in nerve repair and nerve grafting. Hand Clin 2007;23: 73–81.

[4] Chuang DCC. Neurotization and free muscle transfer for brachial plexus avulsion injury. Hand Clin 2007;23:91–104.

[5] Narakas AO. Neurotization or nerve transfer in traumatic brachial plexus lesions. In: Tubiana R, editor. The hand, vol. III. Philadelphia: Saunders; 1988. p. 656–83.

[6] Tsuyama N, Hara T, Nagano A. Intercostal nerve crossing as a treatment of irreparably damaged whole brachial plexus. In: Recent developments in orthopedic surgery. Manchester (England): Manchester University Press; 1987. p. 169–74.

[7] Viterbo F, Trindade JC, Hoshino K, et al. End-to-side neurorrhaphy with removal of the spineurial sheath: an experimental study in rats. Plast Reconstr Surg 1994;94:1038–47.

[8] Watchmaker G, Mackinnon S. Nerve injury and repair. In: Peimer CA, editor. Surgery of the hand and upper extremity. New York: McGraw-Hill; 1996. p. 1262–7, chapter 53.

[9] Chuang DCC. Functioning free muscle transplantation for brachial plexus injury. Clin Orthop Relat Res 1995;314:104–11.

[10] Chuang DCC. Functioning free muscle transplantation. In: Peimer CA, editor. Surgery of the hand and upper extremity. New York: McGraw-Hill; 1996. p. 1901–10.

[11] Chuang DCC. Nerve transfers. In: Boome RS, editor. The brachial plexus. The hand and upper extremity, vol. 14. New York: Churchill Livingstone; 1997. p. 51–62.

[12] Chuang DCC. Functioning free muscle transplantation for the upper extremity. Hand Clin 1997;13:279–89.

[13] Chuang DCC, Cheng MH, Ma HS. Clinical application of functioning free muscle transplantation (FFMT) in the late obstetrical brachial plexus palsy (OBPP). J Plast Surg Association (ROC) 2006;15: 211–28.

[14] Oberlin C, Beal D, Leechavengvongs S, et al. Nerve transfer to biceps muscle using a part of ulnar nerve for C5-6 avulsion of the brachial plexus- anatomical studies and report of four cases. J Hand Surg [Am] 1994;19:232–7.

[15] Brandt KE, Mackinnon SE. A technique for maximizing biceps recovery in brachial plexus reconstruction. J Hand Surg [Am] 1993;18:726–33.

[16] Mackinnon SE, Novak CB, Myckatyn TM, et al. Results of reinnervation of the biceps and brachialis muscles with a double fascicular transfer for elbow flexion. J Hand Surg [Am] 2005;30: 978–85.

[17] Chuang DCC, Wei FC, Norrdhoff MS. Cross-chest C7 nerve grafting followed by free muscle transplantations for the treatment of total avulsed brachial plexus injuries: a preliminary report. Plast Reconstr Surg 1993;92:717–25.

[18] Manketelow RT, Zuker RM. The principles of functioning free muscle transplantation: application to the upper arm. Ann Plast Surg 1989;22:275–82.

[19] Doi K, Hattori Y, Tan SH, et al. Basic science behind functioning free muscle transplantation. Clin Plast Surg 2002;29:483–95.

[20] Chuang DCC. Adult brachial plexus injuries. In: Mathes SJ, Hentz VR, editors. Plastic surgery, vol. 7. Philadelphia: Saunders Elsevier; 2006. p. 515–38.

[21] Doi K. Brachial plexus: free composite tissue transfers. In: Berger R, Weiss AP, editors. Hand surgery. Philadelphia: Lippincott Williams & Wilkins; 2004. p. 1041–53.

[22] Chuang DCC. Contralateral C7 transfer (CC-7T) for avulsion injury of the brachial plexus. The Journal of Plastic Surgical Association Republic of China 1999;3:185–92.

[23] Frey M, Giovanoli P. End-to-side neurorrhaphy of motor nerve: reinnervation of free muscle transplants, first clinical application. Eur J Plast Surg 2003;26:89–94.

Contralateral C7 Transfer in Adult Plexopathies

Julia K. Terzis, MD, PhD[a],*, Zinon T. Kokkalis, MD[b],
Epaminondas Kostopoulos, MD[a]

[a]Department of Surgery, Division of Plastic and Reconstructive Surgery, Eastern Virginia Medical School,
700 Olney Road, LH 2055, Norfolk, VA 23501, USA
[b]Department of Surgery, Eastern Virginia Medical School, Microsurgical Research Center,
LH 2055, Norfolk, VA 23501, USA

Global paralysis of the arm caused by a traction injury of the brachial plexus is a very grave affair [1]. Brachial plexus avulsion injuries are usually caused by high-velocity motor vehicle and motorcycle accidents. In such cases the resulting deficit is devastating, and the aim of functional restoration challenging and difficult for the reconstructive surgeon. The ultimate outlook of the patient is improved drastically if the interval between injury and definitive treatment of the frail upper extremity is short [2].

The treatment of brachial plexus avulsion lesions invariably involves the use of neurotization procedures [3,4]. Modern-day management of root avulsions advocates the combination of various neurotizations with ipsilateral and contralateral intraplexus and extraplexus nerve donors, use of vascularized nerve grafts, and secondary reconstruction with a plethora of musculotendinous transfers, including free muscle transplantation [5,6]. In cases of global root avulsion (five avulsions), intraplexus donors obviously are not available, and all reconstruction is performed from extraplexus donors [7]. Options include cervical plexus motors, the spinal accessory, the phrenic nerve, ipsilateral intercostal nerves, and the contralateral C7. The distal spinal accessory nerve is usually used for direct neurotization of the suprascapular nerve [8,9]. Intercostal nerves have yielded acceptable results, especially for the reconstruction of the musculocutaneous nerve [10,11]. Intercostal

nerves are challenging and time consuming to harvest, and each one has approximately 1,300 axons [12,13].

A nerve transfer from the contralateral healthy C7 root could provide a powerful source of motor nerve fibers. The number of motor fibers is greater than the total number of all extraplexus motor donors available for transfer. The total axonal count for the C7 averaged about 24,000 [12]. Gu and colleagues [14] reported the contralateral C7 root for the first time in 1991. The selective contralateral C7 technique was introduced by the senior author (JKT) in 1992 [15]. Using intraoperative microstimulation and microdissection techniques, selective neurectomies deprive only certain components of the C7 divisions (anterior or posterior division) and rarely the entire root; thus, the functional donor deficit is minimal. Since then, this procedure has been increasingly adopted because it provides a large source of motor nerve fibers without permanent damage of the donor limb function [16–23].

In the current study, we present a retrospective review of 56 patients with root avulsions who underwent contralateral C7 transfer. The purpose of this report is to present the authors' experiences with the selective contralateral C7 technique for reinnervation of various nerve targets above and below the elbow of the injured upper limb. The surgical results of the various neurotizations as well as the potential adverse effects of the procedure are reported. Outcomes are related to patient age, the denervation time, and the type of neurotization.

---

* Corresponding author.
  E-mail address: jktmd1@aol.com (J.K. Terzis).

0749-0712/08/$ - see front matter © 2008 Elsevier Inc. All rights reserved.
doi:10.1016/j.hcl.2008.04.003

Materials and methods

Patients

Between 1979 and 2004, a total of 394 patients with posttraumatic brachial plexus lesions underwent surgical exploration and reconstruction of the brachial plexus. Of these, 62 patients underwent reconstruction with the use of the selective contralateral C7 technique, which the senior author (JKT) introduced in 1991. Evaluation of the final outcomes was performed in 56 patients with a minimum follow-up of 2.5 years after surgery. The mean follow-up period was 6.1 years (range, 2.5 years to 14 years).

The right brachial plexus was involved in 27 patients, and the left plexus was involved in 29 patients. The mean age at surgery was 22.5 ± 9.8 years (range, 5 to 50 years); four patients under the age of 14 sustained traumatic brachial plexus palsy caused by traffic collisions and thus were included in our study. The average period between injury and plexus reconstruction (ie, denervation time, DT) was 29.8 months or 2.5 years (range, 3 to 93 months).

High-velocity motor vehicle accident was the most frequent cause of brachial plexus injury and accounted for injury in 86% of patients (Table 1). The average speed at which the accidents occurred was reported to be 55 mph (range, 30 to 115 mph). Coexistent fractures or dislocations of the involved upper extremity and vascular injuries correlated with severe lesions of the brachial plexus components. Thirty-four patients (61%) had some type of fracture in the involved extremity, and 18 patients (32%) required emergency surgery to repair an injured subclavian or axillary artery.

Evaluation

Clinical examination of the involved upper extremity muscles was always performed in

Table 1
Type of accident for 56 posttraumatic brachial plexus patients

Type of accident	No. of patients	Percent
Motorcycle accident	23	41
Motor vehicle accident	25	45
Snowmobile accident	3	5
Fall from height	1	2
Sports-related accident	2	4
Boat accident	1	2
Tumor resection	1	2

comparison with the contralateral normal side. The British Medical Research Council grading system, further modified by Terzis and colleagues [24] with intermediate grades of (+) and (−), was used for the motor assessment. The muscle grading was recorded on a brachial plexus chart with the rest of the clinical examination.

A complete sensory evaluation was performed including touch, pain, two-point discrimination (2PD), and joint position sense (proprioception). A ninhydrin sweat test of the palms was also performed to measure sudomotor function.

Moreover, a detailed documentation of the motor and sensory functional status of the donor upper extremity was performed before and after the C7 nerve root transfer.

Electrodiagnostic evaluation included needle electromyography and nerve conduction studies, which were obtained in all patients at the first and on each of the follow-up office visits. Inspiratory/expiratory chest x-rays and fluoroscopic studies determined if the diaphragm (phrenic nerve) was paralyzed. A combination of myelography and CT scan of the cervical spine (CT/myelography) was used to rule out avulsions. The avulsion of the lower nerve roots was also confirmed by the presence of Horner's sign.

Intraoperative findings of the involved brachial plexus

All the patients had a supraclavicular and infraclavicular exploration of the involved brachial plexus, as previously described [7,24]. An intraoperative severity score assessment of the brachial plexus lesion, developed by the senior author (JKT), was performed. Each root was graded as follows: 0, avulsion; 1, avulsion/rupture; 2, rupture; 3, rupture/traction; 4, traction; and 5, normal [24]. A normal brachial plexus has a severity score of 25. The lower the severity score, the greater the numbers of avulsed roots present. Identification of sensory versus motor nerve fibers, ganglion cells, or scar tissue was used in each case using intraoperative histochemistry [25].

The severity score was established at the completion of the brachial plexus exploration and after the entire lesion was diagnosed. In this population, the mean severity score was 5.59 ± 5.1. The intraoperative findings regarding each root in all cases are presented in Table 2.

It is noteworthy that among the 280 (5 × 56) cervical roots, 70% (196 of 280) were found to be

Table 2
Intraoperative findings in 56 reconstructed brachial plexuses

Root	Type of lesion						No. of plexuses
	A	A/R	R	R/T	T	N	
C5	21	3	27	1	1	3	56
C6	38	2	12	3		1	56
C7	51	2	1	2			56
C8	45		3	1	3	4	56
T1	41			4	2	9	56
Total	196	7	43	11	6	17	

Abbreviations: A, avulsion injury; A/R, avulsion/rupture; N, normal; R, rupture; R/T, rupture/traction; T, traction.

avulsed from the spinal cord. Avulsion of all five roots was found in 29% (16 of 56) of the patients. Also, in 46 patients (82%) all the roots were involved, whereas in the remaining patients, one or two roots were spared from the injury.

Surgical technique

Contralateral C7 transfer is performed simultaneously with or 4 to 12 weeks after other ipsilateral intraplexus or extraplexus nerve transfers; thus, the selective contralateral C7 transfer is a contralateral intraplexus transfer procedure. The patient is placed in the supine position with a soft roll along the vertebral spine and under the neck. The affected upper extremity is abducted on an arm table. The sterile field includes bilateral upper extremities, both sides of the neck up to the mandible, the anterior and posterior chest to the midline, and bilateral lower extremities. The surgery is performed simultaneously by two teams: one team explores and identifies the normal contralateral plexus, and the other harvests the saphenous nerve grafts from both lower extremities or a vascularized ulnar nerve graft from the affected arm (Fig. 1); both teams use 4x wide field loupe magnification.

For exposure of the normal supraclavicular plexus, the incision is made parallel to the posterior border of the sternocleidomastoid muscle then turned laterally for 2 to 3 cm over the clavicle raising thus a posteriorly based triangular flap (Fig. 2A). The supraclavicular sensory nerves and the external jugular vein are preserved. The phrenic nerve is identified on the anterior surface of the anterior scalene muscle and protected. The dissection proceeds in a caudal direction to expose the C5, C6, and C7 spinal nerves (Fig. 2B). As the C7 root is approached,

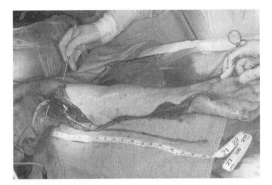

Fig. 1. Harvesting of the left vascularized ulnar nerve graft in a left global plexopathy case with C8 and T1 avulsions. Usually, 56 cm of vascularized trunk graft can be harvested. If the superior ulnar collateral vascular pedicle is high, near the left axilla, the vascularized ulnar graft can be used as a pedicle graft. If the vascular pedicle is more distal, close to the elbow, then the ulnar nerve needs to be transferred as a free vascularized graft with microvascular anastomoses between the superior ulnar collateral vessels and the transverse cervical vessels of the contralateral side.

the transverse cervical vessels and the inferior belly of the omohyoid muscle are isolated and retracted. Then, the C7 is exposed proximally, and it is carefully followed distally to the level of the middle trunk and its divisions.

The first step is to isolate the anterior division (AD) and posterior division (PD). To get enough length of each division exposed, the clavicle needs to be retracted firmly caudally until at least a centimeter of each division is isolated. A blue vessel loop is passed carefully around the AD, and a yellow vessel loop is passed around the PD (see Fig. 2B). At this point, the operating microscope is brought into the operating field. The epineurial sheath of both divisions is split longitudinally with the diamond knife. With the use of intraoperative electrical microstimulation, each fascicle is stimulated, and fascicles that innervate the latissimus dorsi and triceps muscles are isolated from the PD for the nerve transfer procedure. In the AD, fascicles that innervate the pectoralis major are demarcated, and microloops are passed around them. Motor fibers that innervate the pectoralis major are used as donors for contralateral flexors, whereas bundles that innervate the latissimus and triceps are used for the extensors. To avoid donor morbidity, the fascicles of the C7 root that supply wrist extensors are preserved. Depending on the contralateral deficit, usually only a component of the contralateral anterior or PDs is used.

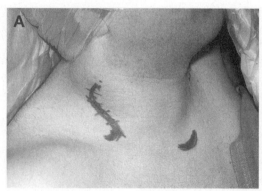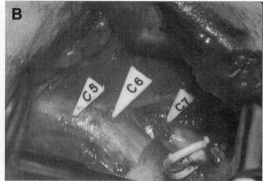

Fig. 2. (*A*) Typical S-incision for exposure of the normal right supraclavicular plexus in a patient with left posttraumatic plexopathy. The "half-moon" marking indicates the sternal notch. (*B*) Exploration of the normal right supraclavicular plexus. The head of the patient is left and the clavicle is on the right. The phrenic nerve can be seen clearly on the anterior surface of the anterior scalene muscle. The distal part of the C7 root is divided in the AD (blue vessel loop) and the PD (yellow vessel loop).

Using atraumatic microdissection techniques, selective neurectomies are performed of components of the anterior and PD to match the cross-sectional area of the interposition cross-chest nerve grafts (sural, saphenous nerves, or vascularized ulnar nerve). To pass the nerve grafts across the anterior chest wall, a subcutaneous tunnel is prepared from the neck incision to the opposite axilla using custom made flexible metal passers (Fig. 3A, B). After the cross-chest nerve grafts have been tunneled to the contralateral paretic side, the selected fascicles of each division of the C7 are coapted with the nerve grafts under high magnification of the operating microscope using 10-0 microsutures (Fig. 4).

At the completion of surgery and before extubation, a custom-made brace with a halo is applied to the patient. This brace keeps the arm abducted 45° and in anterior flexion. The halo prevents lateral movement of the head, reducing the risk of injury to the coaptation sites. The brace is removed 6 weeks later, and the patient's arm is placed in a sling for an additional 4 weeks. Physical therapy with passive range of motion and slow-pulse electrical stimulation [26] starts 6 weeks after the removal of the brace. Home electrical stimulation is provided to all patients with a portable slow pulse stimulation device that the patient is instructed to use for 5 to 6 hours per day for a minimum of a year or until antigravity motor recovery occurs. The physical therapist is made aware of all the new neurotizations in the reinnervated muscles and trains the patient accordingly.

Beginning in the early postoperative period (ie, before the patient is discharged), a detailed neurologic assessment of the donor upper extremity is always performed. Any sensory or motor deficit is documented carefully. The first follow-up visit is arranged at 3 months after surgery and subsequently every 6 months thereafter.

Reconstruction methods

In the current series, the AD alone was used as donor in five patients (9%); the PD alone in 16 patients (29%); and both divisions were used in all other 35 cases (62%). Overall, 148 neurotizations were performed; thus, 148 nerve grafts were used as cross-chest grafts in 56 patients (an average of 2.65 grafts per case). The type of nerve graft used and the selected donor (AD or PD) are presented in Table 3. In the majority of cases, saphenous nerve grafts (67%) are used as interposition grafts, because both sural nerves usually have been used previously in the first stage of Brachial Plexus reconstruction. Vascularized nerve grafting is performed routinely if indicated using the ulnar nerve of the affected extremity, based on the superior ulnar collateral vessels (see Fig. 1).

The recipient nerves—targets—included the axillary, the musculocutaneous, the median (Fig. 5), and the radial nerves. In many cases, selective neurotizations to the branch for the biceps muscle and to the branch to the long or the lateral head of triceps were performed. In cases with longer denervation time, during the first-stage reconstruction, nerve grafts are banked

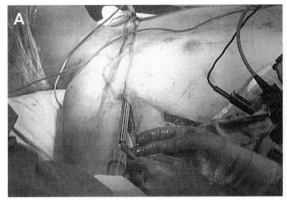
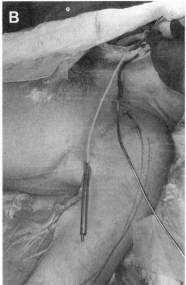

Fig. 3. (*A*) Intraoperative photograph of the tunneling of the vascularized ulnar nerve graft across the chest. The syringe (*lower center*) carrying normal saline is used to irrigate the nerve and make the passing easier. (*B*) The metal passers have been tunneled across the chest and are ready to receive the cross-chest nerve grafts. The thicker passer (*on the left*) will carry the vascularized ulnar nerve graft, whereas the thinner passer (*on the right*) will transfer the saphenous nerve across the chest.

at the elbow level ("banked" nerve grafts), so that they can be used later in a second-stage reconstruction for the innervation of free muscles.

The recipient targets neurotized by selective donors from the contralateral C7 are shown in Table 4. Careful view of this table reveals that contralateral flexors and median nerve neurotizations were performed from the AD, whereas contralateral extensor targets were neurotized from

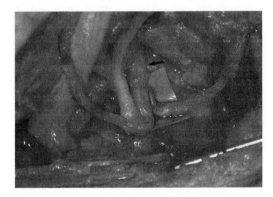

Fig. 4. The PD (*arrow*) of the right C7 root is the donor for multiple contralateral targets in this patient (axillary and radial nerve), whereas the entire AD was used to neurotize the vascularized ulnar nerve graft (*seen on the left*).

the PD. It should be noted that sometimes the PD was the single donor for multiple targets (see Fig. 4), such as the radial nerve and triceps branch, whereas the AD was primarily the donor for both the musculocutaneous and median nerves.

Thirty free muscles were transferred after the first stage of brachial plexus reconstruction to enhance or substitute upper extremity function. Muscles that were used included the contralateral latissimus dorsi, the gracilis, and the rectus femoris. Usually, neurotizations for the free muscles for elbow flexion or finger flexion were performed from the AD (16 cases), whereas free

Table 3
Selected donor (AD or PD) and the type of the nerve graft

| Donor | Type of nerve graft | | | | |
	Sural	Saphenous	Vascularized ulnar	MAC	Total (%)
AD	11	30	19	1	41
PD	11	69	5	2	59
Total (%)	15	67	16	2	

Abbreviation: MAC, medial antebrachial cutaneous nerve.

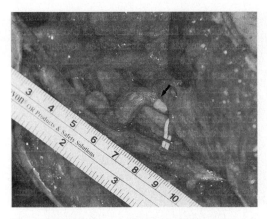

Fig. 5. The left vascularized ulnar is coapted to the left median nerve (*arrow*) of the paralyzed extremity. It is being neurotized from the AD of the right C7 root.

muscles for elbow or finger extension were neurotized from the PD (14 cases) (see Table 4).

Statistical analysis

Comparisons between pre- and postoperative groups were performed using Wilcoxon signed rank test. Comparisons between two postoperative groups were performed using Mann-Whitney test. *P* values were two-tailed, and *P* values of <.05 were considered significant. All the analysis was performed in SAS 9.1.3 (Cary, NC).

Results

The postoperative motor results for each target were assessed as follows: a poor result was a grade of M0 to M2; M2+ to M3 was a fair result; M3+ to M4- indicated a good result; and M4 to M5- was an excellent result [8].

In the entire population (n = 56), all patients had significant motor improvement in the muscle targets above and below the elbow following the contralateral C7 transfer (Wilcoxon signed rank test, *P*<.05). Particularly, for all the neurotizations above the elbow the overall improvement was very significant (*P*<.003).

Surgical results showed good and fair results (>M2+) in 50% of cases for *deltoid* neurotization (20% good results or ≥ M3+); 74% of cases for *biceps* neurotization (52% good and excellent results); 57% of cases for *triceps* neurotization (33% good results); 62% of patients for *wrist and finger flexors* (34% good results); and 50% of patients for *wrist and finger extension* (20% good results). All the postoperative results with regard to each specific neurotization are presented in Table 5.

Additionally, in patients who had neurotizations of the free muscle transfers from the AD or the PD of the contralateral C7 the surgical outcomes were as follows: good and fair results were achieved in 78% of cases for *biceps* free muscle transfer (22% good results); 67% of cases for *finger flexion* restoration (interphalangeal [IP] flexion) (33% good results); 50% of cases for *finger flexion* restoration (metacarpophalangeal [MP] flexion) (17% good results); and in 43% for finger extension restoration (14% good results). The results are shown in Table 6.

Twelve of 29 patients (41%) who underwent median nerve reconstruction achieved S3 sensory recovery in the median nerve area, 10 patients (35%) had S2 recovery, and 7 patients (24%) had no sensory recovery. Thus, protective sensibility (≥S2) was achieved in 76% of patients.

Of the 56 patients, 40 (71%) experienced short-term paresthesia in the median nerve area of the donor hand after the surgery, mainly on the index pulp. The sensory deficit recovered spontaneously in all cases. The recovery time ranged from 2 weeks to 6 months with an average of 3 months. At 6 months, there was no discernible sensory deficit in the contralateral normal limb. Motor deficit such as elbow extension, wrist extension, or extensor digitorum communis weakness, was never encountered in any patient.

Our population was divided in two groups regarding the denervation time (DT). Thirteen of 56 patients underwent contralateral C7 reconstruction within 9 months (average DT, 7.5 months), and the other 43 patients had reconstruction later

Table 4
Type of neurotization: donors and targets

| Donors | Targets | | | | | | | | |
	AX	MC	Median	Radial	Triceps	Ulnar	Free muscles	"Banked"	Other (SS, LT)
AD	1	21	25				16	5	
PD	9	2	4	10	21	1	14	10	2

Abbreviations: AX, axillary nerve; LT, long thoracic nerve; MC, musculocutaneous nerve; SS, suprascapular nerve.

Table 5
Postoperative results per muscle target

Results	Deltoid (n = 10)		Biceps (n = 23)		Triceps (n = 21)		Wrist and finger flexors (n = 29)		Wrist and finger extensors (n = 10)	
	N	%	N	%	N	%	N	%	N	%
Poor (M0 to M2)	5	50	6	26	9	43	11	38	6	60
Fair (M2+ to M3)	3	30	5	22	5	24	8	28	3	30
Good (M3+ or M4−)	2	20	10	43	7	33	10	34	2	20
Excellent (M4 to M5−)	—	0	2	9	—	0	—	0	—	0

Abbreviation: N, number of patients.

than 9 months (average DT, 36 months). In the first group (≤9 months), the outcomes were significantly better than in the latter group (Mann-Whitney test, $P<.05$). Additionally, patients younger than 18 years (18 cases, average 13 years) had significantly better results than older patients (38 cases, average 27 years, $P<.05$). Exemplary cases are presented in Figs. 6–8.

Discussion

Avulsion plexopathies always carry the worst prognosis and make the reconstruction of the plexus more challenging. A variety of intraplexus and extraplexus donors should be recruited in these cases to reconstruct the distal plexus components. Shoulder and elbow functions have been restored successfully by the spinal accessory, intercostal, and phrenic nerve transfer [4,27,28]. However, attempts to restore hand function by neurotization of the median nerve with intercostal and spinal accessory nerves have yielded uncertain results. Especially in multiple avulsions, the lack of adequate ipsilateral intraplexus donors leads the surgeon to seek all alternative donors.

Contralateral C7 root has greater number of axons than all the extraplexus donors and, most importantly, is not involved in the initial injury. Because of its large thickness, it is also a reasonable donor for multiple targets because it can be coapted with several cross-chest nerve grafts.

Adverse factors include the great distances that elongating axons need to travel, long denervation time, and the invasion of the contralateral healthy extremity. The donor morbidity can be minimized substantially by taking only the number of donor fibers needed and by using donors that have adequate overlap from neighboring myotomes [29]. Most of the surgeons use the entire C7 root [14,17,30].

Gu and colleagues [18] and Chuang and colleagues [16] separately reported results of the contralateral C7 to several recipient nerves for treatment of root avulsion brachial plexus injuries with a considerable degree of motor and sensory recovery and a moderate degree of donor deficit. These investigators reported their results using the entire C7 nerve transfer elongated by a pedicled or free vascularized ulnar nerve graft. The contralateral C7 was reported to be a better alternative for transfer to the median nerve than the previously used donor nerves. Songcharoen and colleagues [19] used half the normal C7 and a vascularized pedicle interposition ulnar graft to neurotize the median nerve. They used fascicles that innervated the shoulder muscles, provided from the posterosuperior half of the C7 root, leaving the fascicles on the anteroinferior half of the C7 root that supply the elbow, intact. However, this selective technique was used only to neurotize one specific target nerve, the median nerve.

Table 6
Outcomes of neurotization of the free muscle transfers from the contralateral C7

Results	Biceps (n = 9)		EDC (n = 7)		FDS (MP flexion) (n = 6)		FDP (IP flexion) (n = 6)	
	N	%	N	%	N	%	N	%
Poor (M0 to M2)	2	22	4	57	3	50	2	33
Fair (M2+ to M3)	5	56	2	29	2	33	2	33
Good (M3+ or M4−)	2	22	1	14	1	17	2	33
Excellent (M4 to M5−)	—	0	—	0	—	0	—	0

Abbreviations: EDC, extensor digitorum communis; FDP, flexor digitorum profundus; FDS, flexor digitorum sublimis; N, Number of patients.

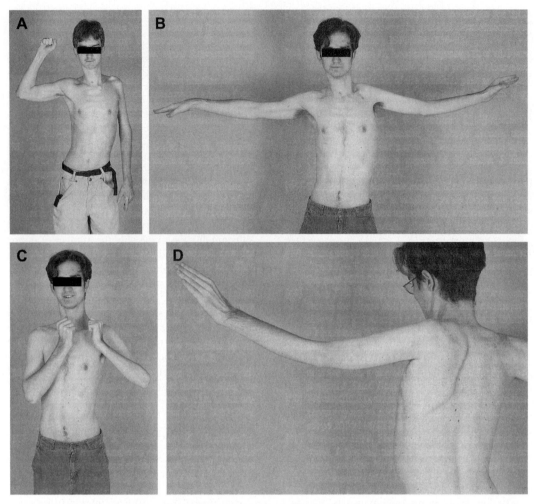

Fig. 6. A 17-year-old boy who was tubing on a lake at high speed, when the tuber struck a pier. He had loss of consciousness and suffered multiple injuries, including fractures of C2 and C3 vertebrae and a left brachial plexus injury. He was referred to our center 7 months later (*A*), where he had exploration of the left brachial plexus. The findings were C5 rupture/avulsion; C6, C7, C8 avulsion; and T1 rupture. He had multiple extraplexus neurotizations, including direct neurotization of the distal accessory to the suprascapular and ipsilateral intercostals to the left musculocutaneous nerve. Four months later, he had exploration of the right C7 root and cross-chest saphenous nerve grafts from the right PD of C7 to left triceps and left deltoid. The patient on recent follow-up exhibits excellent shoulder abduction (*B*), elbow flexion (*C*), and strong elbow extension from the PD of the contralateral C7 (*D*).

In our center, the senior author (JKT) introduced, in 1991, the selective contralateral C7 technique, the aim of which was to neurotize as many targets as possible with the least morbidity. The rationale was, in addition to neurotizing the "traditional" nerve targets such as the median nerve, to neurotize or to strengthen the function of previously reinnervated but weak muscles that are not the first priority, such as the triceps, deltoid, and the finger extensors. Another rationale was to provide motor fibers

for future free muscle transplantation because the most widely used motor donors, such as the spinal accessory or the intercostals, are usually "consumed" for shoulder and elbow reconstruction.

Of paramount importance was the intraoperative mapping of the contralateral C7 root with the aid of intraoperative electrical stimulation and the subsequent use of selective bundles for synergistic muscles of the involved upper limb (ie, the AD was usually used as motor donor for the contralateral flexors, whereas the PD was used for

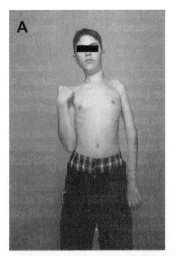

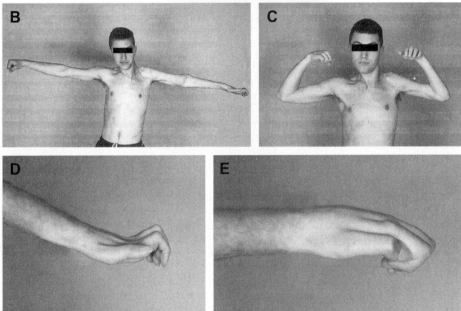

Fig. 7. A 19-year-old man that, in August 1996, was riding his bicycle out of a driveway and was struck by an oncoming car. He was not wearing a helmet and had loss of consciousness. He suffered a left global avulsion plexopathy, with avulsion of all five roots, C5 through T1. He was referred to our center for brachial plexus reconstruction 8 months later (A). In May 1997, he had first-stage reconstruction, which consisted of contralateral C7 AD via a vascularized ulnar nerve graft to the left median nerve. The contralateral PD neurotized two saphenous cross-chest nerve grafts for reconstruction of the left axillary and left radial nerves. The patient is seen in follow-up exhibiting nearly 90° shoulder abduction (B), over 100° elbow flexion (C) and adequate finger and thumb extension (D) and finger flexion (E).

the extensors). The same policy was performed for the neurotization of the free muscles that were transferred in later stages, usually for reanimation of the hand. This "intelligent" plan of reconstruction minimized the possibility of cocontractions between flexors and extensors (eg, between the biceps and triceps), allowing for easier patient reeducation during the rehabilitation phase. In the current series, cocontractions between antagonistic muscles were very rare because of careful preoperative and intraoperative planning.

The postoperative morbidity of the donor limb after selective contralateral C7 technique in our series was very limited; 71% of patients experienced

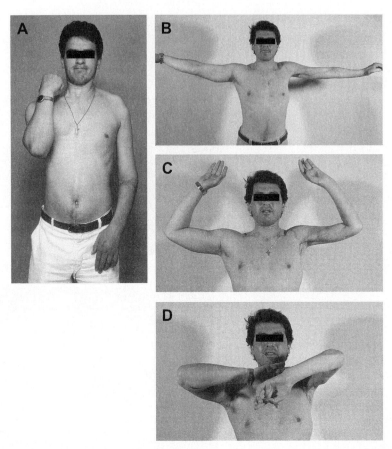

Fig. 8. A 25-year-old man suffering from left brachial plexus paralysis after a motorcycle accident. He was going 120 km/h and was wearing a helmet. He encountered a bus, and to avoid collision he turned and hit the road divider. He was referred for surgery to our center 6 months later (*A*). Exploration at that time revealed avulsion of C8 and T1 and rupture of C5, C6, and C7. The distal brachial plexus was reconstructed with multiple interposition nerve grafts from intraplexus donors. On follow-up, elbow flexion was judged inadequate, and he underwent cross-chest saphenous nerve grafts, which, a year later, neurotized a free muscle for augmentation of elbow flexion. The patient is seen 3 years after the free muscle transfer, exhibiting excellent shoulder abduction (*B*) and external rotation (*C*) and adequate elbow flexion (*D*).

numbness in the median nerve area of the donor hand after the surgery, and motor deficit was never encountered. By 6 months, there was no discernible motor or sensory deficit in the contralateral normal limb. The study of Chuang and colleagues [16] of the entire C7 transection showed a sensory deficit in 52% of patients, which resolved spontaneously, and a motor deficit in 19% of patients. Their only longer persistent abnormality was the triceps reflex, which became weak or absent. In the series by Songcharoen and colleagues [19], 3% of cases had motor deficits: 2% temporary mild triceps weakness and 1% permanent weakness in the extensor digitorum communis. Nearly all (97%) had sensory

deficits transiently, most commonly in the index finger, which resolved completely by 7 months.

Comparison of the outcomes of this series with those of others proved difficult because of the different methods used and because that in most of the series usually a single target was reconstructed, such as the median nerve. In a relatively recent study, Gu and colleagues [30] presented their results in a population of 32 patients with an adequate follow-up (>2 years). They used the entire C7 root in most of their patients (17 cases), followed by the PD (12 cases) and the AD (three cases). Their neurotizations were directed to musculocutaneous, radial, and median nerves. Functional recovery reached ≥M3 in 80% of patients (8 of 10) for the biceps; in 66% (4 of 6) for the wrist and finger extensors; in 50% (7 of 14) for finger flexors; and ≥S3 in 12 patients (85.7%) after median nerve neurotization. Possible explanations for these noteworthy results could be the short denervation time (ie, 75% of their patients had posttraumatic intervals of less than 12 months) and the reason that the entire C7 root was sacrificed in the majority of cases.

Songcharoen and colleagues [19] reported that 29% of their patients (6 of 21 cases) obtained at least M3 recovery of the wrist and finger flexors and sensory recovery ≥S2 in 81% (17 of 21) of cases. Waikakul and colleagues [17] reported the results of contralateral C7 transfer to the median nerve in 96 cases, with a follow-up period of more than 3 years. The AD was used for neurotization of the median nerve via a vascularized ulnar nerve graft. Satisfactory recovery of sensation was achieved in 83% of the patients, whereas muscle power of wrist flexors reached M3 in 29% of the series and in 21% of finger flexors.

In the current study, motor recovery reached a level of ≥M3+ in 20% (2 of 10) of cases for the deltoid, 52% (12 of 23) for the biceps, 24% (5 of 21) for the triceps, 34% (10 of 29) for the wrist and finger flexors, and 20% (2 of 10) for the wrist and finger extensors. Additionally, sensory recovery of ≥S2 was achieved in 76% of patients. It is evident that the motor results were less rewarding for the reconstructions of the deltoid, triceps, and wrist and finger extensors. For some reason, certain muscle groups, such as the abductors, external rotators, and extensors, yield inferior response to reconstructive microsurgery. This finding was collaborated by observations made by Narakas and Hentz [3], who mentioned that this paradox can be explained partially on the basis of the embryologic origin of the various muscles.

Functioning free-muscle transplantation has become a reconstructive option in cases of delayed patient presentation with long denervation time or in cases of global root avulsions, especially when the lower roots of the plexus that innervate the hand are involved [7]. Although our surgical results with free muscle transfers have been encouraging, we believe that this technique should be reserved for late cases or those that have failed attempts at nerve reconstruction.

Factors that influenced the final outcome in our series were the age of the patient, the interval between trauma and surgery, and the type of reconstruction. Other studies came to similar conclusions [17,23,31]. Waikakul and colleagues [17] stated that acceptable motor function was found in only 50% to 60% of the patients aged 18 years or younger with a surgical delay of 3 months or shorter. In a recent report of 12 infants and children, Chen and colleagues [23] stated that the relatively satisfactory results of their series might be attributable to better nerve regeneration and functional remodeling within the central nervous system in children. In our series, patients with a surgical delay within 9 months, and patients aged 18 years or younger achieved significantly better results.

Summary

We conclude from this study that the selective contralateral C7 transfer technique appears to be a safe procedure in adult plexopathies and may augment motor and sensory recovery for those with brachial plexus root avulsions. With the selective contralateral C7 technique, minimal morbidity and more efficiency in the management of brachial plexus avulsion injuries could be accomplished.

Results of this series also showed that contralateral C7 root cannot be transferred only to a single nerve, but it can be applied successfully for simultaneous reconstruction of several different targets in adults, whereas this method was used already in children. This approach allowed the ability to reconstruct additional targets, with lesser morbidity to the normal limb and the possibility of improved outcomes.

References

[1] Yeoman PM, Seddon HJ. Brachial plexus injuries: treatment of the flail arm. J Bone Joint Surg [Br] 1961;43:493–500.

[2] Hentz VR, Narakas A. The results of microneurosurgical reconstruction in complete brachial plexus palsy. Assessing outcome and predicting results. Orthop Clin North Am 1988;19(1):107–14.

[3] Narakas AO, Hentz VR. Neurotization in brachial plexus injuries: indications and results. Clin Orthop 1988;237:43–75.

[4] Midha R. Nerve transfers for severe brachial plexus injuries: a review. Neurosurg Focus 2004;16(5):E5.

[5] Terzis JK, Kostopoulos VK. The surgical treatment of brachial plexus injuries in adults. Plast Reconstr Surg 2007;119(4):73e–92e.

[6] Terzis JK, Vekris MD, Soucacos PN. Brachial plexus root avulsions. World J Surg 2001;25(8): 1049–61.

[7] Terzis JK, Papakonstantinou KC. The surgical treatment of brachial plexus injuries in adults. Plast Reconstr Surg 2000;106(5):1097–122.

[8] Terzis JK, Kostas I. Suprascapular nerve reconstruction in 118 cases of adult posttraumatic brachial plexus. Plast Reconstr Surg 2006;117(2): 613–29.

[9] Terzis JK, Kostas I, Soucacos PN. Restoration of shoulder function with nerve transfers in traumatic brachial plexus palsy patients. Microsurgery 2006; 26(4):316–24.

[10] Malessy MJ, Thomeer RT. Evaluation of intercostal to musculocutaneous nerve transfer in reconstructive brachial plexus surgery. J Neurosurg 1998;88: 266–71.

[11] Nagano A. Intercostal nerve transfer for elbow flexion. Tech Hand Up Extrem Surg 2001;5(3):136–40.

[12] Chuang DC. Neurotization procedures for brachial plexus injuries. Hand Clin 1995;11:633–45.

[13] Gutowski KA, Orenstein HH. Restoration of elbow flexion after brachial plexus injury: the role of nerve and muscle transfers. Plast Reconstr Surg 2000; 106(6):1348–57.

[14] Gu YD, Zhang GM, Chen DS, et al. Cervical nerve root transfer from contralateral normal side for treatment of brachial plexus root avulsions. Chin Med J 1991;104(3):208–11.

[15] Terzis JK. Selective contralateral C7 technique. Presented at the 12th Congress of the International Society for Reconstructive Microsurgery. Singapore, February 6–10, 1996.

[16] Chuang DC, Cheng SL, Wei FC, et al. Clinical evaluation of C7 spinal nerve transection: 21 patients with at least 2 years' follow-up. Br J Plast Surg 1998;51:285–90.

[17] Waikakul S, Orapin S, Vanadurongwan V. Clinical results of contralateral C7 root neurotization to the median nerve in brachial plexus injuries with total root avulsion. J Hand Surg Br [Br] 1999;24: 556–60.

[18] Gu YD, Chen DS, Zhang GM. Long-term functional results of contralateral C7 transfer. J Reconstr Microsurg 1998;14:57–9.

[19] Songcharoen P, Wongtrakul S, Mahaisavariya B, et al. Hemi-contralateral C7 transfer to median

nerve in the treatment of root avulsion brachial plexus injury. J Hand Surg [Am] 2001;26:1058–64.

[20] Shin AY, Spinner RJ, Steinmann SP, et al. Adult traumatic brachial plexus injuries. J Am Acad Orthop Surg 2005;13(6):382–96.

[21] Spinner RJ, Shin AY, Bishop AT. Update on brachial plexus surgery in adults. Tech Hand Upper Extrem Surg 2005;9:220–30.

[22] Xu JG, Wang H, Hu SN, et al. Selective transfer of the C7 nerve root: an experimental study. J Reconstr Microsurg 2004;20:463–70.

[23] Chen L, Gu YD, Hu SN, et al. Contralateral C7 transfer for the treatment of brachial plexus root avulsions in children—a report of 12 cases. J Hand Surg [Am] 2007;32(1):96–103.

[24] Terzis JK, Vekris MD, Soucacos P. Outcomes of brachial plexus reconstruction in 204 patients with devastating paralysis. Plast Reconstr Surg 1999; 104:1221–40.

[25] Carson KA, Terzis JK. Carbonic anhydrase histochemistry. A potential diagnostic method for peripheral nerve repair. Clin Plast Surg 1985;12(2): 227–32.

[26] Liberson WT, Terzis JK. Contribution of clinical neurophysiology and rehabilitation medicine in the management of brachial plexus palsy. In: Terzis JK, editor. Microreconstruction of nerve injuries. Philadelphia: Saunders; 1987. p. 555–70.

[27] Songcharoen P, Mahaisavariya B, Chotigavanich C. Spinal accessory neurotization for restoration of elbow flexion in avulsion injuries of the brachial plexus. J Hand Surg [Am] 1996;21(3): 387–90.

[28] Nagano A, Tsuyama N, Ochiai N, et al. Direct nerve crossing with the intercostal nerve to treat avulsion injuries of the brachial plexus. J Hand Surg [Am] 1989;14:980–5.

[29] Dykes RW, Terzis JK. Spinal nerve distributions in the upper limb: the organization of the dermatome and afferent myotome. Philos Trans R Soc Lond B Biol Sci 1981;293:509–59.

[30] Gu Y, Xu J, Chen L, et al. Long term outcome of contralateral C7 transfer: a report of 32 cases. Chin Med J (Engl) 2002;115(6):866–8.

[31] Gu YD, Zhang GM, Chen DS, et al. Seventh cervical nerve root transfer from the contralateral healthy side for treatment of brachial plexus root avulsion. J Hand Surg [Br] 1992;17:518–21.

Measuring Outcomes in Adult Brachial Plexus Reconstruction

Keith A. Bengtson, MD[a], Robert J. Spinner, MD[b],
Allen T. Bishop, MD[c], Kenton R. Kaufman, PhD[c],
Krista Coleman-Wood, PhD[c], Michelle F. Kircher, RN[c],
Alexander Y. Shin, MD[c],*

[a]Department of Physical Medicine and Rehabilitation, Mayo Clinic, Rochester, MN 55905, USA
[b]Department of Neurosurgery, Mayo Clinic, Rochester, MN 55905, USA
[c]Department of Orthopaedic Surgery, Division of Hand Surgery, Mayo Clinic, 200 First Street SW,
Rochester, MN 55905, USA

Adult brachial plexus injuries are devastating, life-altering injuries that are a reconstructive challenge for the patient and the surgeon [1]. Quantifying the result of a surgical intervention has become a major focus of surgeons and researchers over the past several decades, especially with the recent focus on evidence-based medicine. More recently, attempts have been made to measure outcomes based on multiple criteria. Some measures of outcome focus solely on surgeon evaluation of functional motor recovery (eg, British Medical Research Council (BMRC or MRC) muscle grading scale [2]), whereas others are patient-related outcomes (eg, Disability of the Arm, Shoulder and Hand [DASH] [3]). Other measures focus on quality of life, the ability to return to previous occupations, or the general medical health of patients (eg, Short Form 36 [SF-36]). Despite having been validated by talented and thoughtful researchers, each only addresses a portion of the complex and dynamic results of surgical reconstruction. The need to quantify subjective and objective data in a heterogeneous group of patients and injuries is needed for us to truly determine the outcomes of surgical intervention. The focus of this article is on evaluating the various outcome measures, with perspectives on past and present

techniques, and to assess the challenges and opportunities for the future in this unique and highly diverse patient population.

Goals of surgical reconstruction

To determine how to measure outcomes, the goals of surgical reconstruction of the adult patient who has a brachial plexus injury need to be defined. From a surgeon's perspective, the goals of surgery have largely focused on the return of motor function and restoration of protective sensation. A tremendous volume of literature exists on methods of reconstruction that range from neurolysis to nerve grafting and transfer, to free functioning muscle transfers [1,4–31]. From a patient's perspective, although restoration of function is one of the primary goals, alleviation of pain, cosmesis, return to work and a preinjury lifestyle, and emotional state are also important. Finally, from a society perspective, the need to determine the cost effectiveness of such procedures should also be addressed.

To measure outcomes of brachial plexus reconstruction, we need to understand what the objectives of treatment are, from the patient's and the surgeon's point of view.

Problems with current outcome measures: case illustration

Although as surgeons we would like to simplify measurement of outcomes to a single parameter,

---

* Corresponding author.

E-mail address: shin.alexander@mayo.edu
(A.Y. Shin).

such as strength of elbow flexion through isolated biceps function, multiple factors affect outcomes in brachial plexus reconstruction. A danger in focusing on a single measurement parameter in the global assessment of a patient is the misrepresentation of outcome. For example, a patient who had an ulnar nerve fascicle transfer to the biceps motor branch [26] as part of a reconstruction for a C5 and C6 avulsion may have regained exceptional biceps bulk and strength, but the transfer has essentially failed because of chronic debilitating neuropathic pain associated with the injury (Fig. 1). If strength of elbow flexion is chosen as the defining measure of outcome, this patient would rate as "excellent." However, when patient-related outcome measures are applied, the surgical procedure has failed because of the neuropathic pain and inability to work. This example also illustrates the difficulty in defining what a "good" result is. From a surgeon's perspective, restoration of functional motion may be a "good" result; however, from a patient's perspective, it is far from "good" because he/she still has significant debilitating neuropathic pain.

Factors affecting outcome

The factors that affect outcomes can essentially be divided into three categories: injury factors, patient factors, and nonbiologic factors. Each of these factors needs to be considered in the development of the optimal outcome measurement tool for brachial plexus reconstruction.

Injury factors include the mechanisms of injury (high energy versus low energy, traction versus laceration), type of brachial plexus injury (preganglionic versus postganglionic), level of injury, type of nerve injured (predominantly sensory versus motor versus mixed), and associated bone and soft tissue trauma, not only to the upper extremity but also to the lower extremity. Injury factors are important to understand because a comparison of surgical techniques to improve function must include patients who have similar types of injuries so that one can extrapolate the true outcome of the intervention. It is difficult to compare a patient who has a brachial plexus injury from a motorcycle accident that occurred at 100 mph with one who had a bicycle injury that occurred at 25 mph, or with one who sustained a fall. The concomitant injures, such as brain, extremity, spine, pelvic, visceral organ, or neurologic injuries, are often ignored when comparing the various types of brachial plexus injuries. Such patients may present with similar (although typically not identical) deficits, but clearly, they are different. They have different mechanisms of injuries and energies, and associated osseous and soft tissue injuries, the effect of which is essentially unknown.

Patient factors are those associated with the demographics and personality of the patient. Demographic factors include the patient's age, sex, and handedness. Although demographic factors are easy to identify and report, personality factors are difficult to categorize. Studies of patients who have spinal cord injuries have demonstrated a commonality among the patients that can affect recovery and rehabilitation [32]. Rohe and Krause [33] evaluated men with spinal cord injuries and found that these patients had

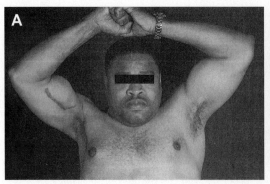
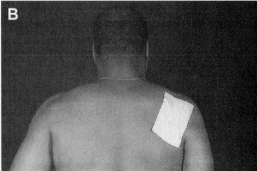

Fig. 1. A 35-year-old man who sustained a C5 and C6 avulsion injury underwent an ulnar nerve fascicle transfer to the biceps motor branch (Oberlin's transfer) in addition to a spinal accessory nerve transfer to the suprascapular nerve. Approximately 2 years after surgery, he demonstrated excellent biceps motor strength and mass (*A*). Unfortunately, he rates his overall success as poor, secondary to significant and debilitating chronic neuropathic pain, requiring multiple medications including transdermal narcotics, despite having a highly successful motor outcome (*B*).

five similar personality types: a tendency toward narcissism, stimulation-seeking behavior, a lower motivation, social isolation, and decreased energy. The effects of these personality traits hamper rehabilitation efforts and significantly affect outcome compared with other patient groups with spinal cord injury. The similarity between male patients who have spinal cord injury and those who have brachial plexus injury is striking, because most of these injuries occur in young men following motor vehicle accidents.

Nonbiologic factors, which are the most difficult to quantify, include the patient's social support system, socioeconomic well-being, perception of cosmesis, and education level. Outcomes can be affected by the degree of social and economic support that the injured patient receives but are nearly impossible to measure other than through salary and educational levels.

When taken all together, these factors have a tremendous effect on how we measure outcomes. Any measurement of outcomes needs to address these factors in a prospective, unbiased fashion.

The ideal outcome measures

The ideal outcome measure should be valid, reliable, responsive, unbiased, appropriate, and easy [34]. Validity indicates that the measurement tool actually measures what it claims to measure, which usually requires some sort of gold standard to measure against. For example, any new measure of blood pressure must be compared with simultaneous blood pressure measurements using an arterial line. Unfortunately, in the realm of brachial plexus reconstruction, the gold standard is unclear. Although most would agree that elbow flexion is the primary objective [1], the secondary objectives are highly debatable. If we did assume that elbow flexion strength is the most important parameter to measure, the method in which it is measured is important. Should strength be measured isometrically at various elbow angles, isokinetically at various angular speeds, or functionally, in relation to how much a subject can lift at a given time? We need to determine if a single measure of strength is adequate to report, or if testing should include measures of endurance, torque, power, and stamina. The answers are not clear, nor are they agreed on. Therefore, validity is difficult to determine in measuring biceps strength or almost any muscle strength.

Reliability indicates that the measurement tool will give consistent answers if repeated by different testers under different circumstances when no change in function has occurred in the subject. Proving reliability requires a large pool of subjects who are willing to submit to repeat testing. Unfortunately, in the case of brachial plexus reconstruction, the number of subjects in any given geographic area is small. Therefore, outcome measures tend to be more empiric in nature. We must use tools that have been tested for reliability on populations that are similar to brachial plexus patients. For example, the DASH questionnaire has been tested on many subjects who have various upper extremity disabilities [3] and, therefore, might be considered reliable for measuring patients who have brachial plexus injuries. Perhaps tools that measure upper extremity function or disability in patients who have stoke or in those who have spinal cord injury may also be used in brachial plexus patients. However, true reliability for measuring outcomes in brachial plexus reconstruction may never be determined because of the small patient population.

Outcomes should have normative data that compare with the general population, and age, gender, and group specific norms. The tool should also have minimal floor and ceiling effects and should provide details along the spectrum of function expected in the studied population. In other words, many participants should not score in either extreme of the measurement. Rather, the scores of the tested population should be well distributed throughout the range of possible scoring. No clumps of scores should be seen on the low or high end of the scoring spectrum.

Other considerations include responsiveness and the general burden on the patient and the tester. If the intervention to the patient produces a response, either positive or negative, an outcome tool must be able to show that response; otherwise, it is not worthwhile. This consideration is especially important if the response to treatment is expected to be small, incremental, or difficult to discern, which is often the case, especially in the early postoperative stage of brachial plexus reconstruction. Therefore, any measurement tool should be sensitive to small changes if it is to be useful.

If a test is too time consuming to take, administer, or evaluate, then it is less likely to be used widely at multiple institutions. Ideally, for example, a questionnaire should be brief, inexpensive, easy to administer, and easy to score. It should not require a highly trained or specialized interviewer or rating expert. Such a tool is likely to be used and accepted widely. Unfortunately, the simplicity of the outcome measure is often inversely proportional to the accuracy and responsiveness of that same measuring tool.

Diagnosis-specific measurement tools are ideal, but these tools are difficult to develop with the small population of brachial plexopathy patients. Additionally, health-related quality of life (HRQOL) scales may be used [34]. Finally, the outcome tool should be adaptable to various languages and cultures so outcomes may be compared on a global scale. Moreover, the tool should not be biased for or against any subgroup or culture [34].

One trend is to consider the patient in a more holistic manner using a generalized model of disablement, such as those proposed by the World Health Organization (WHO), the National Center for Medical Rehabilitation Research, or the American Physical Therapy Association [35–37]. The WHO model has been through various revisions as the International Classification of Impairments, Disabilities, and Handicaps. These models attempt to analyze the patient from many levels of function, beginning at the cellular or "systems" level and progressing up to how the patient functions on a societal level. These models are complex and may be considered still in the early stages of development.

Current outcome measures, their pitfalls and benefits

Current outcome measures can be classified as either surgeon reported or patient reported. Surgeon-reported outcomes are essentially measurements of function (ie, strength, range of motion, sensation), whereas patient-reported outcomes are measures of emotions about their surgery and functional recovery. Surgeon-reported outcomes are typically graded by the surgeon and can be variable and biased, depending on the experience of the surgeon and the surgeon's interpretation of the outcome method. Patient-reported outcome measures are typically in the form of questionnaires that are frequently time-consuming to complete and that ask patients to rate function on a Likert-type scale. A careful review of the literature will demonstrate several commonalities in reporting outcomes. These include studies that are mostly retrospective and are reported by the operating surgeon. Typically, these studies summarize multiple techniques that are performed

simultaneously, making accurate evaluation difficult. These issues have confounded outcomes research (see later discussion).

Measurement of muscle motor function

British Medical Research Council muscle grading

The most widely used outcome measure in brachial plexus surgery has been the BMRC, or MRC (Table 1) [2]. The development of the BMRC has been traced back to the treatment of war injuries and poliomyelitis by Dyck and colleagues [38]. The origins have been traced back to 1917, when R.W. Lovett, a Boston orthopedic surgeon, reported a grading system that was credited to a physical therapist [39]. It was introduced in 1943 [2] and has since been modified multiple times by multiple investigators. The BMRC grading scale has many advantages. It is simple and requires no special equipment to implement [40]. It is well-established and has likely been learned by most practicing physicians sometime in their medical training. It is easy to understand and, once learned, brings a quick and accurate functional picture to mind. However, despite these advantages, the nuances of the differentiating grades can be difficult [40]. The prerequisites for grading include an understanding of the definitions of range of motion. In order for elbow flexion to be a grade 3, full range of motion of the elbow is required, which is complicated with a joint contracture or if full range of motion is not present and the degree of passive motion is not determined. Because of these nuances, different experienced surgeons can give different grades to the same patient.

The BMRC grading scale has other potential pitfalls. Its simplicity is perhaps its biggest limitation. The BMRC scale often measures a single time motion and does not evaluate the muscle for endurance, torque, or stamina. Additionally, it

Table 1
The British Medical Council grading scale

0	No contraction
1	Flicker or trace of contraction
2	Active movement, with gravity eliminated
3	Active movement against gravity
4	Active movement against gravity and resistance
5	Normal power

Data from O'Brien MD. Aids to the examination of the peripheral nervous system. 4th edition. In: Parkinson M, editor. Edinburgh: WB Saunders; 2000. p. 1–62.

measures groups of muscles rather than the isolated function of specific muscles. In the evaluation of elbow flexion, which is affected by the biceps, brachialis, and brachioradialis, it is difficult to determine how much strength is from any of these muscles individually. Similarly, it is difficult to apply the BMRC scale to the shoulder. Isolation and testing of the deltoid, rotator cuff musculature, pectoralis muscles, and trapezius can be difficult. It is not uncommon to have a patient who has a complete axillary nerve injury or a complete suprascapular nerve lesion, but who has full range of motion and slight weakness of abduction. The BMRC grading of his/her deltoid (or supraspinatus) could be misconstrued as a grade 4 (full range of motion, slight weakness) but, in actuality, it is a grade 0 because the deltoid (or supraspinatus) is nonfunctional and the motion and strength are secondary to the supraspinatus (or deltoid) muscle.

Recently, MacAvoy and Green [41], using a cadaveric model, compared the BMRC muscle grading technique with calculated force and torque measurements for biceps strength. These investigators suggested that, although the BMRC scale is good for describing weak muscles, it was completely inadequate for describing any muscle with greater than 4% of normal strength. Specifically, they calculated that "grade 4/5 accounts for 96% of the spectrum of strength" and "the use of the qualifiers (eg, 4+, 4−, 5−) is not new and has represented an attempt to address the inadequacy of the grading system. Rather, the existence of the qualifiers reinforces the inadequacy of the grading system." They go on to conclude that "clinicians have used the MRC scale for decades and will undoubtedly continue to do so. Although many surgeons and investigators may be aware of the wide variability of range of grade 4/5 (manifest by the widespread use of grades 4− and 4+), this skewing of the scale is probably not fully appreciated by all who use it. Clearly, the ideal testing scale would be a method that records a reasonably precise measurement of actual strength for each specific muscle."

Kilogram lifting test

Another popular measure identified in brachial plexus outcomes is "kilogram lifting" [26,42–46], which is another understandable and easily visualized outcome measure. Chammas [42] uses an isometric measurement to define the strength of elbow flexion at 90 degrees, with the upper extremity in "an anatomic neutral position" using an Isobex 2.0 machine. Liverneaux [45] describes the strength of elbow flexion as "flexing the arm to 90 degrees, the maximum weight that patients were able to sustain on the hand." Teboul [46] publishes a picture illustrating the technique of measuring elbow flexion strength, stating that "various weights were placed in the hand, with the elbow extended, and then the patient was asked to flex the elbow once to 90 degrees. The heaviest weight that could be lifted was recorded in kilograms." Clearly, specific protocols must be described to determining the validity and reliability of the measurement. Additionally, the testing must be done in a consistent manner to compare results among patients and across various medical centers.

Quantified electromyography

Quantitative electromyography (EMG) can mean a number of different things, depending on how the motor unit interference pattern is measured. Many investigators have been interested only in the first EMG signs of muscle reinnervation [9,47]. However, those who were truly trying to quantify the EMG results used various methods to do so. For example, Chalidapong [48] recommended a detailed protocol for the measurement of maximum and mean interference pattern activity of various upper extremity movements. These techniques are difficult to perform in a consistent manner, which makes comparisons among institutions difficult, but it is more important to recognize that nascent units and reinnervation potentials do not necessarily correlate with functional recovery [49].

Pinch and grip measurement

Pinch and grip strength testing using various dynamometers, force plates, and other digital or analog instruments is well established and verified in the literature. The techniques are easy to replicate and the results are understandable by most. Unfortunately, most brachial plexus reconstructions involve restoration of elbow flexion and shoulder stability, with restoration of pinch and grip in only the more favorable cases.

Measurement of motion

Measurement of motion as an outcome is a highly used tool in the orthopedic literature and in many ways reflects muscle strength to some degree. Application of a goniometer to active flexion or extension of the elbow, wrist, or fingers can easily convey functional recovery. However, not all joints are as simple as these joints. Shoulder range of motion is clearly an important functional outcome in brachial plexus reconstruction and is one of the most difficult motions to measure accurately. Shoulder motion is an aggregate of glenohumeral and scapulothoracic motion that is affected by the deltoid, supraspinatus, infraspinatus, teres minor, subscapularis, pectoralis major and minor, trapezius, latissimus, rhomboids, levator scapulae, and serratus muscles. Measurement can be overestimated by trunk motion or leaning and by improper inclusion of scapulothoracic motion [50]. Fractures and soft tissue injuries can also affect the way motion is measured or can limit the potential for "true" measurement of movement. A careful review of the literature shows no clear definition of how shoulder motion should be measured (seated versus standing, elbow flexed or extended, composite versus isolated), and a multitude of techniques have been reported. Additionally, various methods measure external rotation (humerus abducted 90 degrees or adducted), internal rotation (by degrees or by which lumbar/thoracic spine one is able to touch), abduction (glenohumeral or scapulo-thoracic motion), and forward flexion. How does one compare these results? Each investigator has his/her own method of measuring shoulder motion. Bertelli [47] writes, "shoulder abduction was evaluated with goniometry,"

without elaboration. Doi [9] reports data on shoulder flexion and external range of motion but does not detail how these were measured. Takka [51] also reports on shoulder abduction and flexion but does not mention how these were obtained. Gu [52], in a similar fashion, tabulates the results of shoulder abduction and external rotation without further details. Rostoucher [53] reports on the presence or absence of shoulder stability, and on active external rotation, abduction, and flexion, but does not elaborate on how they were determined. Terzis [54] is more complete in her description of methods and used video analysis, yet still does not answer the necessary question about how, and which component of, shoulder motion was measured.

Further complicating the measurement of the shoulder is how to address compensation of one muscle group for another. A patient who has a complete axillary nerve lesion, with complete atrophy of the deltoid, may have symmetric equal motion to the uninjured side (Fig. 2). It is the overcompensation of the supraspinatus muscle that allows this to occur. Does it mean the patient's shoulder is normal? Based on the range of motion compared with the opposite side, it is. If a BMRC grade is done, it would be graded as 4, full range of motion, with slightly less than normal strength, yet the deltoid is completely denervated. This situation further begs the question of

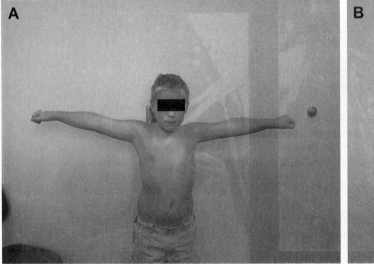
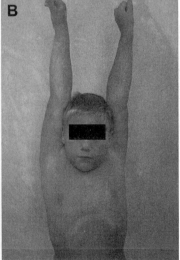

Fig. 2. A 10-year-old boy who sustained a motorcycle accident had an isolated axillary nerve rupture. Despite the rupture, he was able to abduct his arm fully and against gravity (*A*, *B*). His entire arm abduction and forward flexion was secondary to the supraspinatus and infraspinatus muscles.

how a complex joint such as the shoulder, which is affected by multiple muscles and has complex motions, should be evaluated. Simplifications based on a BMRC scale or motion scale are clearly unsuitable. Even with standard methodology, the complexity of the shoulder would be difficult to quantify accurately. It is an area that clearly would benefit from standardization (see later discussion).

Nerve-specific outcomes

The grading of specific nerve function has been proposed. Advocates of this method of grading the entire nerve function include the BMRC system and the American modifications [55]. These grading systems potentially distinguish between strengths of proximally and distally innervated muscles, and gravity and resistance. Full or comparable recovery of nerves to all distal targets seldom occurs. More important, these grading systems do not accurately reflect specific findings or the subtleties of individual nerve injuries or common combinations or nerve injuries. Those types of classification systems have been developed and used extensively by Kline [56].

Global function outcomes

The outcome reports of "poor, fair, good, and excellent" and "satisfied or unsatisfied" clearly have their drawbacks, not the least of which is the lack of a well-established definition of terms. Bentolila [57] uses a patient survey, asking whether the patient was "satisfied, fair, or dissatisfied." Chammas [42] reports on the patient's feeling of "subjective improvement" and his/her "level of satisfaction." Ruhmann [58,59] also uses patients' satisfaction, terming their subjective assessment as poor, good, or excellent. Doi [9,60] defines the patient's elbow flexion strength and ability to position the arm in space, and finger total active range of motion, in terms of "poor, fair, good, or excellent. Kato [61] defines nerve recovery as "good, restoration of functional active movement in at least one axis of a joint; fair, nerve regeneration proven by clinical and neurophysiologic examination, but only little functional worth; and poor, no regeneration." Samardzic [62] reports a separate grading scale of nerve regeneration: "1) *bad* denotes no arm movement or weightless arm movement and usually no trophic changes or alteration observed on electromyographic studies; 2) *fair* denotes arm movement against gravity with the ability to

maintain position and improvement noted with regard to trophic changes and electromyographic studies, active arm abduction up to 45 degrees, and elbow flexion up to 90 degrees; 3) *good* denotes arm movement against resistance with ability to repeat movements in succession and improvement observed with regard to trophic changes and on electromyographic studies, active arm abduction greater than 45 degrees, and full-range elbow flexion: and 4) *excellent* denotes nearly normal function." Once again, standardization is needed to compare results from multiple medical centers.

Return to work

"Return to work" is an important social goal in any type of rehabilitation. However, the range of functions encompassed by "work" is enormous. One would expect that it is easier for a patient who has a brachial plexus injury to return to a sedentary job than a job requiring heavy labor. Therefore, any assessment of "return to work" would have to be specific about the tasks involved. Also, it would be important to note if the patient returned to his/her original, preinjury work or some modified or completely separate vocation.

Sensation and sensibility

Sensation has been used as a measure of outcome but, again, the methods of measuring sensation vary widely. The original BMRC classification for sensation has been less widely adopted, compared with its motor counterpart. Newer methods of testing sensibility have also been developed and reported [63].

Bentolila [57] states that "sensitivity to light touch and to hot and cold was tested, as was stereognosis." However, only the presence or absence of protective sensation was reported. Bertelli [47] is more descriptive in his methodology, stating, "sensory assessments of the hand included assessments of perception of light touch (tested with Semmes-Weinstein monofilaments) and pin pricks (protective sensibility)." Doi [9] also details sensory testing more carefully: "Sensation of vibration was tested with a tuning fork; pain, with pin-prick; sensation of moving touch, with cotton wool; and cutaneous pressure threshold, with Semmes-Weinstein monofilaments. All tests were performed by an experienced hand therapist, and the results of sensory recovery were classified according to the modified Highet scale."

Takka [51] specifies that vibration be measured at 30 and 256 cps, along with touch, pain, and Semmes-Weinstein monofilament tests. Htut [64], in an article devoted to sensory recovery, greatly details the methodology of measuring pinprick and cotton wool sensations, joint position sense, monofilament thresholds, vibration perception thresholds, and thermal thresholds.

Therefore, the measurement of sensation remains confusing, if not controversial. However, sensory recovery is perhaps less important than motor recovery because it is less often one of the main goals of brachial plexus reconstruction.

Patient-related outcomes

Measurement of pain

Pain, as measured by the visual analog scale method, is a valid outcome measure and is a large determinant of patient satisfaction. In general, pain, when recorded, has been assessed using a numeric or a visual analog scale. Htut [64], however, uses an extensive set of measurements, including visual analog scale, McGill Pain Questionnaire, and the patient's description of pain. A task force from the International Association for the Study of Pain suggests that assessing pain should include not only a direct measure of pain such as a visual analog scale, but also a measure of emotional function, such as the Beck Depression Scale and the Profile of Mood States [65]. Additionally, they suggest a record of rescue analgesic use and a measure of patient satisfaction, such as the Patient Global Impression of Change [66]. Pain questionnaires such as the American Academy of Pain Management's Pain Outcomes Profile are also used in some centers [67,68]. Unfortunately, pain may not be directly affected by the primary reconstructive intervention that is being performed.

Patient-related outcomes: disability of the arm, shoulder and hand

Since its introduction in 1996 [3], DASH has become a widely used tool in measuring patient-related outcomes after a surgical intervention. It is a questionnaire that asks general questions regarding function, based on a Likert scale. The total score is converted to a 100 point scale, where 0 is no disability and 100 is complete disability. In its ideal application, individuals take the DASH before a surgical intervention and at the end of treatment. However, the DASH is one of the most abused outcome measures in our literature. It is mostly used as single-point measurement after intervention and the scores among the cohort are typically averaged. It is the difference between the preoperative score and the postoperative score that is the actual measure of the effect of the surgical treatment, not the average of postoperative scores that measures the effect of the surgical treatment. Determining what change in score is "significant" remains debatable. A patient who has a preoperative DASH score of 90 that diminished to an 80 after surgery is still disabled, compared with a patient who dropped the same amount whose preoperative DASH score was 20. A recent publication highlights this inappropriate use of the DASH [69]. In this retrospective study of 31 brachial plexus patients who underwent reconstruction, a follow-up DASH is used and reported to have an average of 70.15. This result was compared with the normalized general population and the conclusion was that patients who have brachial plexus injuries were more disabled than the general population. The study further compared a group of patient follow-up DASH scores in those who had surgery before and 6 months after injury. Without knowing the preoperative scores or the change in scores, the investigators conclude that differences were statistically significant if early surgery was done. The variability in DASH scores in brachial plexus patients is tremendous, which further emphasizes the need to obtain pre- and postoperative scores.

Studies have also demonstrated the effect of lower extremity injuries on DASH scores [70]. This effect further complicates measurement of outcome because many patients who have brachial plexus injuries also have concomitant lower extremity fractures or injuries.

Normative data for different groups of patients is also needed to make accurate comparisons. No normative data exist for patients who have various types of brachial plexus injuries. Davidson [71] demonstrated that the average DASH score for patients who had unilateral upper arm amputation was 39 ± 20, compared with those with brachial plexus injury (type of injury not reported) whose score was 65 ± 15, a difference which was statistically significant. When surgery was performed on the patients who had brachial plexus (n = 3), their DASH scores dropped 25 points, which was also significant. What was not addressed was the type of injury, concomitant injuries, or the effect of pain and other nonbiologic factors on outcomes.

The SF-36 is a 36-item questionnaire that measures generic HRQOL outcomes [34]. Questions are answered using a five-item scale. Results are divided into eight different scales, including physical function, physical role, bodily pain, general health, mental health, emotion role, social function, and vitality.

Generally, the questionnaire takes 5 to 10 minutes to fill out and may be administered by phone or computer. Extensive studies have shown the SF-36 to be reliable and valid. It is a multipurpose health survey that has proved useful in surveys of general and specific populations, comparing the relative burden of diseases, and differentiating the health benefits produced by a wide range of different treatments [72]. Recently, Katajima [73] reported on the use of the SF-36 in brachial plexus–injured patients and demonstrated that in Japanese patients, the SF-36 was not sensitive enough to evaluate regional conditions, and SF-36 scores and objective evaluations of joint function had little correlation.

How has outcome been reported in the literature?

The current literature on brachial plexus outcomes reveals that many measuring tools have been used. The preponderance of published reports typically has been based solely on the BMRC grading scale. A review of multiple investigators, or groups of investigators, who have published reports on outcomes following brachial plexus reconstruction shows that nearly three quarters of them report their outcomes in terms of BMRC muscle grades. However, seven of these groups report on shoulder active range of motion, and seven use some version of a poor/fair/good/excellent scale (defined in varying ways). Six mention some measurement of sensation, five report on grip or pinch strength, and four mention some variation on how many kilograms may be lifted by the patient's affected arm. The remaining measuring tools that are used include return to work status, quantitative EMG, and a visual analog scale of pain (see Refs. [1,9,15,26,29,42–45,47,48,51,53,54, 57–61,64,74–89]). The use of the DASH has gained popularity in reporting brachial plexus surgery outcomes. However, most of the studies report a postoperative DASH score and perform a comparison to normative data. This inappropriate use of the DASH continues to be promoted in the effort to obtain "patient-related outcomes data."

Few studies of quality of life and functional outcome of brachial plexus surgery adequately address the important issues discussed previously. In 1997, Choi and colleagues [90] reported on the quality of life and functional outcome of 34 patients who had undergone treatment of brachial plexus injuries. These patients were sent a 78-item questionnaire that was developed by the investigators that covered injury, treatment course, present status, education, employment, social history, discrimination, harassment, and quality of life. It was adapted to a questionnaire form from an interview form of the US General Social Survey. Sixty-one patients were identified from their database but only 34 were able to be contacted for the survey. The investigators reported that overall life satisfaction was moderate in 78%, 54% were able to return to work, and impact of injury did not affect overall quality of life in 31%. They concluded that despite the devastating nature of the injury, patients reported good quality of life. This study was one of the first to quantify these issues and clearly was ahead of its time. However, the loss of nearly one half of the patients identified, the potential bias of not knowing the results of this one half of the patients, and the use of an invalidated study are limitations.

Agreement does not exists on what tools should be used to measure the effectiveness of brachial plexus reconstruction. Ideally, every surgical group that performs brachial reconstruction should use the same outcome measuring tools, which would make comparisons of surgical techniques possible. Considering the expense and effort in brachial plexus reconstruction, the urgency of such uniformity seems more pressing.

Biomechanical evaluation

One method worthy of consideration for measuring outcomes from brachial plexus reconstruction is three-dimensional kinematic motion analysis. Kinematic upper extremity analysis could become a useful clinical tool because it solves many of the issues affecting quantifying movement in patients who have brachial plexus injuries. Motion analysis uses surface markers, which are lightweight and allow for natural subject movement without constraint [91]. Limb segments are identified by markers placed on the skin, and movement between segments is used to define joints and motions (Fig. 3). Movements that are difficult to measure and differentiate with goniometry can be quantified by appropriate

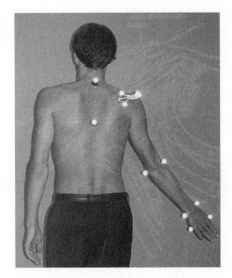

Fig. 3. Using gait motion analysis techniques, the ranges of motion of the upper extremity, in particular the shoulder, can be measured more accurately. Illustrated here is the placement of registration markers along the bony prominences in preparation for measurement of shoulder and elbow motion.

segment identification and joint definition [92]. For example, shoulder abduction can be defined as occurring between the trunk segment and the humeral segment or it can be more appropriately defined as occurring between the scapular and humeral segments. Similarly, the scapulothoracic joint is defined as motion between the trunk and scapular segments. With appropriate segment identification and joint definitions, atypical and normal movements can be isolated, quantified, and attributed to specific anatomic joints. In addition, subjects can move freely using correct and compensatory movements and the kinematic analysis can subdivide the movements and ascribe the motion to the correct joints [93]. Studies in the Mayo Clinic Motion Analysis Laboratory using mechanical representations of the shoulder girdle have demonstrated good accuracy, with an error of less than 2.2% of full-scale range of motion with accuracy for locating individual markers within 1.3 mm during dynamic motion.

Some pitfalls do exist and should be considered before implementing upper extremity kinematics as a standard outcome measurement. Three-dimensional movement analysis systems are expensive to acquire and require skilled personnel to have accurate and reliable data. Ideally, a movement quantification system should be in a fixed location with consistent personnel maintaining the

equipment and acquiring motion data. An engineer is required to work on the biomechanical model and maintain the equipment. Personnel must be skilled in palpation, to place the marker set on the appropriate anatomic locations, and must be able to place markers consistently, to have repeatable results. The amount of time needed to obtain the kinematic results is longer than that for goniometric measurements because of the need to process the data.

The large working range of motion of the shoulder complex complicates the mathematic modeling and calculation of kinematics. Many different biomechanical models are being used to process the data and provide appropriate kinematic data in all planes of movement of the shoulder. An additional problem is that the output from the mathematic models does not readily translate into terminology used by clinicians, which makes simple reporting difficult. For example, shoulder movement that occurs between the flexion and abductions planes (sometimes referred to as occurring within the plane of the scapula) is difficult to convey when using standard planes but can easily be expressed in spherical coordinates. To date, no standardized report formats are available.

At present, no standardized set of upper extremity kinematic data acquisition procedures exists. A plethora of unconstrained movements and tasks simulating activities of daily living have been shown to be reproducible with small standard deviations, although a standardized and meaningful set of movements has not been defined [94].

Once a consistent set of movements is defined and a uniform report format is created, upper extremity kinematic analysis may become a standard for measuring function in persons who have brachial plexus injuries. It can depict the natural history of recovery from the injury or the recovery from reconstruction surgery.

An alternative to estimating strength using the BMRC scale is the quantification of muscle strength using instrumented methodology. Instrumented methods have been documented as more accurate in measuring strength and more sensitive to differences in strength [95]. Several methodologies with some demonstrated validity and reliability could be valuable in quantifying strength of shoulder and upper extremity muscles.

A hand-held dynamometer is a load-registering device that is interposed between the limb of the subject and the hand of the person performing the testing. Strength testing is performed with the patient and examiner in standardized positions similar to those used for muscle grading using the BMRC scale. During testing, the patient exerts a maximum effort and the examiner meets and blocks all resistance created by the patient, preventing movement and giving an isometric contraction. Hand-held dynamometers have been shown to have reasonable intrarater and interrater reliability in strength measurements of the biceps and deltoid muscles [96].

Problems with use of hand-held dynamometers are many and result in incorrect measurements. Studies have shown that measurements of strength in external rotation muscles are lower when determined by hand-held dynamometry as compared with isometric Cybex measurements [97]. If the patient exerts effort greater than the examiner can block, an isotonic contraction will occur and the patient will move out of the testing position without having his/her maximum strength measured; thus, the strength for that muscle group will be underreported. This problem occurs especially when measuring the uninvolved upper extremity, which is required for comparison with the involved side. If the examiner exerts more force than the patient, an eccentric contraction will occur as the patient moves out of the testing position, which will be reflected in a reported strength greater than the standard isometric contraction [98]. Another problem with hand-held dynamometry is the need for the examiner to provide stabilization of the patient to prevent any compensatory or undesirable body movements. With one hand occupied holding the dynamometer, the examiner must control all other test components with his/her remaining hand, which is difficult in the best circumstances and impossible most of the time.

Another option for quantifying strength is instrumentation with fixed load cells. This option uses a load cell attached to an immobile frame that is positioned to allow the patient to push or pull against the load cell while the force generated by each isometric contraction is recorded by a computer. Fixed load cell systems free the examiner to use both hands to stabilize and maintain patient positioning. Stefanova-Uzunova [99] reported using a fixed load cell system to measure upper extremity muscles in children who had brachial plexus birth injuries.

Limitations with the fixed load cell systems include the purchase cost and the cost of testing staff and engineering support for the equipment. Training is required to position patients properly and measure strength appropriately. Each muscle test requires repositioning the patient to interface with the load cell. The system must be calibrated before each use to assure accuracy of measurements. Fixed load cell systems are less common in clinical settings and generally only have protocols for testing shoulder and elbow flexion/extension in the upper extremity.

An alternative strength quantification system is isokinetic dynamometers. These systems have an armature which can be aligned with the patient limb to measure torque generation by various muscle groups of the shoulder and elbow. One advantage of the isokinetic systems is the ability to examine isometric and dynamic strength. Isokinetic testing examines the strength of a muscle group through a predefined range of movement and can be performed by way of either concentric or eccentric muscle contractions. The system can easily test opposite motions (such as flexion and extension) without changing patient positions or repositioning the dynamometer. Excellent stabilization is provided for all body parts by straps that fixate the patient to the testing seat. For each contraction, most isokinetic systems report peak and average torque, work, and power; a coefficient of variability of repeated efforts; and a ratio between agonist and antagonist muscles. Isokinetic testing is considered the gold standard of strength assessment.

Despite having the reputation of being the best technique for testing strength, isokinetic dynamometry does have some problems that limit use of the system. The system is expensive to acquire and requires some expertise to use and engineering support to maintain the equipment. It is cumbersome to adjust to accommodate each patient and can only be used to test the forearm (pronation/supination) and wrist (flexion/extension) movements if the patient has full handgrip strength.

In summary, no single biomechanical system can provide quantification of upper extremity strength testing that is valid, reliable, and readily available.

Opportunities for the future

Based on the authors' experience and the data in the literature, it appears that the field of reporting outcomes for brachial plexus injuries has some significant challenges that need to be overcome. Methods of measurement of muscle, joint motion, and forces need to be performed in a standardized format that is simple to use and reproducible. Isokinetic motor force measurement that isolates muscle groups and evaluates for single force strength, torque, and endurance normalized to the uninjured extremity will become a necessity to compare the outcomes of surgical procedures. By combining biomechanical gait laboratory measurements of joint motion and the measurement of isokinetic strength, variability in reporting outcomes will be minimized.

Combining this type of mechanical measure of outcome with patient-related outcomes, such as using a pre- and postoperative DASH and pain visual analog scales, and other measure of severity of injury and quality of life surveys, will allow a better comparison of results.

Although the technology for this type of sophisticated testing exists, time, cost, and effort to standardize measurements may never come to fruition unless we all make a concerted effort to unite forces and speak the same language.

References

[1] Shin AY, Spinner RJ, Steinmann SP, et al. Adult traumatic brachial plexus injuries. J Am Acad Orthop Surg 2005;13:382–96.

[2] Aids to the examination of the peripheral nervous system. 4th edition. In: Parkinson M, editor. Edinburgh: WB Saunders; 2000. p. 1–62.

[3] Hudak PL, Amadio PC, Bombardier C. Development of an upper extremity outcome measure: the DASH (disabilities of the arm, shoulder and hand) [corrected]. The Upper Extremity Collaborative Group (UECG). Am J Ind Med 1996;29:602–8.

[4] Allieu Y. Evolution of our indications for neurotization. Our concept of functional restoration of the upper limb after brachial plexus injuries. Chir Main 1999;18:165–6.

[5] Carlstedt T, Grane P, Hallin RG, et al. Return of function after spinal cord implantation of avulsed spinal nerve roots. Lancet 1995;346:1323–5.

[6] Chuang DC. Neurotization procedures for brachial plexus injuries. Hand Clin 1995;11:633–45.

[7] Doi K, Hattori Y, Kuwata N, et al. Free muscle transfer can restore hand function after injuries of the lower brachial plexus. J Bone Joint Surg Br 1998;80:117–20.

[8] Doi K, Kuwata N, Muramatsu K, et al. Double muscle transfer for upper extremity reconstruction following complete avulsion of the brachial plexus. Hand Clin 1999;15:757–67.

[9] Doi K, Muramatsu K, Hattori Y, et al. Restoration of prehension with the double free muscle technique following complete avulsion of the brachial plexus. Indications and long-term results. J Bone Joint Surg Am 2000;82:652–66.

[10] Doi K, Sakai K, Kuwata N, et al. Double free-muscle transfer to restore prehension following com-

plete brachial plexus avulsion. J Hand Surg [Am] 1995;20:408–14.

[11] Fletcher I. Traction lesions of the brachial plexus. Hand 1969;1:129–36.

[12] Frampton VM. Management of brachial plexus lesions. J Hand Ther 1988;1:115–20.

[13] Frampton VM. Management of brachial plexus lesions. Physiotherapy 1984;70:388–92.

[14] Grundy DJ, Silver JR. Problems in the management of combined brachial plexus and spinal cord injuries. Int Rehabil Med 1981;3:57–70.

[15] Gu YD, Zhang GM, Chen DS, et al. Seventh cervical nerve root transfer from the contralateral healthy side for treatment of brachial plexus root avulsion. J Hand Surg [Br] 1992;17:518–21.

[16] Hendry HAM. The treatment of residual paralysis after brachial plexus lesions. J Bone Joint Surg Br 1949;31:42.

[17] Kline DG. Perspectives concerning brachial plexus injury and repair. Neurosurg Clin N Am 1991;2:151–64.

[18] Leechavengvongs S, Witoon CK, Uerpairojkit C, et al. Nerve transfer to biceps muscle using a part of the ulnar nerve in brachial plexus injury (upper arm type): a report of 32 cases. J Hand Surg [Am] 1998;23:711–6.

[19] Leffert R. Brachial plexus injuries. New York: Churchill Livingstone; 1985.

[20] Leffert R, Seddon H. Infraclavicular brachial plexus injuries. J Bone Joint Surg Br 1965;47:9–22.

[21] Malone J, Leal J, Underwood J, et al. Brachial plexus injury management through upper extremity amputation with immediate postoperative prostheses. Arch Phys Med Rehabil 1982;63:89–91.

[22] Merrell GA, Barrie KA, Katz DL, et al. Results of nerve transfer techniques for restoration of shoulder and elbow function in the context of a meta-analysis of the English literature. J Hand Surg [Am] 2001;26: 303–14.

[23] Millesi H. Brachial plexus injuries: management and results. Clin Plast Surg 1984;11:115–20.

[24] Narakas A. Surgical treatment of traction injuries of the brachial plexus. Clin Orthop Relat Res 1978;71.

[25] Narakas AO, Hentz VR. Neurotization in brachial plexus injuries. Indication and results [Review] [47 refs]. Clin Orthop Relat Res 1988;43.

[26] Oberlin C, Beal D, Leechavengvongs S, et al. Nerve transfer to biceps muscle using a part of ulnar nerve for C5-C6 avulsion of the brachial plexus: anatomical study and report of four cases. J Hand Surg [Am] 1994;19:232–7.

[27] Rorabeck C. The management of flail upper extremity in brachial plexus injuries. J Trauma 1980;20:491–3.

[28] Shin AY. 2004-2005 Sterling Bunnell Traveling Fellowship report. J Hand Surg [Am] 2006;31:1226–37.

[29] Songcharoen P. Brachial plexus injury in Thailand: a report of 520 cases. Microsurgery 1995;16:35–9.

[30] Wynn P. Brachial plexus injuries. Br J Hosp Med 1984;32:130–9.

[31] Yeoman PM, Seddon HJ. Brachial plexus injuries: treatment of the flail arm. J Bone Joint Surg Br 1961;43:493–500.

[32] O'Donnel JJ, Cooper JE, Gessner JE, et al. Alcohol, drugs, and spinal cord injury. Alcohol Health Res World 1981;6:27–9

[33] Rohe DE, Krause JS. The five-factor model of personality: findings in males with spinal cord injury. Assessment 1999;6:203–14.

[34] Andersen EM. Criteria for assessing the tools of disability outcomes research. Arch Phys Med Rehabil 2000;81:S15–20.

[35] World Health Organization. ICIDH-2: International classification of functioning and disability. Beta-2 draft, short version. 1999.

[36] International classification of functioning, disability, and health (ICF). 2001;1.

[37] Research plan for the Nation Center for Medical Rehabilitation Research. U.S. Department of Health and Human Services NIH Publication No. 93-3509:23, 1993.

[38] Dyck PJ, Boes CJ, Mulder D, et al. History of standard scoring, notation, and summation of neuromuscular signs. A current survey and recommendation. J Peripher Nerv Syst 2005;10:158–73.

[39] Hislop HJ, Montgomery J. Daniels and Worthingham's muscle testing; techniques of manual examination. In: Daniels, Worthington, editors. 7th edition. Philadelphia: W.B. Saunders Co.; 2002. p. 1–10.

[40] James MA. Use of the Medical Research Council muscle strength grading system in the upper extremity. J Hand Surg [Am] 2007;32:154–6.

[41] MacAvoy MC, Green DP. Critical reappraisal of Medical Research Council muscle testing for elbow flexion. J Hand Surg [Am] 2007;32:149–53.

[42] Chammas M, Goubier JN, Coulet B, et al. Glenohumeral arthrodesis in upper and total brachial plexus palsy. A comparison of functional results. J Bone Joint Surg Br 2004;86:692–5.

[43] Chuang DC, Yeh MC, Wei FC. Intercostal nerve transfer of the musculocutaneous nerve in avulsed brachial plexus injuries: evaluation of 66 patients. J Hand Surg [Am] 1992;17:822–8.

[44] Dai SY, Han Z, Zhoug SZ. Transference of thoracodorsal nerve to musculocutaneous or axillary nerve in old traumatic injury. J Hand Surg [Am] 1990;15:36–7.

[45] Liverneaux PA, Diaz LC, Beaulieu JY, et al. Preliminary results of double nerve transfer to restore elbow flexion in upper type brachial plexus palsies. Plast Reconstr Surg 2006;117:915–9.

[46] Teboul F, Kakkar R, Ameur N, et al. Transfer of fascicles from the ulnar nerve to the nerve to the biceps in the treatment of upper brachial plexus palsy. J Bone Joint Surg Am 2004;86:1485–90.

[47] Bertelli JA, Ghizoni MF. Brachial plexus avulsion injury repairs with nerve transfers and nerve grafts directly implanted into the spinal cord yield partial recovery of shoulder and elbow movements. Neurosurgery 2003;52:1385–90.

[48] Chalidapong P, Sananpanich K, Klaphajone J. Electromyographic comparison of various exercises to improve elbow flexion following intercostal nerve transfer. J Bone Joint Surg Br 2006;88:620–2.

[49] Spinner RJ, Kline DG. Surgery for peripheral nerve and brachial plexus injuries or other nerve lesions. Muscle Nerve 2000;23:680–95.

[50] Malessy MJ, de Ruiter GC, de Boer KS, et al. Evaluation of suprascapular nerve neurotization after nerve graft or transfer in the treatment of brachial plexus traction lesions. J Neurosurg 2004;101:377–89.

[51] Takka S, Doi K, Hattori Y, et al. Selection of grip function in double free gracilis transfer procedures after complete paralysis of the brachial plexus. Ann Plast Surg 2005;54:610–4.

[52] Guan SB, Hou CL, Chen DS, et al. Restoration of shoulder abduction by transfer of the spinal accessory nerve to suprascapular nerve through dorsal approach: a clinical study. Chin Med J (Engl) 2006;119:707–12.

[53] Rostoucher P, Alnot JY, Touam C, et al. Tendon transfers to restore elbow flexion after traumatic paralysis of the brachial plexus in adults. Int Orthop 1998;22:255–62.

[54] Terzis JK, Kostas I, Soucacos PN. Restoration of shoulder function with nerve transfers in traumatic brachial plexus palsy patients. Microsurgery 2006;26:316–24.

[55] Peripheral nerve regeneration: a follow-up study of 3656 World War II injuries. Washington, DC: US Government Printing Office; 1956.

[56] Kline DG, Hudson AR. Basic consideration: peripheral nerve regeneration. In: Kline DG, Hudson AR, editors. Nerve injuries. Philadelphia: W.B. Saunders; 1995. p. 87.

[57] Bentolila V, Nizard R, Bizot P, et al. Complete traumatic brachial plexus palsy: treatment and outcome after repair. J Bone Joint Surg Am 1999;81:20–8.

[58] Ruhmann O, Schmolke S, Bohnsack M, et al. Trapezius transfer in brachial plexus palsy. Correlation of the outcome with muscle power and operative technique. J Bone Joint Surg Br 2005;87:184–90.

[59] Ruhmann O, Wirth CJ, Gosse F, et al. Trapezius transfer after brachial plexus palsy. Indications, difficulties and complications. J Bone Joint Surg Br 1998;80:109–13.

[60] Doi K, Hattori Y, Ikeda K, et al. Significance of shoulder function in the reconstruction of prehension with double free-muscle transfer after complete paralysis of the brachial plexus. Plast Reconstr Surg 2003;112:1596–603.

[61] Kato N, Htut M, Taggart M, et al. The effects of operative delay on the relief of neuropathic pain after injury to the brachial plexus: a review of 148 cases. J Bone Joint Surg Br 2006;88:756–9.

[62] Samardzic M, Rasulic L, Bacetic D. Transfer of the medial pectoral nerve: myth or reality. Neurosurgery 2002;50:1277–82.

[63] Birch R, Bonney G, Wynn Parry CB, et al. Surgical disorders of the peripheral nerves. In: Birsch R, Bonney G, Wynn Parry CB, editors. 1st edition. Philadelphia: W.B. Saunders; 1998. p. 81–96.

[64] Htut M, Misra P, Anand P, et al. Pain phenomena and sensory recovery following brachial plexus avulsion injury and surgical repairs. J Hand Surg [Br] 2006;31:596–605.

[65] Cruccu G, Anand P, Attal N, et al. EFNS guidelines on neuropathic pain assessment. Eur J Neurol 2004; 11:153–62.

[66] Dworkin RH, Turk DC, Farrar JT, et al. Core outcome measures for chronic pain clinical trials: IMMPACT recommendations. Pain 2005;113:9–19.

[67] Clark ME, Gironda RJ, Young RW. Development and validation of the pain outcomes questionnaire-VA. J Rehabil Res Dev 2003;40:381–95.

[68] Gironda RJ, Clark ME. Cluster analysis of the pain outcomes questionnaire. Pain Med 2008;(Suppl): 1–16.

[69] Ahmed-Labib M, Golan JD, Jacques L. Functional outcome of brachial plexus reconstruction after trauma. Neurosurgery 2007;61:1016–23.

[70] Dowrick AS, Gabbe BJ, Williamson OD, et al. Does the disabilities of the arm, shoulder and hand (DASH) scoring system only measure disability due to injuries to the upper limb? J Bone Joint Surg Br 2006;88:524–7.

[71] Davidson J. A comparison of upper limb amputees and patients with upper limb injuries using the Disability of the Arm, Shoulder and Hand (DASH). Disabil Rehabil 2004;26:917–23.

[72] Brazier JE, Harper R, Jones NM, et al. Validating the SF-36 health survey questionnaire: new outcome measure for primary care. BMJ 1992;305:160–4.

[73] Kitajima I, Doi K, Hattori Y, et al. Evaluation of quality of life in brachial plexus injury patients after reconstructive surgery. Hand Surg 2006;11:103–7.

[74] Bertelli JA, Ghizoni MF. Improved technique for harvesting the accessory nerve for transfer in brachial plexus injuries. Neurosurgery 2006;58: 366–70.

[75] Birch R. Brachial plexus injuries. J Bone Joint Surg Br 1996;78:986–92.

[76] Chalidapong P, Sananpanich K, Kraisarin J, et al. Pulmonary and biceps function after intercostal and phrenic nerve transfer for brachial plexus injuries. J Hand Surg [Br] 2004;29:8–11.

[77] Chuang ML, Chuang DC, Lin IF, et al. Ventilation and exercise performance after phrenic nerve and multiple intercostal nerve transfers for avulsed brachial plexus injury. Chest 2005;128:3434–9.

[78] Eggers IM, Mennen U. The EFFUL (Evaluation of Function in the Flail Upper Limb) system. A ranking score system to measure improvement achieved

by surgical reconstruction and rehabilitation. J Hand Surg [Br] 1997;22:388–94.

[79] Eggers IM, Mennen U. The evaluation of function of the flail upper limb classification system: its application to unilateral brachial plexus injuries. J Hand Surg [Am] 2001;26:68–76.

[80] Gu YD, Cai PQ, Xu F, et al. Clinical application of ipsilateral C7 nerve root transfer for treatment of C5 and C6 avulsion of brachial plexus. Microsurgery 2003;23:105–8.

[81] Mackinnon SE, Novak CB, Myckatyn TM, et al. Results of reinnervation of the biceps and brachialis muscles with a double fascicular transfer for elbow flexion. J Hand Surg [Am] 2005;30:978–85.

[82] Songcharoen P, Mahaisavariya B, Chotigavanich C. Spinal accessory neurotization for restoration of elbow flexion in avulsion injuries of the brachial plexus. J Hand Surg [Am] 1996;21:387–90.

[83] Songcharoen P, Wongtrakul S, Mahaisavariya B, et al. Hemi-contralateral C7 transfer to median nerve in the treatment of root avulsion brachial plexus injury. J Hand Surg [Am] 2001;26:1058–64.

[84] Terzis JK, Papakonstantinou KC. The surgical treatment of brachial plexus injuries in adults. Plast Reconstr Surg 2000;106:1097–122.

[85] Terzis JK, Vekris MD, Soucacos PN. Outcomes of brachial plexus reconstruction in 204 patients with devastating paralysis. Plast Reconstr Surg 1999; 104:1221–40.

[86] Xu W, Lu J, Xu J, et al. Full-length ulnar nerve harvest by means of endoscopy for contralateral C7 nerve root transfer in the treatment of brachial plexus injuries. Plast Reconstr Surg 2006;118:689–93.

[87] Xu WD, Xu JG, Gu YD. Comparative clinic study on vascularized and nonvascularized full-length phrenic nerve transfer. Microsurgery 2005;25:16–20.

[88] Zhao X, Lao J, Hung LK, et al. Selective neurotization of the median nerve in the arm to treat brachial plexus palsy. An anatomic study and case report. J Bone Joint Surg Am 2004;86:736–42.

[89] Zhao X, Lao J, Hung LK, et al. Selective neurotization of the median nerve in the arm to treat brachial plexus palsy. Surgical technique. J Bone Joint Surg Am 2005;87(Suppl 1):122–35.

[90] Choi PD, Novak CB, Mackinnon SE, et al. Quality of life and functional outcome following brachial plexus injury. J Hand Surg [Am] 1997;22:605–12.

[91] Kohler F, Disselhoret-Klug C, Schmitz-Rode T. A biomechanical body model allowing calculation of anatomical joint angles of upper extremities during unconstrained movements. J Biomech 2006;39: S75–6.

[92] Rab G, Bagley A. A method for determination of upper extremity kinematics. Gait Posture 2002;15: 113–9.

[93] van Andel CJ, Doorenbosch CAM, Veeger DJ, et al. Complete 3D kinematics of upper extremity functional tasks. Gait Posture 2007;27:120–7.

[94] Petuskey K, Abdala E, James MA, et al. Upper extremity kinematics during functional activities: three-dimensional studies in a normal pediatric population. Gait Posture 2007;25:573–9.

[95] Bohannon R. Measurement, nature, and implications of skeletal muscle strength in patients with neurological disorders. Clin Biomech (Bristol, Avon) 1995;10:283–92.

[96] Lennon SM, Ashburn A. Use of myometry in the assessment of neuropathic weakness: testing for reliability in clinical practice. Clin Rehabil 1993;7: 125–31.

[97] Sullivan SJ, Chesley A, Hebert G, et al. The validity and reliability of hand-held dynamometry in assessing isometric external rotator performance. J Orthop Sports Phys Ther 1988;10:213–9.

[98] Burns SP, Spanier DE. Break-technique handheld dynamometry: relation between angular velocity and strength measurements. Arch Phys Med Rehabil 2005;86:1420–6.

[99] Stefanova-Uzunova M, Stamatova L. Dynamic properties of partially denervated muscle in children with brachial plexus birth palsy. J Neurol Neurosurg Psychiatry 1981;44:497–502.

ELSEVIER
SAUNDERS

Hand Clin 24 (2008) 417–423

HAND
CLINICS

Rehabilitation Following Motor Nerve Transfers

Christine B. Novak, PT, MS, PhD(c)

University Health Network, 8N-875, 200 Elizabeth Street, Toronto, Ontario M5G 2C4, Canada

Transfer of an innervated donor nerve to a recipient nerve is performed to provide a source of nerve for sensory or motor innervation. Historically, these transfers have been used as salvage procedures when no proximal nerve source is available and there are limited expectations regarding outcome. Recently, the use of nerve transfers has expanded with a wider range of application, improving the functional outcome, particularly following more proximal nerve injuries [1–10]. Following injury to a motor nerve, there is a critical time period for reinnervation of the motor end plate, after which time the muscle degeneration is not reversible and muscle reinnervation is not possible [11–13]. The distance of the injury from the motor end plate is a significant factor. A nerve transfer can provide a closer source of innervation; therefore, the period of muscle denervation is significantly shortened, providing a greater opportunity for muscle reinnervation.

Although the number of motor axons and the degree of muscle innervation are important factors influencing muscle strength, the importance of cortical changes and plasticity in optimizing the outcome cannot be underestimated. Cortical changes occur following nerve injury and continue through the process of denervation and reinnervation [14–24]. This process is particularly important to recognize for rehabilitation following nerve transfers [14,25–27]. Because new nerves are providing the proximal source of innervation, the previously established motor patterns and cortical maps are not relevant following nerve transfers, and it is necessary to establish new motor patterns and cortical mapping to reestablish functional use of the extremity. Studies have

illustrated the presence and importance of shifting of the cortical mapping following nerve transfers [14,25–28]. Malessy and colleagues [26] evaluated patients following a medial pectoral or an intercostal to musculocutaneous nerve transfer and illustrated a significant increase in motor-evoked potentials as measured with magnetic stimulation with voluntary elbow flexion compared with respiration. Similarly, Chen and colleagues [28] illustrated a shift in cortical mapping following muscle transfer as assessed with transcranial magnetic stimulation. Particularly for nerve transfers, when the source of innervation to the reinnervated muscle is altered, cortical mapping and relearning are key factors in optimizing patient outcome.

The rehabilitation program following motor nerve transfers must include muscle strengthening, with the emphasis on muscle balance, reeducation, cortical mapping, and normal motor patterns.

Early phase rehabilitation

The early phase of rehabilitation is similar to programs following a nerve repair or graft. The main goal is to regain or maintain range of motion following the period of immobilization. Patient education regarding pain and edema control is instituted in the early postoperative phase. To minimize adherence of the nerve to the surrounding soft tissue, the minimum period of immobilization following surgery is recommended. In most cases, there is no tension of the repair site, and 7 to 10 days of immobilization is usually sufficient; however, this time period will depend on other structures that may have been repaired. In surgical exploration of the brachial plexus, the tendinous attachment of the pectoralis major muscle may be detached and repaired. In these cases, the shoulder should be protected in adduction and internal rotation for 4 weeks to allow

E-mail address: christine.novak@utoronto.ca

sufficient time for soft tissue healing of the pectoralis major muscle. During this period of immobilization, range of motion of the hand, wrist, forearm, and elbow should be encouraged to minimize stiffness in these joints and to promote neural mobility and gliding. If a nerve graft is used, assessment should include the donor site and ensure good wound healing and full range of motion of the surrounding joints. Desensitization exercises may also be necessary in patients who experience postoperative allodynia.

Following immobilization, therapy should be resumed to regain full range of motion of the upper extremity. Glenohumeral abduction and external rotation are often particularly restricted and require an experienced physical therapist to restore shoulder and scapular mobility. Once passive range of motion has been regained, the patient may continue with a home program but should be monitored for evidence of muscle reinnervation or soft tissue tightness as may occur with shoulder abduction, shoulder external rotation, or forearm supination due to positioning and to muscle imbalance from the innervated and denervated muscles. With nerve regeneration, muscle reinnervation will occur but will be dependent on the distance to the target motor end plates. Patients with a brachial plexus injury should continue to use a hemi-sling to support the arm and to minimize the downward forces on the glenohumeral joint, minimizing the glenohumeral subluxation. Once the patient has evidence of reinnervation of the supraspinatus muscle and restoration of the integrity of the glenohumeral joint, the hemi-sling can be discontinued. We have found a simple hemi-sling that supports the forearm with the support across the contralateral suprascapular region to be the most comfortable. It provides the required support for the humerus and allows some mobility within the sling. We do not recommend slings that place downward forces on the affected suprascapular region or slings that support the arm circumferentially around the humerus, because they may place compressive forces on the regenerating nerves. Patients are routinely reassessed on a regular basis for evidence of muscle reinnervation.

Late phase rehabilitation

The later phase of rehabilitation begins with evidence of muscle reinnervation. The emphasis of this phase must be on motor reeducation and restoration of muscle balance. In most cases, strengthening exercises will require motor reeducation to learn how to correctly recruit the newly reinnervated muscle and should begin in gravity-assisted or gravity-eliminated positions.

Initially following a nerve transfer, contraction of the reinnervated muscle is initiated with recruitment and contraction of the muscle from the donor nerve. Because the motor pattern has been altered, the newly innervated muscle is not recruited by thinking of the intended action but rather with the "contraction" of the donor muscle. For example, contraction of the elbow flexors following a flexor carpi ulnaris to musculocutaneous nerve transfer is initiated with contraction of the flexor carpi ulnaris muscle. Initial efforts by the patient to flex the elbow will not recruit the intended action because of the alteration of the source of the innervation and motor pattern. The established motor patterns and cortical pathways will permit easier recruitment of the reinnervated target muscle when the newly reinnervated muscle has been innervated with a donor nerve from a muscle with a synergistic action. This recruitment is similar to the relearning associated with a tendon/muscle transfer, such as a triceps to biceps muscle transfer. Nerves that innervate an antagonistic muscle action may be used for the intended donor nerve, but the retraining will require more effort and learning by the patient.

Following an intercostal to musculocutaneous never transfer, standard postoperative therapy usually includes deep breathing exercises to increase the use of the intercostal muscles to initiate a contraction of the biceps and brachialis muscles. Although this action will adequately contract the elbow flexors for short durations, it is difficult to perform prolonged contractions with deep breathing exercises. Stabilization of the trunk uses the core abdominal muscles, the spinal muscles, and the intercostal muscles. Abdominal muscle training will also recruit the intercostal muscles and, in patients with a nerve transfer that has used the intercostal nerves, will effectively recruit the recipient elbow flexor muscles (Fig. 1). Chalidapong and colleagues [29] assessed the muscle activity in the elbow flexors in patients following an intercostal to musculocutaneous nerve transfer. The greatest electromyographic activity in the elbow flexors was found with trunk flexion followed by efforts to flex the elbow; therefore, trunk flexion exercises should be used for strengthening of the elbow flexors in patients following an

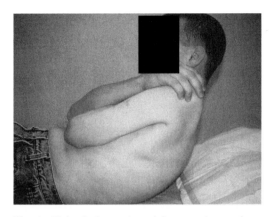

Fig. 1. Abdominal muscle training exercises such as abdominal crunches also recruit the intercostal muscles; therefore, in patients with an intercostal to musculocutaneous nerve transfer, abdominal exercises can be used to recruit the recipient elbow flexor muscles. (*Courtesy of Susan E. Mackinnon, MD, St. Louis, MO.*)

intercostal to musculocutaneous nerve transfer. Abdominal crunches can begin in the early phase of rehabilitation and increase the strength of the biceps and brachialis muscles as reinnervation is progressing.

Motor retraining must use the donor muscle and recipient muscle to recruit the newly innervated muscle and to enhance relearning (Fig. 2). Use of the contralateral uninjured side may also facilitate relearning. As previously stated, use of a synergistic donor nerve will facilitate recruitment of the reinnervated target muscle. Although it is not essential to use a synergistic donor nerve, some patients will not achieve maximal strength in the reinnervated muscle because they cannot "relearn" how to contract the muscle and are unable to recruit the muscle to strengthen it.

Recommended therapy following nerve injury often includes electrical muscle stimulation to prevent muscle degeneration and to enhance motor function; however, the efficacy of electrical muscle stimulation to prevent muscle degeneration remains to be established [30]. Studies using animal models and implanted electrodes have shown that electrical stimulation can preserve some of the normal properties of skeletal muscle [11–13,31,32]. For maximal benefits, the stimulation parameters must be similar to the normal muscle firing pattern if electrical stimulation is used; however, no efficacy trials have verified the use of electrical stimulation using surface electrodes. Recent investigations have illustrated an increase in axonal regeneration following electrical stimulation of the nerve and the potential of electrical stimulation to facilitate muscle recovery following nerve injury [32–34]. This stimulation combined with efforts to improve the regenerative capacity of neurons and the neuromuscular end plates may facilitate muscle reinnervation and prevent irreversible muscle degeneration in the future.

Following muscle reinnervation, electrical muscle stimulation using an alternating current may theoretically be used; however, in many cases there are insufficient reinnervated muscle fibers to produce a contraction, and the stimulation will overflow to an adjacent uninjured muscle. Electrical stimulation as a passive modality to provide contraction of the muscle will not contribute to the relearning of the new motor pattern; therefore, electrical stimulation may be used in conjunction with patient effort and as a sensory and motor stimulus for relearning. One of the main goals of rehabilitation is to improve function, and it is important for the patient to participate in the action and to establish new sensorimotor patterns. Visual and auditory feedback is useful to provide immediate feedback and facilitate relearning. A biofeedback unit using surface electrodes is a useful modality to provide visual and auditory feedback (Fig. 3) and is an excellent relearning tool to provide immediate feedback to enhance muscle activity or to minimize aberrant muscle action. The surface electrodes can be placed on the reinnervated muscle to provide feedback to increase the muscle contraction, or, if an antagonistic muscle is overpowering the newly reinnervated muscle, the electrodes can be used to provide feedback to the patient to minimize the unwanted muscle action. In the author's experience, visual or auditory feedback is useful to facilitate relearning and to recruit newly reinnervated and weak muscles, and electrical muscle stimulation is unnecessary.

Biofeedback using surface electrodes with two-channel or four-channel leads can provide useful immediate feedback to decrease or increase muscle activity. With initiation of a movement, patients often have difficulty isolating the intended muscle contraction and will often co-contract muscles with an antagonistic action. With co-contraction of a stronger uninjured antagonistic muscle action, the weaker reinnervated muscle cannot be strengthened. A four-channel biofeedback unit can be used by placing surface electrodes on the reinnervated muscle and the antagonistic muscle. The patient is then asked

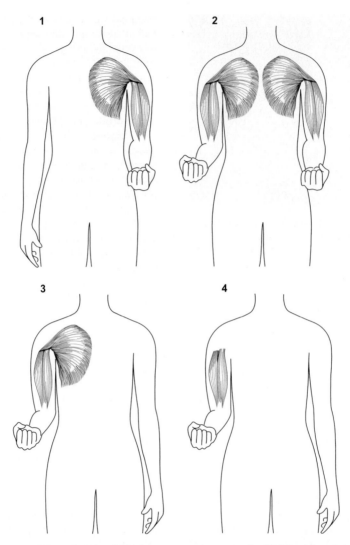

Fig. 2. To facilitate relearning, reeducation following a motor nerve transfer begins with contraction on the normal uninjured side. Following a medial pectoral to musculocutaneous nerve transfer, the patient is asked to begin on the uninjured side with a contraction of the pectoralis major muscle and then to simultaneously contract the biceps muscle (1). This action is then combined with a bilateral contraction of the pectoralis major and biceps muscles (2). The contraction is then isolated to the affected side (3). Once the patient has regained sufficient strength in the reinnervated muscles, the target action is then dissociated from the donor muscle (4).

to increase the muscle activity of the reinnervated muscle while minimizing the action of the antagonistic muscle. This type of immediate biofeedback will facilitate relearning and strengthening of the weaker reinnervated muscle. It is sometimes useful to use simultaneous contraction of the contralateral uninjured side to facilitate relearning. This action provides a "normal" contraction, and, with visual biofeedback, the patient can visualize both the normal contraction and the

reinnervated muscle. Although biofeedback is useful, particularly in the early stages of reinnervation, it is also important for the patient to practice the contraction without the biofeedback to provide the opportunity to perform the exercises more frequently. Once the patient can visualize the muscle contraction, the visual feedback of the muscle is useful for relearning and can be used by the patient to increase the contraction. Because of the muscle weakness and fatigue in the

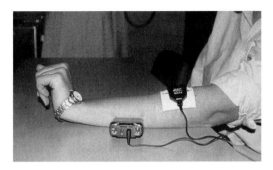

Fig. 3. A simple biofeedback unit using surface electrodes can be used to provide visual or auditory feedback and immediate feedback to enhance muscle activity or to minimize aberrant muscle action. (*Courtesy of* Christine B. Novak, PT, MS, PhD(c), Toronto, Ontario, Canada.)

newly reinnervated muscle, frequent short duration exercise sessions are used, and a slow onset contraction with a long duration hold of 10 to 15 seconds is recommended to minimize muscle fatigue and increase muscle endurance and strength.

Muscle biomechanics should also be considered when constructing exercise programs to strengthen weak reinnervated muscles. More muscle strength is required to perform a contraction at end range against gravity; therefore, the exercises should be based upon the grade of muscle strength and the muscle action. Initially, it is easier to contract the muscle in midrange and to hold the contraction than to initiate the action at the end range of motion. Place and hold exercises can be used in different degrees of range of motion or exercises in gravity-eliminated postures may be used in muscles that are less than a Medical Research Council grade 3 [35]. With good control and increasing muscle strength, strategies are implemented to dissociate the contraction of the donor muscle from the target muscle. When the patient is able to contract the muscle through a full range of motion against gravity, progressive resisted exercises can be implemented. Loading the muscle too early will not assist in strengthening the weak reinnervated muscle because, in most cases, it will result in compensatory muscle contraction by the stronger adjacent muscles, which will perpetuate the problem of muscle imbalance and not correct abnormal movement patterns.

Performance of a motor task requires adaptability, efficiency, and consistency, and improvement requires practice and repetition [36]. These strategies are used for learning any new motor task and should be implemented in the learning associated with nerve transfers. It is also important to incorporate the entire upper extremity and to not isolate the motor pattern to only injured muscles. The surrounding scapular muscles are critical to upper extremity function and, even if uninjured, will be weak from disuse.

Movement of the shoulder requires a combined motor pattern using the glenohumeral and scapular muscles and restoration of normal scapulothoracic rhythm. Although the rotator cuff muscles are important for positioning and movement of the glenohumeral joint, normal shoulder function cannot be achieved without the action of the scapular muscles, particularly the middle/lower trapezius and serratus anterior. Although the scapular muscles may not have been denervated in the original traumatic brachial plexus injury, these muscles will be weak from disuse and will contribute to the muscle imbalance. Good reinnervation of the rotator cuff muscles may be graded as a poor outcome if the scapular muscles are weak and contributing to abnormal scapular movement patterns.

As recovery progresses, patients should be encouraged to perform activities that require use of both extremities for self-care, work, and recreation. Bimanual tasks will integrate both the injured and uninjured limbs and provide the opportunity for input from the contralateral cortical region and to input normal movement patterns. Functional outcome and vocational rehabilitation specialists should be consulted early in the rehabilitation process to assist the patient in future vocational planning, particularly for young patients. An outcome study by Choi and colleagues [37] illustrated that many patients who returned to work following brachial plexus lesions did so within 1 year following injury and emphasizes the need for early integration of long-term goals for patients with nerve injuries.

Summary

To maximize function following nerve transfers, the rehabilitation program must include motor reeducation to initiate recruitment of the weak reinnervated muscles and to establish new motor patterns and cortical mapping. Patient education and a home program are essential to obtain the optimal functional result.

References

[1] Mackinnon SE, Novak CB. Nerve transfers. Hand Clin 1999;15:643–66.

[2] Mackinnon SE, Novak CB, Myckatyn TM, et al. Results of reinnervation of the biceps and brachialis muscles with a double fascicular transfer. J Hand Surg 2005;30A:978–85.

[3] Novak CB, Mackinnon SE. A distal anterior interosseous nerve transfer to the deep motor branch of the ulnar nerve for reconstruction of high ulnar nerve injuries. J Reconstr Microsurg 2002;18: 459–63.

[4] Novak CB, Mackinnon SE. Patient outcome after surgical management of an accessory nerve injury. Otolaryngol Head Neck Surg 2002;127:221–4.

[5] Novak CB, Tung TH, Mackinnon SE. Patient outcome following a thoracodorsal to musculocutaneous nerve transfer for reconstruction of elbow flexion. Br J Plast Surg 2003;55:416–9.

[6] Novak CB, Mackinnon SE. Surgical treatment of a long thoracic nerve injury. Ann Thorac Surg 2002;73:1643–5.

[7] Novak CB, Mackinnon SE. Treatment of a proximal accessory nerve injury with a nerve transfer. Laryngoscope 2004;114:1482–4.

[8] Oberlin C, Beal D, Leechavengvongs S, et al. Nerve transfer to biceps muscle using a part of ulnar nerve for C5–C6 avulsion of the brachial plexus: anatomical study and report of four cases. J Hand Surg 1994; 19A:232–7.

[9] Oberlin C, Teboul F, Severin S, et al. Transfer of the lateral cutaneous nerve of the forearm to the dorsal branch of the ulnar nerve, for providing sensation on the ulnar aspect of the hand. Plast Reconstr Surg 2003;112:1498–500.

[10] Tung TH, Novak CB, Mackinnon SE. Nerve transfers to the biceps and brachialis branches to improve elbow flexion strength after brachial plexus injuries. J Neurosurg 2003;98:313–8.

[11] Fu SY, Gordon T. Contributing factors to poor functional recovery after delayed nerve repair: prolonged denervation. J Neurosci 1995;15:3886–95.

[12] Williams HB. A clinical pilot study to assess functional return following continuous muscle stimulation after nerve injury and repair in the upper extremity using a completely implantable electrical system. Microsurgery 1996;17:597–605.

[13] Williams HB. The value of continuous electrical muscle stimulation using a completely implantable system in the preservation of muscle function following motor nerve injury and repair: an experimental study. Microsurgery 1996;17:589–96.

[14] Anastakis DJ, Chen R, Davis KD, et al. Cortical plasticity following upper extremity injury and reconstruction. Clin Plast Surg 2005;32:617–34.

[15] Bach-Y-Rita P. Brain plasticity as a basis for recovery of function in humans. Neuropsychologia 1990; 28:547–54.

[16] Jenkins WM, Merzenich MM, Ochs MT, et al. Functional reorganization of primary somatosensory cortex in adult owl monkeys after behaviorally controlled tactile stimulation. J Neurophysiol 1990; 63:82–104.

[17] Mano Y, Chuma T, Watanabe I. Cortical reorganization in training. J Electromyogr Kinesiol 2003;13: 57–62.

[18] Merzenich MM, Jenkins WM. Reorganization of cortical representations of the hand following alterations of skin inputs induced by nerve injury, skin island transfers and experience. J Hand Ther 1993; 6:89–104.

[19] Nudo RJ, Milliken GW, Jenkins WM, et al. Use-dependent alterations of movement representations in primary motor cortex of adult squirrel monkeys. J Neurosci 1996;16:785–807.

[20] Pascual-Leone A, Cammarota A, Wassermann EM, et al. Modulation of motor cortical outputs to the reading hand of braille readers. Ann Neurol 1993; 34:33–77.

[21] Pascual-Leone A, Torres F. Plasticity of the sensorimotor cortex representation of the reading finger in Braille readers. Brain 1993;116(Pt 1):39–52.

[22] Pons TP, Garraghty PE, Ommaya AK, et al. Massive cortical reorganization after sensory deafferentation in adult macaques. Science 1991;252: 1857–60.

[23] Remple MS, Bruneau RM, VandenBerg PM, et al. Sensitivity of cortical movement representations to motor experience: evidence that skill learning but not strength training induces cortical reorganization. Behav Brain Res 2001;123:133–41.

[24] Wall JT, Kaas JH. Long-term cortical consequences of reinnervation errors after nerve regeneration in monkeys. Brain Res 1986;372:400–4.

[25] Malessy MJ, Thomeer RT, van Dijk JG. Changing central nervous system control following intercostal nerve transfer. J Neurosurg 1998;89:568–74.

[26] Malessy MJ, van der Kamp W, Thomeer RT, et al. Cortical excitability of the biceps muscle after intercostal-to-musculocutaneous nerve transfer. Neurosurgery 1998;42:787–94.

[27] Malessy MJ, Bakker D, Dekker AJ, et al. Functional magnetic resonance imaging and control over the biceps muscle after intercostal-musculocutaneous nerve transfer. J Neurosurg 2003;98:261–8.

[28] Chen R, Anastakis DJ, Haywood CT, et al. Plasticity of the human motor system following muscle reconstruction: a magnetic stimulation and functional magnetic resonance imaging study. Clin Neurophysiol 2003;114:2434–46.

[29] Chalidapong P, Sananpanick K, Klaphajone J. Electromyographic comparison of various exercises to improve elbow flexion following intercostal nerve transfer. J Bone Joint Surg 2006;88B:620–2.

[30] Eberstein A, Eberstein S. Electrical stimulation of denervated muscle: is it worthwhile? Med Sci Sports Exerc 1996;28:1463–9.

[31] Fu SY, Gordon T. Contributing factors to poor functional recovery after delayed nerve repair: prolonged axotomy. J Neurosci 1995;15:3876–85.

[32] Gordon T, Brushart TM, Amirjani N, et al. The potential of electrical stimulation to promote functional recovery after peripheral nerve injury-comparisons between rats and humans. Acta Neurochir Suppl 2007;100:3–11.

[33] Furey MJ, Midha R, Xu Q-G, et al. Prolonged target deprivation reduces the capacity of injured motoneurons to regenerate. Neurosurgery 2007;60: 723–33.

[34] Geremia NM, Gordon T, Brushart TM, et al. Electrical stimulation promotes sensory neuron regeneration and growth-associated gene expression. Exp Neurol 2007;205:347–59.

[35] Medical Research Council of the U.K. Aids to the examination of the peripheral nervous system. Palo Alto (CA): Pentagon House; 1976.

[36] Duff SV. Impact of peripheral nerve injury on sensorimotor control. J Hand Ther 2005;18:277–91.

[37] Choi PD, Novak CB, Mackinnon SE, et al. Quality of life and functional outcome following brachial plexus injury. J Hand Surg 1997;22A:605–12.

ELSEVIER
SAUNDERS

Hand Clin 24 (2008) 425–444

HAND
CLINICS

Cortical Plasticity Following Nerve Transfer in the Upper Extremity

Dimitri J. Anastakis, MD, MHPE, MHCM, FRCSC, FACS[a],*,
Martijn J.A. Malessy, MD[b], Robert Chen, MBBChir, MSc, FRCPC[c],
Karen D. Davis, PhD[d,e], David Mikulis, MD[f]

[a]Division of Plastic Surgery, University of Toronto, 399 Bathurst Street,
East Wing −2, Toronto, Ontario Canada M5G 2S8
[b]Department of Neurosurgery, Leiden University Medical Centre,
J-11-R-84, Albinusdreef 2, 2300 RC, Leiden, The Netherlands
[c]Division of Neurology, University of Toronto, 399 Bathurst Street,
MP 13-304, Toronto, Ontario, Canada M5G 2S8
[d]Division of Neurosurgery, Institute of Medical Science, University of Toronto,
399 Bathurst Street, MP14-306, Toronto, Ontario, Canada M5T 2S8
[e]Division of Brain, Imaging and Behaviour – Systems
Neuroscience, Toronto Western Research Institute,
University Health Network, 399 Bathurst Street,
MP14-306, Toronto, Ontario, Canada M5T 2S8
[f]Department of Medical Imaging, University of Toronto, 399 Bathurst Street,
MC 3-431, Toronto, Ontario, Canada M5G 2S8

Since first reported by Tuttle in 1913 [1], nerve transfers have become mainstream in the reconstruction of brachial plexus and complex peripheral nerve injuries. Nerve transfers require that the function of an expendable donor nerve be sacrificed to restore function in the recipient nerve and muscle. Nerve transfers represent a major advance in peripheral nerve surgery, with many innovative transfers associated with improved functional results.

The concept that the central nervous system (CNS) needs to adapt or relearn following nerve transfer is not new. The homunculus reminds us that a large region of the sensorimotor cortex (SMC) is dedicated to the hand and upper extremity (Fig. 1). As such, one would expect that peripheral nerve injuries would have a profound effect on the brain. In 1984, Narakas [2]

speculated that there must be a central mechanism related to successful outcomes following transfer of the intercostal nerves (ICN) to the musculocutaneous nerve (MCN) for elbow flexion. With increasing clinical experience, peripheral nerve surgeons have come to appreciate the important role that cortical plasticity and motor relearning play in functional recovery following a nerve transfer. Even with the current state of knowledge, researchers still do not fully understand all that happens to the human SMC following peripheral nerve injury, repair, regeneration, and rehabilitation.

This article provides an overview of the methods used to study cortical plasticity and the current knowledge of cortical plasticity as it relates to upper extremity peripheral nerve lesions, repair, and rehabilitation. The article describes cortical changes seen following ICN–MCN and crossed C7 nerve transfers, and highlights key concepts of cortical plasticity and motor relearning of importance to the peripheral nerve surgeon.

* Corresponding author.

E-mail address: dimitri.anastakis@uhn.on.ca
(D.J. Anastakis).

0749-0712/08/$ - see front matter © 2008 Elsevier Inc. All rights reserved.
doi:10.1016/j.hcl.2008.04.005

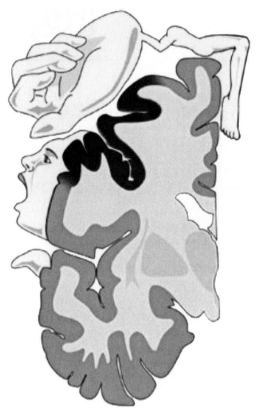

Fig. 1. The homunculus. A large region of the SMC is dedicated to the hand and upper extremity. (*From* Anastakis DJ, Chen R, Davis KD, et al. Cortical plasticity following upper extremity injury and reconstruction. Clin Plast Surg 2005;32:618; with permission.)

conditions may be motor or sensory in nature and adaptation can occur throughout the neuraxis. Cortical plasticity is an intrinsic property of the CNS retained throughout life. For peripheral nerve surgeons, it is impossible to understand normal neuromuscular function or the consequences of peripheral nerve injury and reconstruction without giving thought to the concepts of cortical plasticity and motor relearning.

Human cortical plasticity has been studied using noninvasive techniques, such as transcranial magnetic stimulation (TMS) [3,4], electroencephalography, magnetoencephalography (MEG), functional MRI (fMRI), structural MRI (sMRI), and positron emission tomography (PET) [5–9]. Anastakis and colleagues [10] have summarized the experimental techniques used for studying cortical plasticity. A comparison of PET, MEG, fMRI, and TMS is provided in Table 1. From Table 1 we see that TMS measures different inhibitory and excitatory circuits in the motor cortex not measured by other techniques. Also, we can appreciate that fMRI provides good spatial resolution both in terms of location and extent of activation. However, fMRI provides poor temporal resolution. MEG provides almost real-time temporal resolution and, although it is accurate at localizing centers of activation, the spatial extent of activation can be difficult to assess. Therefore, TMS, fMRI, and MEG measure different aspects of cortical physiology and, when used together, are powerful tools in the study of cortical plasticity.

Experimental techniques for studying cortical plasticity

The word "plastic" is derived from the Greek word *plastikos*, which means to mold or form. In general terms, cortical plasticity is the brain's capability to adapt to varying conditions. These

Structural MRI

Recent technological advances in sMRI now provide an opportunity to study white matter connectivity, gray matter volume (density), and cortical thickness [11–14]. These advances have

Table 1
Comparison among PET, MEG, functional MRI, and TMS

	PET	MEG	fMRI	TMS
Spatial resolution	Fair to good	Excellent	Good to excellent	Poor
Temporal resolution	Poor (min)	Excellent (ms)	Good (s to min)	Excellent (ms)
Measurement	Blood flow	Magnetic field	Deoxyhemoglobin	Neuronal excitability, inhibitory and excitatory circuits
Invasiveness	Intravenous radioactive tracer	None	None	None

Adapted from Anastakis DJ, Chen R, Davis KD, et al. Cortical plasticity following upper extremity injury and reconstruction. Clin Plast Surg 2005;32:619; with permission.

opened the door to the examination of cortical plasticity from an anatomic framework.

White matter can be visualized with diffusion tensor imaging (DTI), a technique that relies on visualization of the diffusion of water molecules in the brain [15]. The dominant direction of water diffusion in the brain tends to be along the long axis of axons in white matter. When water diffusion has a preferred direction, such as along the axons in white matter, DTI can detect and quantitate this diffusion preference in white matter and fiber tract maps can be generated [12,13,16–18]. Fiber tracking with DTI can be used to identify the connections to and from a chosen region of interest in the brain or "seed" area [19,20]. Fiber tracking with DTI cannot, however, distinguish afferent fibers from efferent fibers. Several quantitative parameters of water diffusion in the tissue can be derived, including mean diffusivity and fractional anisotropy. Fractional anisotropy, a measure of the directionality of diffusion, has been used to assess the extent and degree of myelination in white matter [21,22]. DTI tractography and fractional anisotropy measurements have been used to delineate anatomic connections between cortical areas and also to delineate connections between the cortex and subcortical regions (including the brainstem and thalamus) [16,18,23–28] in healthy subjects. Numerous scientific and clinical applications have been reported [11,12,29–31]. Specifically, DTI has been used to examine the integrity of tracts potentially damaged by stroke [32,33], brain injury [34,35], tumors [36,37], and blindness [38], as well as to assess cortical motor recovery following brain injury [35], anatomic changes associated with cognitive decline [39], and recovery from a minimally conscious state [40].

Several approaches have been developed to assess brain volume and morphology. One of the most widely used is voxel-based morphometry (VBM) [41]. VBM tests for statistically significant differences in regional gray matter density between subject groups. The analysis [42] includes spatial normalization of images to a standard space, extraction of the gray matter (segmentation of gray matter, white matter, and cerebrospinal fluid), spatial smoothing, and statistical analysis for identifying group differences. It can also include covariate assessment to determine the effect of specific attributes (eg, age, disease severity) on brain volumes. VBM has identified gray matter differences attributed to psychiatric and neurologic conditions [43–53]; injury states [54,55];

chronic pain [56–61]; personality traits, such as neuroticism and extraversion [62]; gender and aging [63,64]; handedness [65]; and training [66]. Registration, spatial normalization, and statistical issues [67–69] have led to improved VBM, including modulation to compensate for spatial normalization. Complementary to VBM is cortical thickness analysis (CTA), which provides a direct quantitative measure of morphology (cortical thickness in millimeters). Methodological and reliability studies of CTA have been reported extensively [70–77]. CTA has been used to assess cortical thickness in healthy subjects [66,69,71,75,77,78], and in patients with a variety of disorders, including chronic pain [58], schizophrenia [79], and Huntington's disease [80].

Functional MRI

fMRI is a noninvasive neuroimaging technique that provides an indirect measure of neuronal activity based on the relative proportion of oxyhemoglobin to deoxyhemoglobin in the blood and is therefore blood oxygen level–dependent [81,82]. A decrease in deoxyhemoglobin concentration results in increasing signal intensity on fMRI images (Fig. 2). When the cerebral cortex becomes active, oxygen extraction increases by 16%, but blood flow increases by 45% [83]. This

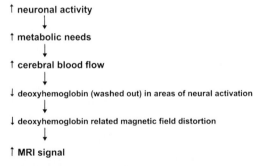

↑ neuronal activity
↓
↑ metabolic needs
↓
↑ cerebral blood flow
↓
↓ deoxyhemoglobin (washed out) in areas of neural activation
↓
↓ deoxyhemoglobin related magnetic field distortion
↓
↑ MRI signal

Fig. 2. Cortical activation and fMRI image. When performing a motor task, cortical activity increases, resulting in increases in metabolic need. The increase in metabolic need results in increased cerebral blood flow, which delivers more oxygen than the tissue can consume even in its activated state. Oxyhemoglobin therefore replaces deoxyhemoglobin in the microcirculation. Hence, the signal-distorting effect of deoxyhemoglobin is diminished and the MRI signal increases. (*From* Anastakis DJ, Chen R, Davis KD, et al. Cortical plasticity following upper extremity injury and reconstruction. Clin Plast Surg 2005;32:619; with permission.)

results in an increase in oxygen concentration, raising the MR signal intensity by 2% to 5% at a field strength of 1.5 T [84]. fMRI can produce activation maps with high spatial resolution by acquiring numerous images in resting and active states and statistically comparing the two states [85–89].

fMRI techniques track signal change over time by acquiring a series of images as subjects are presented with test stimuli or perform experimental tasks during blood oxygen level–dependent image acquisition. In a typical study, the subject alternates between rest and stimulus or task conditions. Because the magnitude of MRI signal changes related to brain activation is small compared with the amount of noise in each image, acquisition of thousands of images in multislice studies of the brain are necessary with multiple iterations of the resting and task cycles before statistically significant regions of brain can be identified. Comparisons of images generated during the rest and active states produce activation

maps with high resolution. fMRI is a proven and effective tool for assessing cortical plasticity.

Transcranial magnetic stimulation

TMS makes use of a brief, high-current electrical pulse through a coil of wire to induce magnetic field lines perpendicular to the coil. An electric field is induced perpendicular to this magnetic field. When applied over the scalp, TMS currents are capable of activating underlying neural structures (Fig. 3). Focal figure-eight magnetic coils can be used to map muscle representations in M1 [90,91]. The optimal position and orientation of the currents necessary to activate corticospinal neurons associated with a specific muscle group can be ascertained.

Another important measure determined through a TMS mapping procedure is the center-of-gravity, an amplitude-weighted position on the motor map. Using surface matching methods, TMS maps have been shown to correlate with

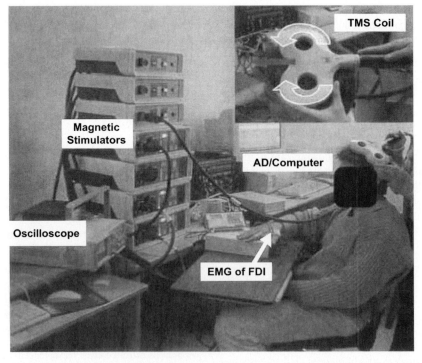

Fig. 3. TMS. The TMS coil is placed over the motor cortex. The magnetic field generated stimulates that hand representation of the motor cortex. Motor-evoked potential in the contralateral first dorsal interosseous muscle (FDI) is recorded with surface electromyographic (EMG) electrodes. In the upper-right insert, the curved arrows represent the direction of the electrical current in the coil and the straight arrow represents the direction of the induced current in the brain. Analogue to digital converter/computer. (*From* Anastakis DJ, Chen R, Davis KD, et al. Cortical plasticity following upper extremity injury and reconstruction. Clin Plast Surg 2005;32:620; with permission.)

areas of cortical activation in PET and fMRI scans taken during hand movements [92,93]. A number of factors contribute to the mapping of the primary motor cortex. Such factors include the precise location of the muscle representations, the excitability of the given representations, and the mapping protocol (eg, coil type and positioning, inducing current). Center-of-gravity measurements, for example, are sensitive to the direction in which motor representations expand [94].

Other measures important in the study of cortical plasticity include motor thresholds, short interval intracortical inhibition, and intracortical facilitation. Anastakis and colleagues [10] defined each of these and described their physiologic importance. This information is summarized in Table 2.

Cortical plasticity following amputation

Much of what we know about the CNS response to peripheral nerve injury comes from MEG, fMRI, and TMS studies done following amputation and nerve injury in human and animal models. Amputations and nerve injuries can result in altered sensorimotor representations. MEG studies have shown that, following hand amputation, sensory representation expands from facial regions into the zone formally represented by the hand [95–97]. Borsook and colleagues [98] used fMRI to study a subject 24 hours after an

arm amputation and 1 month postinjury. They observed that reorganization of sensory pathways developed very soon after amputation in humans and suggested that unmasking of ordinarily silent inputs, rather than sprouting of new axon terminals, was responsible for these changes.

Cortical plasticity following amputation has also been demonstrated using TMS. Identical TMS pulses produced greater motor-evoked potential (MEP) and recruited a larger percentage of the motor neuron pool for resting muscles proximal to the stump than for the same muscles in the intact limb. Furthermore, the cortical motor maps of muscles proximal to the stump were larger than maps corresponding to the same muscles on the intact side [99]. This pattern roughly parallels the results obtained from ischemic nerve block experiments, suggesting that short-term and long-term plastic changes make use of the same fundamental mechanisms. Chen and colleagues [100] have shown that the plasticity is likely due to a decrease in γ-aminobutyric acid–mediated (GABA-mediated) inhibition and increased membrane excitability, as both short interval intracortical inhibition and motor thresholds are decreased on the affected side. In line with the TMS findings, an fMRI study of M1 organization after upper limb amputation early in life [101] found an unusual, broad activation in M1 contralateral to stump movement and speculated that the large activation is not only the result of disinhibition,

Table 2
TMS parameters and definitions

Parameter	Abbreviation	Description
Center-of-gravity	COG	• Amplitude-weighted position on the motor map
Motor thresholds	MT	• Minimum TMS intensity necessary to induce a small motor-evoked potential from a specific muscle • A measure of the inherent excitability of neuronal membranes
Short interval intracortical inhibition	SICI	• Determined by observing the effect of subthreshold conditioning TMS pulses on the amplitude of a test motor-evoked potential induced by suprathreshold TMS pulses • Reduced in representations of muscles engaged in the task, but is elevated in relaxed neighboring muscles [140] • Reflects excitatory and inhibitory networks in the motor cortex [141] • SICI may reflect changes specifically in γ-aminobutyric acid–ergic inhibitory neurons [142] • Voluntary muscle contraction associated with decreased SICI
Intracortical facilitation	ICF	• Determined by observing the effect of subthreshold conditioning TMS pulses on the amplitude of a test motor-evoked potential induced by suprathreshold TMS pulses

Data from Anastakis DJ, Chen R, Davis KD, et al. Cortical plasticity following upper extremity injury and reconstruction. Clin Plast Surg 2005;32:618.

but also the consequence of plastic physiologic differentiation and maturation.

Cortical plasticity following peripheral nerve lesion

Peripheral nerve lesions have immediate and long-lasting consequences on cortical representations [102]. In the rat, expansion of the motor cortex representation of the forelimb occurred within hours of transection of a facial motor nerve and the changes continued to evolve for several weeks [103,104]. In the primate, transection of the median nerve initially results in a silent "black hole" in the somatosensory cortex corresponding to the representations of the thumb and of the index, middle, and ring fingers. Neurons in this silent "black hole" (ie, zone of unresponsive cortex) may become responsive to body regions adjacent to the differentiated hand. Initially, input into this zone of unresponsive cortex is crude and overlapping. However, within 2 to 3 weeks, the topography of representation of the new inputs in this zone is refined and shows sharp borders between the expanding territories and adjacent cortical areas [105,106]. The primate model illustrates topographic reorganization of the somatosensory cortex following a peripheral nerve lesion. Thus, deafferentation following a median nerve lesion results in the rapid invasion of the former median nerve cortical territory by the adjacent cortical areas. After this, the subsequent changes depend on the nature of the nerve lesion and its management.

If the median nerve is not permitted to regenerate (ie, no surgical repair) the extensive reorganization of the cortical map, as described above, persists so that the cortical area, previously receiving input from the median nerve, remains completely occupied by expanding adjacent cortical areas. However, if there is a crush injury, followed by regeneration, the ensuing process is considerably different because regenerating axons can follow their original Schwann cells and reach their original cutaneous locations. The resulting cortical representation of the median nerve innervating cutaneous areas after regeneration is not substantially different from the normal representation.

If the median nerve is transected and then repaired, different cortical changes are seen. Because of random axonal growth following peripheral nerve repair, most of the original cutaneous areas are not reinnervated by their original axons. This results in significant

reorganization changes in the cortex, specifically restricted to those regions where input from the median nerve is normally represented. Over a long period of observation in the primate model, the cortical representation of cutaneous areas appeared to change continuously. Thus, nerve transection results in both immediate and progressively developing changes in the cortical maps of a cutaneous surface.

Mechanisms of cortical plasticity

The mechanisms of cortical plasticity, according to current and widely accepted opinion, involve the unmasking of previously ineffective connections and sprouting of intact afferents from adjacent cortical or subcortical territories. Unmasking can produce changes that occur immediately following deafferentation and are likely caused by reduction of GABA-ergic inhibition to preexisting projections from adjacent cortical regions, or unmasking at subcortical levels leading to activation of thalamocortical projections not previously activated by the deafferented nerves [107]. Immunostaining of the primary somatosensory cortex following peripheral nerve transection reveals a reduction in cellular GABA, supporting the hypothesis that decreased intracortical inhibition leads to unmasking of hidden adjacent inputs [108]. Axonal sprouting at the level of the dorsal horn, dorsal column nuclei, thalamus, or cortex may cause long-term changes, occurring over weeks and months [109–111]. Thus, the mechanisms of cortical plasticity may involve the unmasking of previously hidden or dormant connections, or the axonal sprouting of intact afferents from adjacent cortical or subcortical territories, or both.

Cortical plasticity following intercostal nerve transfers

In severe brachial plexus lesions, ICN–MCN transfers can be used to restore useful biceps function [112]. The ICNs used for nerve transfer innervate five different thoracic respiratory muscles. Some of these respiratory muscles may be active during inspiration and others during expiration. Each muscle plays a role in complex thoracic movements [113,114]. Normally, corticospinal neurons, which ultimately project to the intercostal muscles by way of the intercostal motor neurons, are active during the implementation of central motor programs for respiration or posture control. Following an ICN–MCN transfer, central ICN motor programs for respiration and posture control are both linked to and responsible for biceps control (Fig. 4) [115].

The level of biceps control has been shown to change with time. Electromyography studies have shown that during initial biceps reinnervation, respiratory activity may be present without clinical contraction of the biceps. As reinnervation progresses, patients find they are able to initiate involuntary elbow flexion with respiration. The onset of voluntary control commonly requires a respiratory effort. That is, patients learn a "trick" of flexing their elbow by consciously inhaling deeply. Toward the final stages of reinnervation, voluntary contraction of the biceps can be initiated and sustained independent of respiratory activity (Fig. 5). Most patients achieve volitional biceps control similar to that of the normal limb without the use of any learned tricks. However, a complete loss of respiratory influence does not occur once voluntary control is established. Electromyographic studies have confirmed ongoing respiratory activity during voluntary elbow flexion. In addition, studies using polygraphy have shown that patients can simultaneously keep their elbows flexed and continue breathing. This phenomenon suggests that patients have learned a new way to control elbow flexion. Researchers speculate that, because there is a change in the control of the reinnervated biceps over time, some form of CNS "rewiring" must take place as an adaptation to the altered peripheral nerve connections [115].

The cortical plasticity seen following ICN–MCN transfer suggests that the cortical neurons controlling the biceps must fulfill two important requirements. First, they must respond to a central flexion motor program. The central motor program probably originates in the thalamus, sensory cortex, and sensory association areas [116]. Second, they must link directly or indirectly with ICN α-motor neurons. It has been hypothesized that the necessary reorganization of connectivity may take place in either the cortex or in the spinal cord (Figs. 6 and 7).

In the spinal hypothesis, new cervicothoracic connections are formed between the original MCN α-motor neurons and the original ICN α-motor neurons. Fig. 6 illustrates this reorganization. Theoretically, the corticospinal tract fibers involved in an ICN–MCN transfer are either those projecting to the original MCN α-motor neurons or those projecting to the original ICN

α-motor neurons. The biceps corticospinal tract fibers normally project to α-motor neurons at the C-5 and C-6 levels. The intercostal corticospinal tract fibers normally project to thoracic levels. If the corticospinal tract, which originally participated in normal biceps control, remains involved after the transfer, both groups of α-motor neurons need to be connected for functional control of the reinnervated biceps. Using retrograde nerve tracing, research in primates following ICN–MCN transfer has shown that this type of connectivity or spinal plasticity does not occur [117]. The results of two human studies, in which transcervical and transthoracic magnetic stimulation was used following ICN–MCN transfer, confirmed that spinal plasticity does not occur [118,119]. From both primate and human studies, one can conclude that it is unlikely that new spinal cord neural connections are formed. Therefore, one can speculate that plastic changes must occur in the cerebral cortex enabling the restoration of volitional biceps control.

The cortical areas most likely involved in volitional biceps control include the "biceps area" and the "intercostal area" originally linked to thoracic movements. Both TMS and fMRI have been used to study cortical changes following ICN–MCN transfer. Furthermore, researchers have defined the relationship between the fMRI signal and the underlying neural activity.

Analysis has shown that the fMRI signal actually reflects neural activity related to input and local intracortical processing, rather than output from the area [120]. In those patients with functional biceps reinnervation, activity is induced and localized within the primary motor area (M1). Neither the number of active pixels nor the mean value of their activations differed between reinnervated biceps and control limbs. In addition, the neuronal input activity involved in biceps flexion after successful ICN–MCN reinnervation did not differ in location or intensity between surgically treated and control limbs. The normal cortical "biceps area" appeared to regulate biceps contraction, even though cerebral activity could not reach the biceps by following the normal nervous system pathway. The cortical neurons involved in biceps flexion following successful reinnervation following ICN–MCN transfer are the same as those that are active in normal biceps flexion. From these results one can postulate that, for the initiation of biceps contraction, the denervation after trauma and subsequent ICN–MCN transfer does not lead to

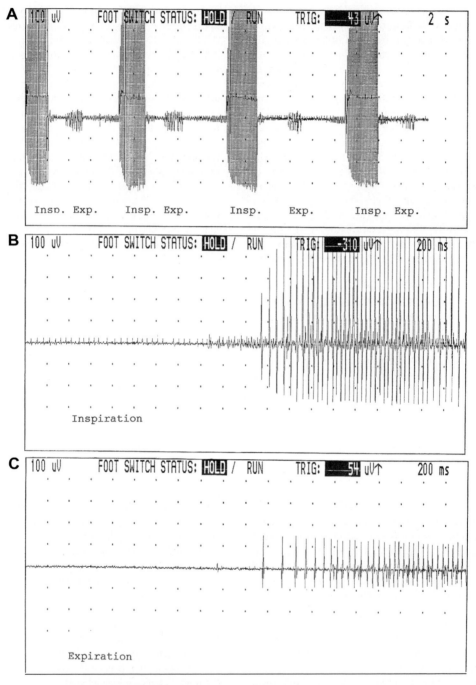

Fig. 4. Needle electromyogram of the biceps following ICN–MCN transfer. (*A*) Activity recorded during deep breath-ing. Higher voltage bursts were seen during inspiration. Lower voltage bursts occurred during expiration. Note time base of 2 seconds per division. Close-up of inspiratory activity (*B*) and expiratory activity (*C*). Each consists of repeated firings of a single motor unit, and different motor units are active in inspiration and expiration. (*From* Malessy MJA, van Dijk JG, Thomeer RTWM. Respiration related activity in the biceps brachii muscle after intercostal–musculocuta-neous nerve transfer. Clin Neurol Neurosurg 1993;95(Suppl):S98; with permission.)

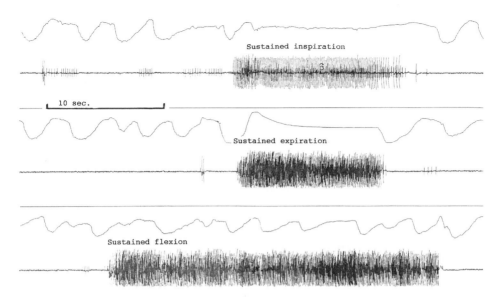

Fig. 5. Polygraphy showing flexion and respiration effects. The figure is restricted to a single strain gauge (expiration is shown upwards) and the biceps electromyographic lead. The top two traces show the amount of activity in the biceps during sustained inspiration. Note the cessation of breathing. The two traces in the middle show a much denser electromyographic pattern in the biceps during sustained expiration. The bottom two traces show a similar electromyographic pattern during attempted flexion of the elbow. Note that the patient can sustain flexion while breathing continues. (*From* Malessy MJA, van Dijk JG, Thomeer RTWM. Respiration related activity in the biceps brachii muscle after intercostal–musculocutaneous nerve transfer. Clin Neurol Neurosurg 1993;95(Suppl):S101; with permission.)

changes in the original neural input activity and local intracortical processing.

An earlier study by Giraux and colleagues [121] supports this hypothesis. After hand transplantation, the original map for hand activation is restored. That is, the original neural network is reactivated. Following hand transplantation, the new peripheral input allowed a global remodeling of the upper extremity's cortical map and reversed the functional reorganization induced by the amputation.

TMS has been used to map the cortex of normal controls and patients having undergone ICN–MCN transfer. TMS studies in normal controls revealed that the cortical map of the intercostal cortical area is localized in the midline, whereas the cortical map of the biceps is located a few centimeters lateral from the midsagittal plane. At the end stage of reinnervation, the cortical areas of the affected upper extremities were smaller and less excitable than in controls. The locations of these areas could not be distinguished from those of the normal cortical biceps area but seemed to differ from those of the intercostal cortical area. The different locations

of maps of the reinnervated biceps and the intercostal cortical area point to cerebral plasticity. That is, a shift in motor control.

Researchers have examined the question of whether the CNS pathways controlling ICN activity after transfer resemble the original connections of the biceps or those of the physiologically controlling intercostal muscles [122,123]. The facilitatory effects of respiration and elbow flexion were used. The amplitudes of MEPs increase and their latencies decrease by slight voluntary contraction of the target muscle, a phenomenon known as "facilitation" (Fig. 8) [122,123]. A facilitatory effect of respiration on MEPs of the reinnervated biceps would point to a close resemblance to the original CNS connections to the donor ICN. Conversely, facilitatory effects of voluntary contraction (flexion or adduction) would point to CNS connections with recipient nerve. At the end stage of recovery, voluntary contraction had a larger facilitatory effect on MEPs of the ICN reinnervated muscles than on respiration. This indicates that CNS connections to the donor ICN have changed from those controlling respiration to those controlling

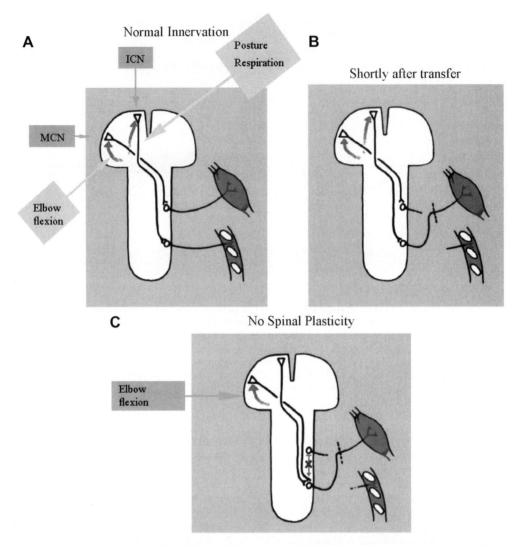

Fig. 6. Schematic representation of ICN–MCN transfer. (*A*) Normal innervation. The central motor program for elbow flexion is connected to the MCN and the central motor program for respiration and/or posture control is connected to the ICN. (*B*) Shortly after transfer, central ICN motor programs become connected to the biceps. Initially, biceps contraction can only be effected by means of a voluntary respiratory effort. Central adaptation is required to regain volitional control. Red arrows represent central input to the pyramidal tract. (*C*) No spinal plasticity. Neural activity in the original biceps area cannot excite ICN α-motor neurons because novel spinal pathways have not been formed. Red arrow shows. Gray arrows show. The "x" through the arrow indicates that such input or connections are not present. (*From* Malessy MJA, Bakker, D, Dekker AJ, et al. Functional magnetic resonance imaging and control over the biceps muscle after intercostal–musculocutaneous nerve transfer. J Neurosurg 2003;98:266; with permission.)

volitional contraction. In addition, from the difference in the effect of facilitation (that of contraction being larger than that of respiration) it follows that the quality of the CNS pathway to ICN motor neurons has changed, tending toward the MCN recipient rather than to the ICN donor.

Cortical plasticity following ICN–MCN transfer

Combining the findings of fMRI and TMS studies [124–126], we are able to hypothesize on the cortical plasticity that occurs following ICN–MCN transfer (see Fig. 7). Neural input for volitional biceps control is reactivated

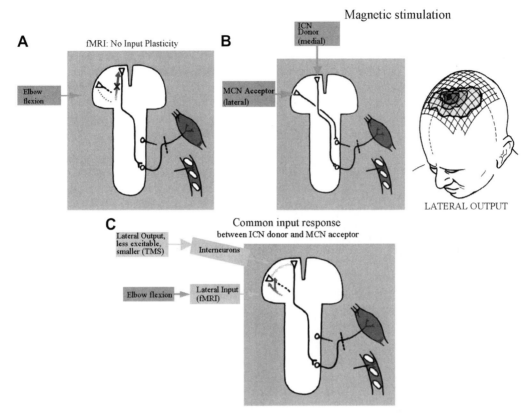

Fig. 7. Schematic of proposed of cortical plasticity following ICN–MCN transfer (based on fMRI and TMS studies). (*A*) Neural input activity for volitional biceps control does not show plastic changes following ICN–MCN transfer according to findings. Red arrows represent central input to the pyramidal tract. The "x" through the arrow indicates that such input or connections are not present. (*B*) The center-of-gravity of the ICN–MCN biceps TMS map is indistinguishable from that of the normal biceps location and is different from that of the medial location of the intercostal muscles. These findings show that plastic changes occur in the neural output activity. (*C*) An interneuronal network between the ICN donor and the MCN acceptor creates an accessible output pathway by mediating the response to a common input. Arrows show. (*From* Malessy MJA, Bakker, D, Dekker AJ, et al. Functional magnetic resonance imaging and control over the biceps muscle after intercostal–musculocutaneous nerve transfer. J Neurosurg 2003;98:267; with permission.)

following functional biceps reinnervation after ICN–MCN transfer. The target of the neural output activity does change from the C5–6 α-motor neuron pool to the thoracic ICN α-motor neuron pool. The CNS changes that occur may be the result of structural plasticity: namely, the formation of new connections between ICN and MCN neurons. Motor cortex mapping has confirmed a lateral shift in the area controlling ICN reinnervated biceps with time. At the end stage of recovery, it resembled the physiologic biceps area [127]. Axonal sprouting is an important element in plastic reorganization [111,128] but may not be of sufficient magnitude to be the major factor [129]. The formation of new direct connections

between flexion and intercostal corticospinal neurons requires axonal sprouting over a span of several centimeters. The change in control from respiratory commands to voluntary flexion takes months rather than years [115], which makes spontaneous axonal sprouting seem unlikely.

The principal mechanism behind cortical reorganization following ICN–MCN transfer may be functional plasticity: namely, the activity-dependent strengthening of previously silent or subthreshold synaptic connections between ICNs and MCN neurons. It has been proposed that the ICN–MCN reinnervated biceps TMS map represents a cortical network of flexion interneurons that connect to the medially located intercostal

Magnetic Stimulator

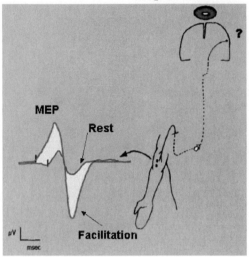

Fig. 8. TMS findings following innervation of biceps following ICN–MCN transfer. Note the facilitatory effect on MEPs during contraction as compared with rest: MEP amplitudes increase and latencies decrease. (*From* Malessy MJA, Thomeer RTWM, van Dijk JG. Changing central nervous system control following intercostal nerve transfer. J Neurosurg 1998;89:569; with permission.)

corticospinal neurons [127]. Flexion interneurons and intercostal corticospinal neurons may have preexisting connections because postural control over the thorax is an essential prerequisite for upper extremity movements. For instance, when flexing the elbow to lift an object, the intercostal muscle must contract simultaneously for thorax stabilization and postural control. Both groups of neurons may be part of a neural network contributing to different aspects of elbow flexion. ICN–MCN transfer may induce changed patterns of stimulus repetition. This may result in increased synaptic effectiveness in cortical networks, in turn strengthening the response coherence between the two groups of neurons [130,131]. The mechanisms of such synaptic changes have in part been elucidated [111]. The presence of intercortical connections between biceps and intercostal corticospinal neurons may also explain the discrepancy between the successful restoration of volitional control over biceps contraction following ICN–MCN transfer and the inability to do so after hypoglossal–MCN transfer [132]. It is unlikely that connections between the tongue and upper limb cortical areas exist, in view of their isolated

movement patterns. The preexisting interneuronal network for coordination of the contraction of upper extremity and thoracic muscles involved in elbow flexion thus creates an accessible output pathway for the control of the reinnervated biceps. The presence of a common input response between the corticospinal neurons of the ICN donor and the MCN acceptor seems crucial to obtain a functional result following ICN–MCN transfer. Moreover, a common input response between donor and acceptor needs to be present in all types of nerve transfer to become functionally effective.

Cortical plasticity following contralateral C7 nerve transfer

Restoration of elbow flexion has been described using the contralateral C7 root as a donor nerve and the MCN or lateral cord as the recipient nerve. Until recently, little was known about how conscious motor cortical control is reorganized in these patients. When the contralateral C7 root is used as a donor nerve, flexion of the reconstructed upper extremity is no longer under the control of the contralateral cortex, but rather under the control of the ipsilateral cortex. The ipsilateral cortex to the reconstructed limb controls extension of the intact limb and flexion of the reconstructed limb. In 2006, Beaulieu and colleagues [133] used fMRI to study cortical activation in seven brachial plexus patients who had undergone biceps reinnervation using a contralateral C7 transfer to the MCN or lateral cord. This study confirmed that normal cortical activation for unilateral elbow flexion occurred in the contralateral cortex in both normal and reconstructed limbs. The investigators showed that flexion of the reconstructed limb (ie, contralateral C7 nerve transfer) was associated with a bilateral cortical network of activation. That is, the contralateral cortex originally involved in control of the reconstructed limb still participated in the control of elbow flexion through the bilateral premotor and primary motor cortex networks. The investigators described the neural network involved in flexion of the reconstructed elbow to include the ipsilateral pathway in the primary motor cortex, premotor cortex, supplementary motor area, posterior parietal areas, and contralateral networks in the same areas. The cortex originally involved in control of elbow flexion in the reconstructed limb is still involved in the control of elbow flexion through the bilateral premotor and primary motor cortex networks.

This study reaffirms the importance and relevance of bilateral hemisphere control of motor movements or skills. It also speaks to the proposed mechanism of cortical plasticity wherein we see the unmasking of previously silent connections or sprouting of intact afferents from adjacent cortical or subcortical territories. Unmasking can produce changes that occur anywhere along the neuraxis. Following contralateral C7 transfer, we may see unmasking and recruitment of bicortical neural networks involved in flexion of the reconstructed limb, including the ipsilateral pathway in the primary motor cortex, premotor cortex, supplementary motor area, posterior parietal areas, and contralateral networks in the same areas.

Unfortunately, little is known about the level of independent control over the reconstructed limb. That is, how well can unrelated bimanual tasks be performed? Since the same hemisphere controls both upper extremities, independent coordination requires specific neural networks to smoothly execute bimanual activities. The level of independence has not been well documented with fMRI and TMS. Anecdotally, we have all heard of unwanted cocontractions of the reconstructed limb during tasks performed by the normal limb and that contraction of the C7 contralateral reinnervated muscle could only be effected by a conscious movement of the normal limb. When independent control of the C7 reinnervated limb does not occur, the value of this transfer is questionable. It is not known whether the level of control that can be attained is predictable and whether the quality of control depends on individual variations in preexisting left–right coordination networks. It would therefore be of interest to develop techniques that allow for the preoperative assessment of left–right coordination networks before using a contralateral C7 transfer.

Cortical plasticity and motor learning

fMRI and other techniques have demonstrated evidence of cortical plasticity during motor skill acquisition. Karni and colleagues [134] demonstrated evidence of adult motor cortex plasticity during motor skill learning in normal subjects using rapid sequences of finger movements. The investigators found a slowly evolving long-term, experience-dependent reorganization of the adult M1, which may underlie the acquisition and retention of motor skills. The influence of training is commonly characterized by adaptive brain changes featuring expansion of those sensory zones most strongly connected to the learned skill. For example, training monkeys to use a single digit more than other digits leads to expansion of the cortical representation for that finger at the expense of the other fingers [135]. Similar results have been seen in humans, including changes among highly trained musicians [136] and blind individuals that have used Braille for a long time [137]. Such work has revealed the potential for adaptive change occurring at the SMC during motor learning.

Motor relearning following nerve transfer

Today's view of the adult CNS is that of an adaptive and responsive system. Cortical plasticity occurs in the SMC in response to anything from learning to use a new thumb following a toe transfer to flexing the elbow with a free functioning muscle transfer or following an ICN–MCN transfer.

The proposed framework for motor skill learning is based on longitudinal fMRI and TMS studies done in patients following toe transfers for thumb reconstruction [138]. In this patient population, fMRI studies have shown that at the onset of learning a new motor skill (eg, thumb flexion), there is an expansion of motor cortical representation (Fig. 9). In addition, TMS studies have also shown an increase in excitability and decreased intracortical inhibition at the onset of learning the new motor skill. This phenomenon may represent a "priming" of the cortex at the onset of learning a new motor skill. fMRI studies have confirmed that, as the patient practices the motor skill, the amount of cortical representation increases. These changes in cortical representation are correlated with specific events in reconstruction, rehabilitation, and functional recovery [138]. As the skill is mastered, the degrees of cortical representation and excitability decrease and approach normal levels. The changes in cortical representation and excitability during motor skills learning, from novice to expert, are illustrated in Fig. 10.

Surgeons are familiar with less than ideal functional results following motor reconstruction. It is hypothesized that sensory input is important in the modulation of cortical plasticity during motor skill learning. In the reconstructive plans for patients with combined motor and sensory

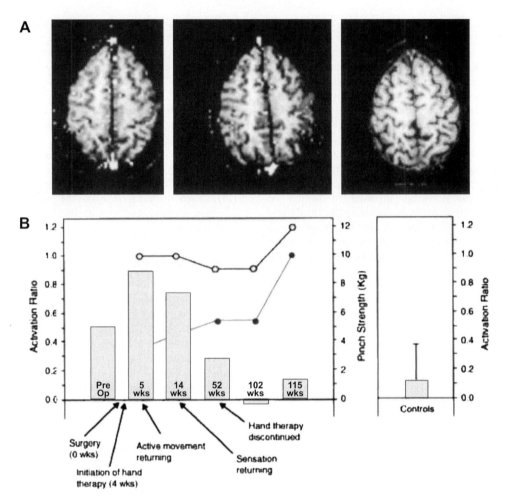

Fig. 9. Activation maps and SMC activation ratios. (*A*) Activation maps showing sequential changes in the contralateral primary somatosensory cortex during the button-press task before and after the toe-to-thumb transfer in the index case. (*Left*) Preoperative. (*Center*) Five weeks postoperative. (*Right*) One-hundred-fifteen weeks postoperative. There are well-defined clusters (*red*) of activation around the central sulcus in the cortical representation of the right upper extremity. Note the visible increase in the extent of activation in the week 5 image (*center*). (*B*) SMC activation ratio and pinch strength in the open circles. Mean SMC activation ratio with standard error bar obtained from eight controls is shown for comparison. The early phase of recovery is characterized by increased left SMC activation coinciding with the return of active movement and sensation. During the later phase of recovery, as pinch strength normalized, SMC activation returned to control levels. (*From* Manduch M, Bezuhly M, Anastakis DJ, et al. Serial fMRI assessment of the primary motor cortex following thumb reconstruction. Neurology 2002;59(8):1280; with permission.)

deficits, ensuring optimal sensory function before motor reconstruction may be more important than previously believed. One may speculate that the absence of sensory input contributes to aberrant cortical plasticity during motor learning, ultimately affecting functional outcomes. If functional gain and motor cortical reorganization are indeed dependent on inputs, such as cutaneous afferents, sensory re-education may not only be important in the recovery of protective sensation,

but may also play a role in optimizing gains in motor function following reconstruction of the upper extremity. Hence, we believe that every effort should be made to restore sensory function in advance of motor reconstruction.

Repetition and practice are fundamental to motor learning and to mastering any motor skill. Manduch and colleagues [138] suggest that repetition and practice may contribute to the decreased amount of cortical representation seen as the new

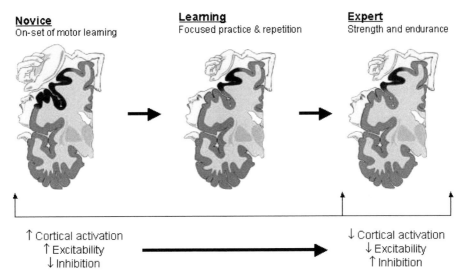

Novice
On-set of motor learning

Learning
Focused practice & repetition

Expert
Strength and endurance

↑ Cortical activation
↑ Excitability
↓ Inhibition

↓ Cortical activation
↓ Excitability
↑ Inhibition

Fig. 10. Cortical activation maps and excitability during motor skills learning. This figure illustrates the proposed changes in cortical activation, excitability, and inhibition as seen in fMRI and TMS during motor skills learning. As the subject learns and becomes an expert, decreased cortical activation, decreased cortical excitability, and increased inhibition occur. (*Adapted from* Anastakis DJ, Chen R, Davis KD, et al. Cortical plasticity following upper extremity injury and reconstruction. Clin Plast Surg 2005;32:618; with permission.)

motor skill is mastered. In addition, fMRI studies in patients following free functioning muscle transfer suggest that motor reorganization continues to evolve and may be modified by training and experience long after motor reconstruction [139]. The investigators suggest that there may be inherent value in increasing the duration of therapy well beyond 2 years after reconstruction to facilitate ongoing cortical reorganization and ultimately improve functional outcome. There may be fundamental differences in the cortical changes that occur between patients undergoing thumb reconstruction with toe transfer and patients undergoing nerve reconstruction with nerve transfers. This being said, the investigators [139] believe that there is capacity for cortical change well beyond the traditional 2-year cut off for rehabilitation, irrespective of reconstruction a patient has undergone.

The temporal pattern of activation observed following thumb reconstruction with toe transfer might in fact represent a "signature" of good functional recovery [138]. Reconstructive failures that occur despite physically and electrophysiologically intact neuromuscular connections in the periphery might be explainable by a lack of cortical sensorimotor network recruitment. That is, there may be a "central" mechanism of treatment failure. Absence of this signature may indicate

maladaptive plasticity. These observations remain speculative.

Motor relearning strategies following nerve transfers

The key motor learning strategies following nerve transfer include:

1. Preoperative training and practice of the movements required to activate the nerve transfer
2. Reinforcement of the importance of practice and repetition
3. Early activation of the motor movement with resistance or gravity removed
4. Focused practice and repetition with a therapist during early stages of motor learning
5. Strengthening and endurance exercises for up to and possibly beyond 2 years following motor reinnervation

Summary

Cortical plasticity is an intrinsic property of the CNS retained throughout life. For peripheral nerve surgeons, it is not possible to understand normal neuromuscular function or the consequences of peripheral nerve injury and reconstruction without giving thought to the concepts of cortical plasticity and motor relearning. Cortical changes, including topographic reorganization of the somatosensory cortex, occur following peripheral nerve lesions. Although significant strides have been made in our understanding of cortical plasticity following nerve transfer and during motor relearning, a great deal remains that we do not understand. Further investigations are required into the cortical plasticity that occurs following peripheral nerve injury, during both motor and sensory recovery and following primary nerve repair or nerve transfer. Greater understanding of the cortical changes that occur in these patients may alter the timing and types of rehabilitation strategies used. In the future, cortical plasticity and its manipulation may be an important contributor to functional outcome following nerve transfer.

References

[1] Tuttle HK. Exposure of the brachial plexus with nerve transplantation. JAMA 1913;61:15–7.

[2] Narakas OA. Thoughts on neurotization or nerve transfers in irreparable nerve lesions. Clin Plast Surg 1984;11:115–20.

[3] Hallett M. Transcranial magnetic stimulation and the human brain. Nature 2000;406:147–50.

[4] Chen R. Studies of human motor physiology with transcranial magnetic stimulation. Muscle Nerve Suppl 2000;9:S26–32.

[5] Barker AT, Jalinous R, Freeston IL. Noninvasive magnetic stimulation of human motor cortex. Lancet 1985;1:1106–7.

[6] Gevins A, Leong H, Smith ME, et al. Mapping cognitive brain function with modern high-resolution electroencephalography regional modulation of high resolution evoked potentials during verbal and non-verbal matching tasks. Trends Neurosci 1995;18:429–36.

[7] Hari R, Lounasmaa OV. Recording and interpretation of cerebral magnetic fields. Science 1989;244: 432–6.

[8] Turner R, Le BD, Chesnick AS. Echo-planar imaging of diffusion and perfusion. Magn Reson Med 1991;19:47–53.

[9] Friston KJ, Frith CD, Liddle PF, et al. Comparing functional (PET) images: the assessment of significant change. J Cereb Blood Flow Metab 1991;11: 690–9.

[10] Anastakis DJ, Chen R, Davis KD, et al. Cortical plasticity following upper extremity injury, repair and reconstruction. Clin Plast Surg 2005;32: 617–34.

[11] Lee SK, Kim DI, Kim J, et al. Diffusion-tensor MR imaging and fiber tractography: a new method of describing aberrant fiber connections in developmental CNS anomalies. Radiographics 2005;25:53–65.

[12] Masutani Y, Aoki S, Abe O, et al. MR diffusion tensor imaging: recent advance and new techniques for diffusion tensor visualization. Eur J Radiol 2003;46:53–66.

[13] Ramnani N, Behrens TE, Penny W, et al. New approaches for exploring anatomical and functional connectivity in the human brain. Biol Psychiatry 2004;56:613–9.

[14] Smith SM, Jenkinson M, Johansen-Berg H, et al. Tract-based spatial statistics: voxelwise analysis of multi-subject diffusion data. Neuroimage 2006; 31:1487–505.

[15] Mori S, Zhang J. Principles of diffusion tensor imaging and its applications to basic neuroscience research. Neuron 2006;51:527–39.

[16] Behrens TE, Johansen-Berg H, Woolrich MW, et al. Non-invasive mapping of connections between human thalamus and cortex using diffusion imaging. Nat Neurosci 2003;6:750–7.

[17] Norris DG. Principles of magnetic resonance assessment of brain function. J Magn Reson Imaging 2006;23:794–807.

[18] Werring DJ, Clark CA, Parker GJ, et al. A direct demonstration of both structure and function in the visual system: combining diffusion tensor imaging with functional magnetic resonance imaging. Neuroimage 1999;9:352–61.

[19] Ding Z, Gore JC, Anderson AW. Classification and quantification of neuronal fiber pathways using diffusion tensor MRI. Magn Reson Med 2003;49: 716–21.

[20] Mori S, Crain BJ, Chacko VP, et al. Three-dimensional tracking of axonal projections in the brain by magnetic resonance imaging. Ann Neurol 1999;45: 265–9.

[21] Basser PJ, Pierpaoli C. Microstructural and physiological features of tissues elucidated by quantitative-diffusion-tensor MRI. J Magn Reson B 1996; 111:209–19.

[22] Moseley M, Bammer R, Illes J. Diffusion-tensor imaging of cognitive performance. Brain Cogn 2002;50:396–413.

[23] Burgel U, Amunts K, Hoemke L, et al. White matter fiber tracts of the human brain: three-dimensional mapping at microscopic resolution, topography and intersubject variability. Neuroimage 2006;29:1092–105.

[24] Hadjipavlou G, Dunckley P, Behrens TE, et al. Determining anatomical connectivities between cortical and brainstem pain processing regions in humans: a diffusion tensor imaging study in healthy controls. Pain 2006;123:169–78.

[25] Johansen-Berg H, Behrens TE, Sillery E, et al. Functional-anatomical validation and individual variation of diffusion tractography-based segmentation of the human thalamus. Cereb Cortex 2005;15:31–9.

[26] Olesen PJ, Nagy Z, Westerberg H, et al. Combined analysis of DTI and fMRI data reveals a joint maturation of white and grey matter in a fronto-parietal network. Brain Res Cogn Brain Res 2003;18:48–57.

[27] Rushworth MF, Behrens TE, Johansen-Berg H. Connection patterns distinguish 3 regions of human parietal cortex. Cereb Cortex 2005;16: 1418–30.

[28] Wakana S, Jiang H, Nagae-Poetscher LM, et al. Fiber tract-based atlas of human white matter anatomy. Radiology 2004;23:77–87.

[29] Bammer R, Acar B, Moseley ME. In vivo MR tractography using diffusion imaging. Eur J Radiol 2003;45:223–34.

[30] Horsfield MA, Jones DK. Applications of diffusion-weighted and diffusion tensor MRI to white matter diseases—a review. NMR Biomed 2002;15: 570–7.

[31] Taber KH, Pierpaoli C, Rose SE, et al. The future for diffusion tensor imaging in neuropsychiatry. J Neuropsychiatry Clin Neurosci 2002;14:1–5.

[32] Seghier ML, Lazeyras F, Vuilleumier P, et al. Functional magnetic resonance imaging and diffusion tensor imaging in a case of central poststroke pain. J Pain 2005;6:208–12.

[33] Werring DJ, Toosy AT, Clark CA, et al. Diffusion tensor imaging can detect and quantify corticospinal tract degeneration after stroke. J Neurol Neurosurg Psychiatry 2000;69:269–72.

[34] Lee JW, Choi CG, Chun MH. Usefulness of diffusion tensor imaging for evaluation of motor function in patients with traumatic brain injury: three case studies. J Head Trauma Rehabil 2006;21: 272–8.

[35] Werring DJ, Clark CA, Barker GJ, et al. The structural and functional mechanisms of motor recovery: complementary use of diffusion tensor and functional magnetic resonance imaging in a traumatic injury of the internal capsule. J Neurol Neurosurg Psychiatry 1998;65:863–9.

[36] Roberts TP, Liu F, Kassner A, et al. Fiber density index correlates with reduced fractional anisotropy in white matter of patients with glioblastoma. Am J Neuroradiol 2005;26:2183–6.

[37] Shinoura N, Suzuki Y, Yamada R, et al. Restored activation of primary motor area from motor reorganization and improved motor function after brain tumor resection. Am J Neuroradiol 2006;27: 1275–82.

[38] Shimony JS, Burton H, Epstein AA, et al. Diffusion tensor imaging reveals white matter reorganization in early blind humans. Cereb Cortex 2006;16(11): 1653–61.

[39] Rose SE, McMahon KL, Janke AL, et al. MRI diffusion indices and neuropsychological performance in amnestic mild cognitive impairment. J Neurol Neurosurg Psychiatry 2006;77(10):1122–8.

[40] Voss HU, Uluc AM, Dyke JP, et al. Possible axonal regrowth in late recovery from the minimally conscious state. J Clin Invest 2006;116:2005–11.

[41] Wright IC, McGuire PK, Poline JB, et al. A voxel-based method for the statistical analysis of gray and white matter density applied to schizophrenia. Neuroimage 1995;2:244–52.

[42] Ashburner J, Friston KJ. Voxel-based morphometry—the methods. Neuroimage 2000;11:805–21.

[43] Betting LE, Mory SB, Li LM, et al. Voxel-based morphometry in patients with idiopathic generalized epilepsies. Neuroimage 2006;32:498–502.

[44] Chen S, Xia W, Li L, et al. Gray matter density reduction in the insula in fire survivors with post-traumatic stress disorder: a voxel-based morphometric study. Psychiatry Res 2006;146:65–72.

[45] De Lange FP, Kalkman JS, Bleijenberg G, et al. Gray matter volume reduction in the chronic fatigue syndrome. Neuroimage 2005;26:777–81.

[46] Etgen T, Draganski B, Ilg C, et al. Bilateral thalamic gray matter changes in patients with restless legs syndrome. Neuroimage 2005;24:1242–7.

[47] Lyoo IK, Pollack MH, Silveri MM, et al. Prefrontal and temporal gray matter density decreases in opiate dependence. Psychopharmacology (Berl) 2006;184:139–44.

[48] Lyoo IK, Sung YH, Dager SR, et al. Regional cerebral cortical thinning in bipolar disorder. Bipolar Disord 2006;8:65–74.

[49] Morgen K, Sammer G, Courtney SM, et al. Evidence for a direct association between cortical atrophy and cognitive impairment in relapsing-remitting MS. Neuroimage 2006;30:891–8.

[50] Protopopescu X, Pan H, Tuescher O, et al. Increased brainstem volume in panic disorder: a voxel-based morphometric study. Neuroreport 2006;17:361–3.

[51] Rusch N, van Elst LT, Ludaescher P, et al. A voxel-based morphometric MRI study in female patients with borderline personality disorder. Neuroimage 2003;20:385–92.

[52] Valente AA Jr, Miguel EC, Castro CC, et al. Regional gray matter abnormalities in obsessive-compulsive disorder: a voxel-based morphometry study. Biol Psychiatry 2005;58:479–87.

[53] Wessels AM, Simsek S, Remijnse PL, et al. Voxel-based morphometry demonstrates reduced grey matter density on brain MRI in patients with diabetic retinopathy. Diabetologia 2006;49(10): 2474–80.

[54] Crawley AP, Jurkiewicz MT, Yim A, et al. Absence of localized grey matter volume changes in the motor cortex following spinal cord injury. Brain Res 2004;1028:19–25.

[55] Jurkiewicz MT, Crawley AP, Verrier MC, et al. Somatosensory cortical atrophy after spinal cord injury: a voxel-based morphometry study. Neurology 2006;66:762–4.

[56] Apkarian AV, Sosa Y, Sonty S, et al. Chronic back pain is associated with decreased prefrontal and thalamic gray matter density. J Neurosci 2004;24: 10410–5.

[57] Draganski B, Moser T, Lummel N, et al. Decrease of thalamic gray matter following limb amputation. Neuroimage 2006;31:951–7.

[58] Davis KD, Pope G, Chen J, et al. Cortical thinning in irritable bowel syndrome: implications for homeostatic, attention and pain processing. Neurology 2008;70:153–4.

[59] Kuchinad A, Schweinhardt P, Seminowicz DA, et al. Accelerated brain gray matter loss in fibromyalgia patients: premature aging of the brain? J Neurosci 2007;27:4004–7.

[60] Schmidt-Wilcke T, Leinisch E, Ganssbauer S, et al. Affective components and intensity of pain correlate with structural differences in gray matter in chronic back pain patients. Pain 2006;125: 89–97.

[61] Schmidt-Wilcke T, Leinisch E, Straube A, et al. Gray matter decrease in patients with chronic tension type headache. Neurology 2005;65:1483–6.

[62] Omura K, Todd CR, Canli T. Amygdala gray matter concentration is associated with extraversion and neuroticism. Neuroreport 2005;16:1905–8.

[63] Lehmbeck JT, Brassen S, Weber-Fahr W, et al. Combining voxel-based morphometry and diffusion tensor imaging to detect age-related brain changes. Neuroreport 2006;17:467–70.

[64] Smith CD, Chebrolu H, Wekstein DR, et al. Age and gender effects on human brain anatomy: a voxel-based morphometric study in healthy elderly. Neurobiol Aging 2006;28(7):1075–87.

[65] Herve PY, Mazoyer B, Crivello F, et al. Finger tapping, handedness and grey matter amount in the Rolando's genu area. Neuroimage 2005;25: 1133–45.

[66] May A, Hajak G, Ganssbauer S, et al. Structural brain alterations following 5 days of intervention: dynamic aspects of neuroplasticity. Cereb Cortex 2007;17(1):205–10.

[67] Ashburner J, Friston KJ. Why voxel-based morphometry should be used. Neuroimage 2001;14: 1238–43.

[68] Bookstein FL. Voxel-based morphometry should not be used with imperfectly registered images. Neuroimage 2001;14:1454–62.

[69] Good CD, Johnsrude IS, Ashburner J, et al. A voxel-based morphometric study of ageing in 465 normal adult human brains. Neuroimage 2001;14: 21–36.

[70] Chung MK, Robbins SM, Dalton KM, et al. Cortical thickness analysis in autism with heat kernel smoothing. Neuroimage 2005;25:1256–65.

[71] Fischl B, Dale AM. Measuring the thickness of the human cerebral cortex from magnetic resonance images. Proc Natl Acad Sci USA 2000;97: 11050–5.

[72] Han X, Jovicich J, Salat D, et al. Reliability of MRI-derived measurements of human cerebral cortical thickness: The effects of field strength, scanner upgrade and manufacturer. Neuroimage 2006;32(1):180–94.

[73] Jones SE, Buchbinder BR, Aharon I. Three-dimensional mapping of cortical thickness using Laplace's equation. Hum Brain Mapp 2000;11:12–32.

[74] Kabani N, Le GG, MacDonald D, et al. Measurement of cortical thickness using an automated 3-D algorithm: a validation study. Neuroimage 2001; 13:375–80.

[75] MacDonald D, Kabani N, Avis D, et al. Automated 3-D extraction of inner and outer surfaces of cerebral cortex from MRI. Neuroimage 2000; 12:340–56.

[76] Lerch JP, Evans AC. Cortical thickness analysis examined through power analysis and a population simulation. Neuroimage 2005;24:163–73.

[77] Schneider P, Sluming V, Roberts N, et al. Structural and functional asymmetry of lateral Heschl's gyrus reflects pitch perception preference. Nat Neurosci 2005;8:1241–7.

[78] Luders E, Narr KL, Thompson PM, et al. Hemispheric asymmetries in cortical thickness. Cereb Cortex 2006;16:1232–8.

[79] Jang DP, Kim JJ, Chung TS, et al. Shape deformation of the insula in schizophrenia. Neuroimage 2006;32(1):220–7.

[80] Rosas HD, Liu AK, Hersch S, et al. Regional and progressive thinning of the cortical ribbon in Huntington's disease. Neurology 2002;58:695–701.

[81] Ogawa S, Tank DW, Menon R, et al. Intrinsic signal changes accompanying sensory stimulation: functional brain mapping with magnetic resonance imaging. Proc Natl Acad Sci USA 1992; 13:5951–5.

[82] Ogawa S, Lee TM, Kay AR, et al. Brain magnetic resonance imaging with contrast dependent on blood oxygenation. Proc Natl Acad Sci USA 1990;87:9868–72.

[83] Davis TL, Kwong KK, Weissfoff RM, et al. Calibrated fMRI: Mapping the dynamics of oxidative metabolism. Proc Natl Acad Sci USA 1998;95(4): 1834–9.

[84] Kwong KK, Belliveau JW, Chesler DA, et al. Dynamic MRI of human brain activity during primary sensory stimulation. Proc Natl Acad Sci USA 1992; 89:5675–9.

[85] Cohen MS, Bookheimer SY. Localization of brain function using magnetic resonance imaging. Trends Neurosci 1994;17:268–76.

[86] Crease RP. Biomedicine in the age of imaging. Science 1993;261:554–61.

[87] DeYoe EA, Bandettini P, Neitz J, et al. Functional magnetic resonance imaging (fMRI) of the human brain. J Neurosci Methods 1994;54:171–87.

[88] Ogawa S, Lee TM, Nayak AS, et al. Oxygenation—sensitive contrast in magnetic resonance image of

rodent brain at high magnetic fields. Magn Reson Med 1990;14:68–78.

[89] Prichard JW, Brass LM. New anatomical and functional imaging methods. Ann Neurol 1992;32: 395–400.

[90] Cohen LG, Bandinelli S, Topka HR, et al. Topographic maps of human motor cortex in normal and pathological conditions: mirror movements, amputations and spinal cord injuries. Electroencephalogr Clin Neurophysiol 1991;43(Suppl):36–50.

[91] Brasil-Neto JP, Cohen LG, Panizza M, et al. Optimal focal transcranial magnetic activation of the human motor cortex: effects of coil orientation, shape of the induced current pulse, and stimulus intensity. J Clin Neurophysiol 1992;9:132–6.

[92] Gevins A, Brickett P, Costales B, et al. Beyond topographic mapping: towards functional-anatomical imaging with 124-channel EEGs and 3-D MRIs. Brain Topogr 1990;3:53–64.

[93] Wasserman EM, Wang W, Zeffiro TA, et al. Locating the motor cortex on the MRI with transcranial magnetic stimulation and PET. Neuroimage 1996; 3:1–6.

[94] Cohen LG, Gerloff C, Faiz L, et al. Directional modulation of motor cortex plasticity induced by synchronicity of motor outputs in humans. Soc Neurosci Abstr 1996;22:1452.

[95] Elbert T, Plor H, Birbaumer N, et al. Extensive reorganization of the somatosensory cortex in adult humans after nervous system injury. Neuroreport 1994;5:2593–7.

[96] Yang TT, Gallen CC, Rivlin AS, et al. Effect of duration of acute spinal cord compression in a new acute cord injury model in the rat. Surg Neurol 1978;10:39–43.

[97] Yang TT, Gallen CC, Ramachandran V, et al. Noninvasive detection of cerebral plasticity in adult human somatosensory cortex. NeuroReport 1994; 5:701–4.

[98] Borsook D, Becerra L, Fishman S, et al. Acute plasticity in the human somatosensory cortex following amputation. Neuroreport 1998;9:1013–7.

[99] Ridding MC, Rothwell JC. Reorganization in human motor cortex. Can J Physiol Pharmacol 1995;73:218–22.

[100] Chen R, Corwell B, Yaseen Z, et al. Mechanisms of cortical reorganization in lower-limb amputees. J Neurosci 1998;18:3443–50.

[101] Dettmer C, Liepert J, Adler T, et al. Abnormal motor cortex organization contralateral to early upper limb amputation in humans. Neurosci Lett 1999; 263:41–4.

[102] Garraghty LB, Muja N. NMDA receptors and plasticity in adult primate somatosensory cortex. J Comp Neurol 1996;367:19–26.

[103] Sanes JN, Suner S, Donoghue JP. Dynamic organization of primary motor cortex output to target muscle in adult rats. Long-term patterns of

reorganization following motor or mixed peripheral nerve lesion. Exp Brain Res 1990;79:479–91.

[104] Sanes JN, Suner S, Lando JF, et al. Rapid reorganization of adult rat motor cortex somatic representation after motor nerve injury. Proc Natl Acad Sci USA 1988;85:2003–7.

[105] Merzenich MM, Jenkins WM. Reorganization of cortical representations of the hand following alterations of skin inputs induced by nerve injury, skin island transfers and experience. J Hand Ther 1993;6:89–104.

[106] Wall JT, Kaas JH, Sur M, et al. Functional reorganization in somatosensory cortical areas 3b and 1 of adult monkeys after median nerve repair: possible relationships to sensory recovery in humans. J Neurosci 1986;6:218–33.

[107] Buonomano DV, Merzenich MM. Cortical plasticity: from synapses to maps. Annu Rev Neurosci 1998;21:149–86.

[108] Garraghty PE, LaChica EA, Kaas JH. Injury-induced reorganization of somatosensory cortex is accompanied by reductions in GABA staining. Somatosens Mot Res 1991;8:347–54.

[109] Sengelaub DR, Muja N, Mills AC, et al. Denervation-induced sprouting of intact peripheral afferents into the cuneate nucleus of adult rats. Brain Res 1997;769:256–62.

[110] Wall JT, Xu J, Wang X. Human brain plasticity: an emerging view of the multiple substrates and mechanisms that cause cortical changes and related sensory dysfunctions after injuries of sensory inputs from the body. Brain Res Brain Res Rev 2002;39:181–215.

[111] Florence SL, Kaas JH. Large-scale reorganization at multiple levels of the somatosensory pathway follows therapeutic amputation of the hand in monkeys. J Neurosci 1995;15:8083–95.

[112] Malessy MJA, Thomeer RTWM. Evaluation of intercostal to musculocutaneous nerve transfer in reconstructive brachial plexus surgery. J Neurosurg 1998;88:266–71.

[113] Taylor A. The contribution of the intercostal muscles to the effort of respiration in man. J Physiol 1960;151:390–402.

[114] De Troyer A, Estenne M. Functional anatomy of the respiratory muscles. Clin Chest Med 1988;9:175–93.

[115] Malessy MJA, van Dijk JG, Thomeer RTWM. Respiration related activity in the biceps brachii muscle after intercostal-musculocutaneous nerve transfer. Clin Neurol Neurosurg 1993;95(Suppl): S95–102.

[116] Ghez C. Voluntary movement. In: Kandel ER, Schwartz JH, Jessell TM, editors. Principles of neural science. New York: Elsevier; 1991. p. 609–25.

[117] Cheng H, Shoung HM, Wu ZA, et al. Functional connectivity of the transected brachial plexus after intercostal neurotization in monkeys. J Comp Neurol 1997;380:155–63.

[118] Kawai H. Intercostal nerve transfer. In: Kawai H, Kawabata H, editors. Brachial plexus palsy. Singapore: World Scientific; 2000. p. 161–236.

[119] Kawai H, Murase T, Shibuya R, et al. Magnetic stimulation of biceps after intercostal cross-innervation for brachial plexus palsy. A study of motor evoked potentials in 25 patients. J Bone Joint Surg Br 1994;76:666–9.

[120] Logothetis NK, Pauls J, Augath M, et al. Neurophysiological investigation of the basis of the fMRI signal. Nature 2001;412:150–7.

[121] Giraux P, Sirigu A, Schneider F, et al. Cortical reorganization in motor cortex after graft of both hands. Nat Neurosci 2001;4:691–2.

[122] Ravnborg M, Blinkenberg M, Dahl K. Standardization of facilitation of compound muscle action potentials evoked by magnetic stimulation of the cortex. Results in healthy volunteers and in patients with multiple sclerosis. Electroencephalogr Clin Neurophysiol 1991;81:195–201.

[123] Rothwell JC, Thompson PD, Day BL, et al. Stimulation of the human motor cortex through the scalp. Exp Physiol 1991;76:159–200.

[124] Malessy MJA, Bakker D, Dekker AJ, et al. Functional magnetic resonance imaging and control over the biceps muscle after intercostal–musculocutaneous nerve transfer. J Neurosurg 2003;98:261–8.

[125] Malessy MJA, Thomeer RTWM, van Dijk JG. Changing central nervous system control following intercostal nerve transfer. J Neurosurg 1998;89:568–74.

[126] Malessy MJA, van der Kamp W, Thomeer RTWM, et al. Cortical excitability of the biceps muscle after intercostal-to-musculocutaneous nerve transfer. Neurosurgery 1998;42:787–95.

[127] Mano Y, Nakamuro T, Tamura R, et al. Central motor reorganization after anastomosis of the musculocutaneous and intercostal nerves following cervical root avulsion. Ann Neurol 1995;38:15–20.

[128] Florence SL, Jain N, Pospichal MW, et al. Central reorganization of sensory pathways following peripheral nerve regeneration in fetal monkeys. Nature 1996;381:69–71.

[129] Kaas JH. Plasticity of sensory and motor maps in adult mammals. Annu Rev Neurosci 1991;14:137–67.

[130] Kandel ER, Hawkins RD. The biological basis of learning and individuality. Sci Am 1992;267:53–60.

[131] Merzenich MM, Sameshima K. Cortical plasticity and memory. Curr Opin Neurobiol 1993;3:187–96.

[132] Malessy MJA, Hoffmann CF, Thomeer RTWM. Initial report on the limited value of hypoglossal nerve transfer to treat brachial plexus root avulsions. J Neurosurg 1999;91:601–4.

[133] Beaulieu J-Y, Blustajn J, Teboul F, et al. Cerebral plasticity in crossed C7 grafts of the brachial plexus: an fMRI study. Microsurgery 2006;26:303–10.

[134] Karni A, Meyer G, Jezzard P, et al. Functional MRI evidence for adult motor cortex plasticity during motor skill learning. Nature 1995;377(6545):155–8.

[135] Jenkins WM, Merzenich MM, Ochs MT, et al. Functional reorganization of primary somatosensory cortex in adult owl monkeys after behaviorally controlled tactile stimulation. J Neurophysiol 1990;63:82–104.

[136] Elbert T, Pantev C, Wienbruch C, et al. Increased cortical representation of the fingers of the left hand in string players. Science 1995;270:305–7.

[137] Pascual-Leone A, Torres F. Plasticity of the sensorimotor cortex representation of the reading finger in Braille readers. Brain 1993;116:39–52.

[138] Manduch M, Bezuhly M, Anastakis DJ, et al. Serial fMRI assessment of the primary motor cortex following thumb reconstruction. Neurology 2002;59(8):1278–81.

[139] Chen R, Anastakis DJ, Haywood CT, et al. Plasticity of the human motor system following muscle reconstruction: a magnetic stimulation and functional magnetic resonance imaging study. Clin Neurophysiol 2003;114(12):2434–46.

[140] Liepert J, Classen J, Cohen LG, et al. Task-dependent changes in intracortical inhibition. Exp Brain Res 1998;118:421–6.

[141] Kujirai T, Caramia MD, Rothwell JC, et al. Corticocortical inhibition in human motor cortex. J Physiol (Lond) 1993;471:501–19.

[142] Ziemann U, Corwell B, Cohen LG. Modulation of plastic changes in human motor cortex after forearm ischemic nerve block. J Neurosci 1998;18:1115–23.

Optimizing Skeletal Muscle Reinnervation with Nerve Transfer

Samuel C. Lien, BS, Paul S. Cederna, MD,
William M. Kuzon, Jr, MD, PhD*

Department of Surgery, Section of Plastic and Reconstructive Surgery, University of Michigan,
2130 Taubman Center, 1500 East Medical Center Drive, Ann Arbor, MI 48109-0340, USA

Peripheral nerve injuries are common—and sometimes devastating—sequelae of blunt or penetrating trauma. Although the central and peripheral nervous systems have remarkable capacity for regeneration and adaptation, most patients with nerve injuries do not regain full motor or sensory ability and, under many conditions, experience significant and permanent functional disability despite the best efforts of reconstructive surgeons. The consequences of skeletal muscle denervation and the incomplete and imprecise process of muscle reinnervation are the prime contributors to the disability that patients experience after peripheral nerve injury. A complex cascade of events occurs in skeletal muscle immediately after nerve transection, leading to profound, short-term, largely reversible structural and functional changes in the denervated muscle.

If the muscle is rapidly supplied with a large number of regenerating motor axons, synaptogenesis proceeds and results in a reasonable recovery of motor activity. If the axons are motion-specific, meaning that they produce contractile activity resulting in movement with appropriate volitional control, useful integrated motor function can be recovered. If the number of motor axons is insufficient, if the denervation interval is prolonged beyond a short time period, or if the motor axons are not motion-specific, the functional result is compromised, often significantly. Although numerous strategies exist to

prevent or ameliorate intramuscular changes when reinnervation is compromised, no method rivals prompt reinnervation with a sufficient number of motion-specific motor axons. We argue that from a clinical outcome standpoint, nerve transfer is the best strategy to reinnervate distal muscle groups after proximal nerve injury. This punch line cannot be overemphasized: The best recovery after a motor nerve injury is achieved only if an abundant supply of motion-specific motor axons is rapidly provided to the muscles denervated as a result of the nerve transection. This is precisely what makes nerve transfers the current leader among the available strategies for the surgical management of nerve injuries in the proximal portions of the extremities.

Sequelae of denervation

With axotomy, muscle fibers previously innervated by the affected nerve undergo a process properly called denervation atrophy. It is important to recognize that because of synaptic instability and limited, ongoing axonal dropout, a small percentage of the skeletal muscle fibers in all muscles are in the process of becoming denervated and reinnervated. This cycle of denervation and reinnervation continues throughout life. The short-term, atrophic changes that occur as a result of these brief periods of denervation are completely reversible with reinnervation and should be considered physiologic in nature. As the length of time that the muscle is denervated increases, there is a progressive series of detrimental changes that eventually results in

* Corresponding author.
E-mail address: wkuzon@med.umich.edu
(W.M. Kuzon).

0749-0712/08/$ - see front matter. Published by Elsevier Inc.
doi:10.1016/j.hcl.2008.08.001

a muscle recalcitrant to reinnervation. Use of the term "denervation atrophy" to describe this series of pathologic changes that occur with long-term denervation has caused significant confusion and has led to the widespread belief that all denervation is pathologic. The importance of distinguishing physiologic, reversible, short-term denervation atrophy from irreversible, pathologic, long-term atrophy in the context of attempting to restore the function of a denervated muscle is obvious.

Immediately after denervation, muscle fibers remain viable, myosin and actin filaments are catabolized, myofibrils are reabsorbed, muscle cells shrink in size, and the enlarging extracellular space fills with collagen (Fig. 1). The mediators of this atrophic process are mainly proteases associated with the ubiquitin-proteosome pathway. Research has been shown that inhibition of these proteases reduces the extent of short-term denervation atrophy while facilitating axonal regeneration and muscle reinnervation [1].

If enough time is allowed to elapse before reinnervation, a small proportion of individual muscle cells may undergo a process similar to apoptosis. The progressive malalignment and disorganization of myofibrils that occur after denervation eventually leave entire regions within the muscle cell void of myofibrils; these changes signal the imminent death of the muscle cell [2]. The extent to which this occurs seems to depend highly on species. Muscle fiber loss with prolonged denervation is marked in some strains of rats, whereas recent work with rabbits suggests that even up to 1 year after denervation there is no evidence of muscle fiber necrosis [3]. It is not clear to what extent this mechanism applies to humans.

Changes in fiber-type composition also occur after denervation. Although the changes that occur in myosin heavy chain (MHC) expression in muscle fibers after denervation are complex, it is fair to say that under most circumstances, a shift from a mix of slow-twitch (type I) and fast-twitch (type II) fibers to a predominance of type II fibers is seen beginning within the first week after denervation. Studies on rat hind leg muscles have shown that after 1 year of denervation,

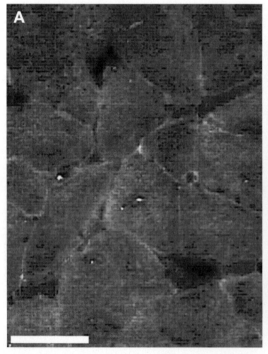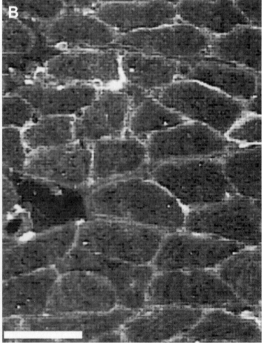

Fig. 1. Histologic section of (*A*) normal rat extensor digitorum longus (EDL) muscle and (*B*) denervated rat EDL muscle. Note the large fibers of uniform size and minimal connective tissue between fibers in the normal muscle. In denervated muscle, the diameter of the fibers is markedly reduced and the connective tissue surrounding each fiber is more prominent. Calibration bar = 50 μM.

muscles almost exclusively contain type II fibers, regardless of their original ratio of type I to type II fibers. These muscles also have nearly identical contractile properties and similar susceptibilities to fatigue and manage intracellular calcium within the sarcoplasmic reticulum in similar ways regardless of their original composition [4,5]. As muscle cells shift expression from type I to type II MHCs, there is a concurrent expression of multiple different kinds of the type II MHC isoform not usually seen in adult muscle. It seems as if muscles reset their MHC isoform expression to a certain predetermined ratio of isoforms when denervated; at least in rodents, this seems to be predominately type II isoforms [6]. This finding suggests that intrinsic properties of the muscle, combined with input from the motor neuron, determine the ultimate expression of MHC isoforms in a mature muscle cell. Without input from the motor nerve, muscle cells are left to express MHC fiber types according to their intrinsic program.

Changes within the denervated muscle do not occur uniformly across all muscle fibers, resulting in topographic changes within the muscle as reinnervation occurs. This is true especially under circumstances of partial nerve injury. Under normal circumstances, the muscle fibers of a given motor unit are dispersed spatially within the muscle, with two fibers from a given motor unit rarely being in direct physical contact. With partial denervation, muscle fibers may be reinnervated shortly after denervation by sprouts from remaining intact motor axons. These fibers are then recruited into the adjacent, healthy motor unit and shift their MHC isoform expression accordingly, which results in the phenomenon of fiber type grouping. With complete nerve division and wholesale reinnervation, nearly all of the muscle fibers in the vicinity of a regenerating axon are reinnervated by its sprouts. Large islands of muscle fibers of a certain type form in the newly reinnervated muscle and compromise the previously heterogenous mixture of fiber types. Functionally, the process of fiber type grouping produces a latent period between reinnervation and functional recovery of the muscle's contractile capabilities that can last as long as 30 days [7]. The latent period persists for the length of time required by muscle fibers to alter their expression of fiber types to conform to their new motor unit.

Besides the changes within the muscle fibers themselves, denervation also affects capillary blood flow within the muscle. In the first 7 months after denervation, the ratio of the number of capillaries to the number of muscle fibers decreases precipitously to nearly 10% of the original ratio. After that, the loss of capillaries slows, leaving the atrophic muscle with what little blood supply it needs to sustain its reduced metabolic activity [8]. As much as 40% of the muscle can be essentially avascular by 18 months after denervation [9]. Many of the capillaries that remain intact are sequestered among the thick bands of collagen that invade the extracellular matrix. With time, collagen deposition advances and capillary necrosis continues, which decreases the potential of the denervated muscle to regain its contractile properties should it be reinnervated [10].

Synchronous with these atrophic processes, significant changes occur within the muscle to optimize the environment for reinnervation. During embryogenesis, muscle fibers are covered homogenously by acetylcholine receptors (AChRs). With synaptogenesis, there is a phenotypic change in the fiber surface, with AChRs becoming concentrated solely under the motor endplate, leaving the rest of the muscle surface devoid of AChRs. With the loss of the presynaptic terminal that occurs after nerve transection, proliferation of AChRs occurs; soon the muscle surface is again covered by a wide distribution of receptors all awaiting contact from the tip of a regenerating nerve. When regenerating nerves reach the target muscle, the presynaptic terminal is reformed and again the AChRs proliferate within the synaptic cleft, thereby restoring their heterogenous distribution. In a similar fashion, neural cell adhesion molecules are widely expressed on the whole sarcolemma of the primitive muscle fiber and play a role in guiding the growth of the incoming motor axon. Once a motor endplate has been established, neural cell adhesion molecules are expressed only in the vicinity of the neuromuscular junction. With denervation, neural cell adhesion molecules are again expressed as a generalized sarcolemma protein and likely play a role in allowing new motor axons to form synapses [11]. These changes in the expression and distribution of AChRs, neural cell adhesion molecules, and other postsynaptic membrane proteins "hypersensitize" the surface of the muscle to regenerating axons.

Denervation induces a profound effect in the active mechanical properties of skeletal muscle. Early on, most of the contractile deficit is caused by the decrease in the total cross-sectional area of muscle fibers. The maximum tension generated by tetanic contractions of the denervated muscle falls in proportion to the decrease in total muscle cross-sectional area. As denervation is prolonged, progressive disorganization of the myofibrils and replacement of muscle fibers with collagen results in a decrease in the specific force capacity. Specific force is best thought of as the force per unit muscle tissue, so a specific force deficit indicates that an intrinsic defect in contractile capacity is present. Two general classes of mechanisms impact skeletal muscle contractility after denervation and reinnervation: (1) mechanisms that affect primarily muscle mass and (2) mechanisms that affect muscle force capacity independent of muscle mass. Mechanisms that result in muscle atrophy result in deficits in whole muscle force. Mechanisms that affect force capacity independent of muscle mass result in deficits in specific force. The former of these deficits is amenable to remediation via reinnervation and physical training; the latter deficit is permanent.

In addition to changes in maximum force, virtually all other characteristics of muscle mechanical function are altered with denervation. There is a decrease in the power output of the muscle and an increase in the time to peak contractile force and relaxation. A reduction in the speed of contraction, which occurs between 2 and 6 days after denervation, occurs to a similar degree in types I and II muscle fibers [12]. One week after denervation, these parameters are partially restored because of changes in the excitability of the muscle cells and changes in the baseline level of cellular repolarization after contraction [12]. In the later stages of denervation, however, force, specific force, and power all continue to fall as the structure of the muscle continues to degrade.

Process of reinnervation and recovery

Skeletal muscle reinnervation requires axonal elongation, synaptogenesis, and resumption of contractile function. The quality of the recovery of structural integrity, gross mechanical properties, and integrated motor function after skeletal muscle reinnervation depend on several variables that affect these basic processes. These variables include the length of the denervation interval (discussed in detail in the next section), the path that the axons take to reach the muscle fibers, the number of reinnervating axons relative to the number that originally innervated the muscle, and the specificity of the reinnervating axons. Axonal regeneration has been described extensively elsewhere and is not reviewed in this article.

When regenerating motor neurons gain proximity to denervated muscle fibers, cholinergic synapses are formed. Growth cones at the tip of the regenerating nerves are stimulated to form synapses by chemical factors on the basal lamina surrounding the muscle fibers and neural cell adhesion molecules expressed on the muscle fiber surface. This is followed by widening of the axon terminal over the muscle membrane, the production of vesicles of ACh to store in the presynaptic terminal, and the attraction of AChRs to the surface of the muscle fiber at the motor endplate. Initially, there is a transient period of hyperinnervation. Recent work done with the rat tibialis anterior muscle has shown that after inflicting a crush injury to the sciatic nerve, there is partial reinnervation of the muscle at 2 weeks. From 3 to 4 weeks after nerve injury, there is a period of hyperinnervation in which the axon/motor endplate ratio exceeds 1:1. This is followed by restoration of a 1:1 ratio by 6 weeks [13].

The importance of nerve regeneration onto the sites of the original motor endplates is highlighted by comparing the success of muscle grafts containing motor endplates to those that have been stripped of them. Muscle grafts void of endplates show a significant decrease in contractile ability and fiber type differentiation compared with grafts with intact endplates. From a functional standpoint, this reiterates the importance of conduits left by the original motor nerve to guide the regenerating axons to the original motor endplates [14].

Studies that involve nerve-intact and lidocaine-degenerated muscle grafts demonstrate the potential for full recovery of mechanical properties and integrated muscle function if appropriate criteria are fulfilled. Nerve-intact grafts involve the autologous transplant of a muscle after tenotomy and disruption of its blood supply but preservation of its innervation. The tendons are attached elsewhere, and the muscle's blood supply is restored through an anastomosis to an adjacent vessel. The temporary disruption of perfusion causes the muscle fibers and the intramuscular portions of the motor axons to degenerate. A similar set of conditions can be achieved by using lidocaine to degenerate the muscle cells. The undamaged, extramuscular portion of the nerve is able to regenerate along the original axonal conduits, which provides for rapid reinnervation, ample numbers of axons, and maintenance of the original neural circuitry. In rat hindlimb muscles, nerve-intact muscle grafts can fully recover their original mass, motor unit properties (including motor unit numbers), and whole-muscle functional capacity [15].

So-called "standard" muscle grafts, in which the motor nerve is severed and repaired in addition to the tendons and blood vessels, recover only 35% to 50% of their original mass and functional ability [16]. The only difference between standard and nerve-intact grafts is disruption of the endoneurial conduits in the standard grafts. Because the regenerating axons must cross the nerve coaptation site, there is a reduction of axon numbers entering the muscle, and the neural circuitry is not precisely restored. Reinnervation of the target muscle is inefficient and disorganized, with significant fiber type grouping, loss of muscle mass, and functional disability. Even under conditions of rapid reinnervation, a substantial functional disability can be engendered by altering the number and circuitry of the reinnervating axons.

Available data clearly indicate that a reduction in the number of reinnervating motor axons leads to a substantial reduction in the recovery of force capacity. For example, studies that use nerve-muscle neurotization (implanting the end of a severed nerve within the belly of a denervated muscle) uniformly report dismal functioning of the reinnervated muscle, likely because the axons are forced to regenerate outside endoneurial conduits, which reduces the number of axons that reach muscle fibers and substantially impacts neural circuitry [17,18]. Strong, direct evidence indicates that muscles reinnervated by a reduced number of axons experience a reduction in their force-generating capabilities, most likely because of residual denervated muscle fibers that persist among the fibers that have been reinnervated (Fig. 2) [19]. In these studies, a linear decrease in whole muscle and specific forces was observed as the number of axons available for reinnervation was reduced.

Rapid versus delayed reinnervation

It is a widely held belief that the reversal of the changes that occur in skeletal muscle with denervation and the recovery of contractile function upon reinnervation tend to be unsatisfactory when the denervation period is extended because of either a long period of time required for axonal regeneration or a delay before surgical nerve

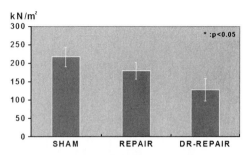

Fig. 2. Rat extensor digitorum muscle (EDL) force is plotted on the y axis. Compared with EDL forces from animals in the SHAM (control) group, EDL muscles that were reinnervated by a large number of motor axons demonstrate diminished force output (REPAIR group). If the number of axons available to reinnervate the muscle is deliberately reduced (DR-REPAIR group), the force deficit after reinnervation is increased. This demonstrates the importance of providing large numbers of motor axons for skeletal muscle reinnervation.

repair [20–24]. Surprisingly few experimental studies have focused on the functional recovery of skeletal muscle reinnervated after prolonged denervation. The studies that are available are consistent in finding that even a brief delay in reinnervation is detrimental to the recovery of mechanical function. Changes in the axotomized nerve and in the muscle both contribute to the functional deficits observed.

After tibial nerve transection and reconstruction in the rat hindlimb, recovery of whole muscle force in the gastrocnemius muscle was inversely proportional to the denervation interval [25]. In keeping with the concept that atropic and atrophy-independent mechanisms contribute differentially to force deficits after prolonged denervation, the observed specific force deficit was not proportional to the denervation interval (Fig. 3). In contrast to the roughly linear decline in whole muscle force as the time of reinnervation progressively lengthened, all groups in which the nerve reconstruction was delayed for a month or longer manifested a specific force deficit of 30% to 50%. Other experimental studies are consistent with these findings [26], and abundant clinical evidence supports these experimental observations [20–22].

The mechanisms responsible for the observed deficits include a diminishing affinity between regenerating muscle and nerve fibers with increasing denervation time. Denervation of skeletal muscle results in a phenotypic change in the expression of surface proteins. Other proteins,

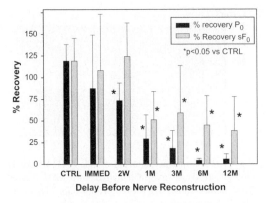

Fig. 3. Percent recovery of rat medial gastrocnemius force with increasing denervation interval. Rats underwent transection of the tibial nerve, and the interval before nerve reconstruction is indicated on the x axis. Medial gastrocnemius muscle force was measured after an appropriate recovery interval. The recovery of whole muscle force progressively decreases as the denervation interval is increased. Specific force recovery is markedly decreased if nerve reconstruction is delayed for a month or longer. (*From* Kobayashi J, Mackinnon SE, Watanabe O, et al. The effect of duration of muscle denervation on functional recovery in the rat model. Muscle & Nerve 1997;20(7):858–66; with permission. Copyright © 1997, John Wiley & Sons, Inc.)

including myogenic transcription factors such as MRF4, Myf-5, Id-1, MyoD, and myogenin are up-regulated. This leads to dramatic alterations in the isoform expression and spatial distribution of numerous structural and functional molecules, such as neural cell adhesion molecule, ciliary neurotrophic factor receptors, and nicotinic AChR [27]. This embryonic state, which is optimal for new synapse formation, returns to the refractory pattern of adulthood when the denervation exceeds 1 to 2 months [24]. The result of this return to a phenotype refractory to reinnervation is that a synaptic relation cannot be resumed even if regenerating axons make contact with the muscle fibers. There is a progressive replacement of the contractile tissue by connective tissue and fatty tissue, progressive intramuscular fibrosis, and permanent ultrastructural changes in the muscle fibers themselves. These wholesale structural and functional changes underscore the importance of rapid reinnervation in the setting of a clinical nerve injury.

Strategies to prevent long-term "denervation atrophy"

Numerous strategies have been proposed to prevent long-term denervation atrophy, including electrical stimulation, trophic support, sensory protection, and "babysitting." Extensive investigations in animal models and injured patients have demonstrated a wide spectrum of outcomes using these various approaches.

Electrical stimulation

The lack of contractile activity in denervated or paralyzed skeletal muscle seems to be a critical element in initiating and maintaining the many adaptive changes seen in the structural and functional properties of muscle [28–31]. Research has demonstrated that when the level of contractile activity in a muscle is either increased or decreased (even if the muscle remains innervated), significant alterations occur in the contractile properties, phenotype, and levels of gene expression in that muscle [28,30,32–38]. These changes are most clearly demonstrated with exercise training [33], electrical stimulation [30,32,35–38], clinical nerve conduction blocks [28], and cross-innervation experiments [34]. Specifically, contractile activity elicited by electrical stimulation can partially reverse the effects of denervation on skeletal muscle [37,39]. Electrically generated tetanic contractions of denervated muscles reduce the loss of mass, maximum force [36,37,39], and fiber cross sectional area [40–42] and partially suppress the up-regulation of transcripts for α, β, γ, and δ subunits of nAChR [43,44], MyoD, and myogenin [45].

Different protocols of electrical stimulation result in the maintenance of different levels of mass and contractile properties [32]. These observations demonstrate the importance of the specific stimulation parameters, including pulse width and amplitude, frequency of pulses [26,36], number of pulses per contraction [37,38], and number of contractions per day [38]. Prior studies typically altered several stimulation parameters simultaneously, thus obscuring the physiologic effect of each of the independent stimulation variables [46]. Optimal maintenance of other aspects of muscle structure or function may require different protocols of stimulation. Such an optimized protocol may help differentiate the roles of contractile activity and trophic factors released from intact motor neurons in the regulation of the contractility, morphology, and molecular expression of muscle fibers. An optimized stimulation protocol that maintains the structure and contractility of stimulated-denervated muscles may enable the following clinical applications: (1) enhance the recovery of motor function of muscles that have been denervated for a prolonged period of time before reinnervation and (2) maintain the contractile properties of denervated muscles for the restoration of motor function with functional electrical stimulation of muscles.

Several investigators have systematically evaluated the various stimulation parameters to determine the optimal protocol for maintenance of muscle mass and force over prolonged periods of denervation. Dow and colleagues [46] demonstrated that 200 to 1200 contractions per day maintained muscle mass, mean muscle fiber cross sectional area, maximum force, and mRNA expression of myogenin, MyoD, and α-nAchR levels. These results seem promising and demonstrate that muscle mass and force can be maintained over prolonged periods of denervation with electrical stimulation. Unfortunately, to date, no animal studies have demonstrated improved muscle mass and force after muscle reinnervation when electrical stimulation is used as a bridge to reinnervation. The simple maintenance of muscle mass and force through use of electrical stimulation alone does not provide the optimal recovery of muscle function after prolonged periods of denervation.

Trophic support

One method of encouraging muscle to maintain its structural and contractile characteristics in the setting of denervation is to allow the muscle to be temporarily reinnervated by an adjacent sensory nerve. The idea is that the sensory nerve provides trophic support to the muscle during the time period required by the original motor nerve to regenerate and reinnervate the muscle itself. Studies performed on the rat hindlimb demonstrate that compared with controls, muscles that receive trophic support during a period of denervation weigh more, have better preservation of their microscopic structure and fiber type, and maintain a higher isometric force generating capability [47,48]. It seems that trophic support modifies denervation atrophy by altering the expression of neurotrophic factors within the muscle fibers. Although the expression of one factor in particular, glial cell line–derived neurotrophic factor, is transiently down-regulated by trophic support, the mechanism of trophic support has yet to be firmly established [49]. Other experiments involving the rat model have been less promising, with the benefits of trophic support demonstrated early in the motor neuron

reinnervation period but disappearing with time to the point at which functionally there is no significant difference between control and trophic support groups [50].

An analogous theory of trophic support exists for transected motor neurons. The idea is similar: if an environment that supports survival and growth can be maintained for the nerve, it will be more successful at reinnervating its target muscle. Along these lines, the effect of exogenously and endogenously delivered glial cell line–derived neurotrophic factor on transected motor neurons has been studied. Research has demonstrated that neuronal cell death and atrophy are delayed with glial cell line–derived neurotrophic factor administration [51]. Unfortunately, these effects are transient, and by addressing the motor neuron instead of the muscle, this method does little by itself to combat denervation atrophy. Overall, trophic support seems to be of limited benefit in the early time period after denervation and of little to no benefit after 1 to 2 months of denervation.

"Babysitting" procedure and sensory protection

The "babysitting" procedure has been introduced to provide temporary motor innervation during periods of prolonged denervation [52–56]. Motor nerve babysitting was originally described in the treatment of unilateral facial paralysis; temporary innervation of the facial muscles was achieved and maintained through an ipsilateral nerve transfer until axons from a cross facial nerve graft could be used to reinnervate the paralyzed face. Sensory nerve protection also has been used to preserve muscle mass; transient innervation of muscles is preserved through sensory nerve axons until axons from the transected and repaired motor nerve reach the target muscle [57–59]. Unfortunately, the innervated muscle does not become reinnervated by the native motor nerve as long as it is innervated by the "babysitter" or the sensory nerve [60–63]. For motor nerve babysitting and sensory protection, a second episode of denervation and reinnervation is required to permit successful reinnervation by the intended motor nerve. Experiments have demonstrated that two episodes of denervation and reinnervation are deleterious to the recovery of skeletal muscle contractile function (Fig. 4).

Summary

The punch line has not changed: The best recovery after a motor nerve injury is achieved

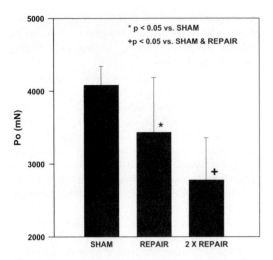

Fig. 4. Force generation in rat extensor digitorum longus (EDL) muscle is plotted on the y axis. Animals in the SHAM group underwent exposure of the peroneal nerve only. In the REPAIR group, the peroneal nerve was cut and repaired and EDL muscle force was measured 60 days later. In the 2xREPAIR group, the peroneal nerve was cut and repaired. Sixty days later, the peroneal nerve was cut and repaired again, and EDL muscle force was measured after a subsequent 60-day recovery. The markedly reduced force in EDL muscles of animals in the 2xREPAIR group indicates that clinical strategies that rely on two cycles of denervation and reinnervation are suboptimal.

only if an abundant supply of motion-specific motor axons is rapidly provided to the muscles denervated as a result of the nerve transection. Denervation results in substantial changes in muscle structure and significant impairments in muscle function. Despite these profound changes, denervated skeletal muscle can become reinnervated as regenerating axons contact denervated muscle fibers and re-establish synaptic function. Atrophy-dependent and atrophy-independent mechanisms contribute to the dysfunction noted in reinnervated muscle; these mechanisms are progressive as denervation time increases. Phenotypic changes in long-term denervated muscle render the muscle fibers unreceptive to the process of synaptogenesis. The clinical consequence is that the quality of recovery in reinnervated muscle is inversely proportional to the denervation interval.

Evidence also demonstrates that the recovery of contractile function depends on an abundant supply of regenerating motor axons. Under circumstances in which the axonal supply is reduced below an ill-defined, "critical" threshold, the

recovery of mechanical function is markedly impacted. Reductions in axonal supply occur clinically when axons are asked to regenerated in an extra-endoneurial environment or across more than one nerve coaptation site. The volitional control of muscles depends on appropriate neural circuitry. Although it cannot be re-established with great precision after peripheral nerve injuries, a significant adaptive capacity of the peripheral and central nervous systems provides for the recovery of useful volitional function if motion-specific axons are provided. For proximal nerve injuries, the long regeneration distances make it difficult or impossible to achieve rapid reinnervation. The complex topography of nerves in the upper portions of the limb makes it difficult, via either nerve repair or nerve grafting, to direct motion-specific axons to specific distal targets. As a consequence, nerve repair and nerve grafting in the proximal extremity have been a great disappointment as strategies for the restoration of distal-limb motor function. Distal nerve transfers allow surgeons to fulfill the optimum conditions for skeletal muscle reinnervation and represent the best current strategy for motor restoration in the setting of proximal limb nerve injuries.

References

[1] Badalamente MA, Hurst LC, Stracher A. Neuromuscular recovery using calcium protease inhibition after median nerve repair in primates. Proc Natl Acad Sci U S A 1989;86(15):5983–7.

[2] Borisov AB, Carlson BM. Cell death in denervated skeletal muscle is distinct from classical apoptosis. Anat Rec 2000;258(3):305–18.

[3] Ashley Z, Sutherland H, Lanmuller H, et al. Atrophy, but not necrosis, in rabbit skeletal muscle denervated for periods up to one year. Am J Physiol Cell Physiol 2007;292(1):440–51.

[4] Lieber RL, Friden JO, Hargens AR, et al. Long-term effects of spinal cord transection on fast and slow rat skeletal muscle. II. Morphometric properties. Exp Neurol 1986;91(3):435–48.

[5] Margreth A, Salviati G, Di Mauro S, et al. Early biochemical consequences of denervation in fast and slow skeletal muscles and their relationship to neural control over muscle differentiation. Biochem J 1972; 126(5):1099–110.

[6] Patterson MF, Stephenson GM, Stephenson DG. Denervation produces different single fiber phenotypes in fast- and slow-twitch hindlimb muscles of the rat. Am J Physiol Cell Physiol 2006;291(3):518–28.

[7] Warszawski M, Telerman-Toppet N, Durdu J, et al. The early stages of neuromuscular regeneration after crushing the sciatic nerve in the

rat: electrophysiological and histological study. J Neurol Sci 1975;24(1):21–32.

[8] Carpenter S, Karpati G. Necrosis of capillaries in denervation atrophy of human skeletal muscle. Muscle Nerve 1982;5(3):250–4.

[9] Borisov AB, Huang SK, Carlson BM. Remodeling of the vascular bed and progressive loss of capillaries in denervated skeletal muscle. Anat Rec 2000;258(3): 292–304.

[10] Lu DX, Huang SK, Carlson BM. Electron microscopic study of long-term denervated rat skeletal muscle. Anat Rec 1997;248(3):355–65.

[11] Sanes JR, Covault J. Axon guidance during reinnervation of skeletal muscle. Trends Neurosci 1985;8: 523–8.

[12] Finol HJ, Lewis DM, Owens R. The effects of denervation on contractile properties of rat skeletal muscle. J Physiol 1981;319:81–92.

[13] Magill CK, Tong A, Kawamura D, et al. Reinnervation of the tibialis anterior following sciatic nerve crush injury: a confocal microscopic study in transgenic mice. Exp Neurol 2007;207(1):64–74.

[14] Bader D. Reinnervation of motor endplate-containing and motor endplate-less muscle grafts. Dev Biol 1980;77(2):315–27.

[15] Cederna PS, Asato H, Gu X, et al. Motor unit properties of nerve-intact extensor digitorum longus muscle grafts in young and old rats. J Gerontol A Biol Sci Med Sci 2001;56(6):B254–8.

[16] Cote C, Faulkner JA. Characteristics of motor units in muscles of rats grafted with nerves intact. Am J Physiol 1986;250(6 Pt 1):828–33.

[17] Brunelli GA, Brunelli GR. Direct muscle neurotization. J Reconstr Microsurg 1993;9(2):81–90.

[18] Mackinnon SE, McLean JA, Hunter GA. Direct muscle neurotization recovers gastrocnemius muscle function. J Reconstr Microsurg 1993;9(2):77–80.

[19] Cederna PS, Youssef MK, Asato H, et al. Skeletal muscle reinnervation by reduced axonal numbers results in whole muscle force deficits. Plast Reconstr Surg 2000;105(6):2003–9.

[20] Aird RB, Naffziger HC. The pathology of human striated muscle following denervation. J Neurosurg 1953;10:216–27.

[21] Birch R, Raji AR. Repair of median and ulnar nerves: primary repair is best. J Bone Joint Surg 1991;73:154–7.

[22] Bowden REM, Gutman E. Denervation and reinnervation of human voluntary muscle. Brain 1944; 67:273.

[23] Gordon T, Stein RB. Time course and extent of recovery in reinnervated motor units of cat triceps surae muscles. J Physiol 1982;323:307–23.

[24] Gutmann E, Young JZ. The reinnervation of muscle after various periods of atrophy. J Anat 1944;78: 15–43.

[25] Kobayashi J, Mackinnon SE, Watanabe O, et al. The effect of duration of muscle denervation on functional recovery in the rat model. Muscle Nerve 1997;20(7):858–66.

[26] Fu SY, Gordon T. Contributing factors to poor functional recovery after delayed nerve repair: prolonged denervation. J Neurosci 1995;15:3886–95.

[27] Grinnell AD. Dynamics of nerve-muscle interaction in developing and mature neuromuscular junctions. Physiol Rev 1995;75:789–834.

[28] Buffelli M, Pasino E, Cangiano A. Paralysis of rat skeletal muscle equally affects contractile properties as does permanent denervation. J Muscle Res Cell Motil 1997;18:683–95.

[29] Gundersen K. Determination of muscle contractile properties: the importance of the nerve. Acta Physiol Scand 1998;162:333–41.

[30] Pette D, Vrbova G. Adaptation of mammalian skeletal muscle fibers to chronic electrical stimulation. Rev Physiol Biochem Pharmacol 1992;120:115–202.

[31] Reid J. On the relation between muscular contractility and the nervous system. The London and Edinburgh Monthly Journal of Medical Science 1841;1:320–9.

[32] Al-Amood WS, Lewis DM. Fast-to-slow transition in myosin heavy chain expression of rabbit muscle fibres induced by chronic low-frequency stimulation. J Physiol 1987;392:377–95.

[33] Andersen JL, Klitgaard H, Saltin B. Myosin heavy chain isoforms in single fibres from m. vastus lateralis of sprinters: influence of training. Acta Physiol Scand 1994;151:135–42.

[34] Buller AJ, Pope R. Plasticity in mammalian skeletal muscle. Philos Trans R Soc Lond B Biol Sci 1977; 278:295–305.

[35] Dennis RG, Dow DE, Faulkner JA. An implantable device for stimulation of denervated muscles in rats. Med Eng Phys 2003;25(3):239–53.

[36] Eken T, Gundersen K. Electrical stimulation resembling normal motor-unit activity: effects on denervated fast and slow rat muscles. J Physiol 1988; 402:651–69.

[37] Gundersen K, Eken T. The importance of frequency and amount of electrical stimulation for contractile properties of denervated rat muscles. Acta Physiol Scand 1992;145:49–57.

[38] Westgaard RH, Lomo T. Control of contractile properties within adaptive ranges by patterns of impulse activity in the rat. J Neurosci 1988;8:4415–26.

[39] Kern H, Hofer C, Strohhofer M, et al. Standing up with denervated muscles in humans using functional electrical stimulation. Artif Organs 1999;23:447–52.

[40] Girlanda P, Dattola R, Vita G, et al. Effect of electrotherapy on denervated muscles in rabbits: an electrophysiological and morphological study. Exp Neurol 1982;77:483–91.

[41] Pachter BR, Eberstein A, Goodgold J. Electrical stimulation effect on denervated skeletal myofibers in rats: a light and electron microscopic study. Arch Phys Med Rehabil 1982;63:427–30.

[42] Schmalbruch H, Al-Amood WS, Lewis DM. Morphology of long-term denervated rat soleus muscle and the effect of chronic electrical stimulation. J Physiol 1991;441:233–41.

[43] Goldman D, Brenner HR, Heinemann S. Acetylcholine receptor alpha-, beta-, gamma-, and delta-subunit mRNA levels are regulated by muscle activity. Neuron 1988;1:329–33.

[44] Neville CM, Schmidt M, Schmidt J. Response of myogenic determination factors to cessation and resumption of electrical activity in skeletal muscle: a possible role for myogenin in denervation supersensitivity. Cell Mol Neurobiol 1992;12(6):511–27.

[45] Eftimie R, Brenner HR, Buonanno A. Myogenin and MyoD join a family of skeletal muscle genes regulated by electrical activity. Proc Natl Acad Sci U S A 1991;88:1349–53.

[46] Dow DE, Cederna PS, Hassett CA, et al. Number of contractions to maintain mass and force of denervated rat EDL muscles. Muscle Nerve 2004;30: 77–86.

[47] Bain JR, Veltri KL, Chamberlain D, et al. Improved functional recovery of denervated skeletal muscle after temporary sensory nerve innervation. Neuroscience 2001;103(2):503–10.

[48] Veltri K, Kwiecien JM, Minet W, et al. Contribution of the distal nerve sheath to nerve and muscle preservation following denervation and sensory protection. J Reconstr Microsurg 2005;21(1):57–70 [discussion: 71–4].

[49] Zhao C, Veltri K, Li S, et al. NGF, BDNF, NT-3, and GDNF mRNA expression in rat skeletal muscle following denervation and sensory protection. J Neurotrauma 2004;21(10):1468–78.

[50] Papakonstantinou KC, Kamin E, Terzis JK. Muscle preservation by prolonged sensory protection. J Reconstr Microsurg 2002;18(3):173–82 [discussion: 183–4].

[51] Hottinger AF, Azzouz M, Deglon N, et al. Complete and long-term rescue of lesioned adult motoneurons by lentiviral-mediated expression of glial cell line-derived neurotrophic factor in the facial nucleus. J Neurosci 2000;20:5587–93.

[52] Endo T, Hata J, Nakayama Y. Variations on the "baby-sitter" procedure for reconstruction of facial paralysis. J Reconstr Microsurg 2000;16:37–43.

[53] Kalantarian B, Rice DC, Tiangco DA, et al. Gains and losses of the XII-VII component of the "baby-sitter" procedure: a morphometric analysis. J Reconstr Microsurg 1998;14:459–71.

[54] Mersa B, Tiangco DA, Terzis JK. Efficacy of the "baby-sitter" procedure after prolonged denervation. J Reconstr Microsurg 2000;16:27–35.

[55] Terzis JK. "Babysitters": an exciting new concept in facial reanimation. In: Castro D, editor. Proceedings of the sixth international symposium on the facial nerve. Rio de Janeiro (Brazil): Kulger and Ghedini; 1988.

[56] Terzis JK, Sweet RC, Dykes RW, et al. Recovery of function in free muscle transplants using microneurovascular anastomoses. J Hand Surg [Am] 1978;3: 37–59.

[57] Hynes NM, Bain JR, Thoma A, et al. Preservation of denervated muscle by sensory protection in rats. J Reconstr Microsurg 1997;13:337–43.

[58] Ochi M, Kwong WH, Kimori K, et al. Delay of the denervation process in skeletal muscle by sensory ganglion graft and its clinical application. Plast Reconstr Surg 1996;97:577–86.

[59] Zhang F, Lineaweaver WC, Ustuner T, et al. Comparison of muscle mass preservation in denervated muscle and transplanted muscle flaps after motor and sensory reinnervation and neurotization. Plast Reconstr Surg 1997;99:803–14.

[60] Elsberg CA. Experiments on motor nerve regeneration and the direct neurotization of paralysed muscles by their own and foreign nerves. Science 1917; 45:318–20.

[61] Bennett MR. Development of neuromuscular synapses. Physiol Rev 1983;63:915–1048.

[62] Covault J, Sanes JR. Neural cell adhesion molecule (N-CAM) accumulates in denervated and paralyzed skeletal muscles. Proc Natl Acad Sci U S A 1985;82: 4544–8.

[63] Lieber RL. Skeletal muscle structure and function. Baltimore (MD): Williams and Wilkins; 1992 248–57.

End-to-Side Nerve Repair: Review of the Literature and Clinical Indications

Linda T. Dvali, MD[a],*, Terence M. Myckatyn, MD[b]

[a]Division of Plastic and Reconstructive Surgery, University of Toronto, University Health Network,
Toronto Western Division, 2-400, 399 Bathurst Street, Toronto, Ontario, M5T 2S8, Canada
[b]Division of Plastic and Reconstructive Surgery, Washington University School of Medicine, Suite 17424 East Pavilion,
One Barnes Jewish Hospital Plaza, St. Louis, MO 63110, USA

End-to-side (ETS) nerve repair involves coapting the distal stump of a transected nerve to the side of a donor nerve. Attachment to the donor nerve may occur either without alteration of the donor nerve or in conjunction with the creation of some form of injury (deliberate or nondeliberate) to the donor nerve. This technique was described over a century ago as a reconstructive strategy for facial nerve injury and brachial plexus avulsion injuries [1–3]. However, the technique never gained wide popularity. The introduction of the microscope and improving microscopic techniques revolutionized the methods of primary repair and interpositional nerve grafting and likely explain why ETS techniques were not initially adapted [4,5]. The ETS technique was revived in the early 1990s when Viterbo and colleagues [6–8] demonstrated histologic and electrophysiologic evidence of reinnervation into the distal stump in a rat model. The benefits of reviving the ETS technique seem obvious given its use where traditional nerve repair and grafting are unavailable or likely to result in poor functional outcomes. For example, it can be used in injuries where the proximal stump of an injured nerve is unavailable or distant to its end target, or in the case of a long nerve gap. Additionally donor site morbidity associated with nerve graft harvest can be avoided. This article evaluates recent studies on ETS repair, focusing on evidence for collateral sprouting, the role of the epineurial or perineurial windows in ETS repairs, sensory versus motor regeneration after ETS repair, and recommendations regarding the current clinical applications for ETS techniques.

The exact cellular processes that occur in the donor nerve after ETS nerve repair are the subjects of continued controversy. The main area of controversy concerns the proposed source of regenerating axons into the distal nerve following ETS repair. In general, there are three possibilities: (1) invasion from the transected proximal stump of the injured nerve, (2) regeneration from donor nerve axons that were damaged during nerve preparation, or (3) regeneration from true "collateral sprouting" from the ETS site.

The term "collateral sprouting" implies spontaneous, de novo sprouting of nerve axons in the absence of nerve injury. The concept of axonal sprouting in the absence of injury is controversial but, in mylenated nerves, it is thought to arise from the nodes of Ranvier just proximal to the level of the coaptation. "Regenerative sprouting," in contrast, occurs in response to nerve injury and, according to widely accepted opinions, in both ETS and end-to-end models of nerve reconstruction. For the purposes of this article, we will specifically refer to "spontaneous collateral sprouting" if no nerve injury is implied, and "regenerative sprouting" when axonal disruption is suspected. Spontaneous collateral sprouting, without any evidence of nerve injury, is yet to be conclusively proven in the literature.

The presence of axons within a recipient nerve after ETS repair is often presented as supporting evidence for collateral sprouting. While these axons may represent true collateral sprouting, they may also be false-positive results. Other

* Corresponding author.
E-mail address: linda.dvali@uhn.on.ca (L.T. Dvali).

sources of regenerating axons include contamination from the proximal stump in experimental models, or "regenerative sprouts" from inadvertent axonal injury. ETS repairs have been primarily studied in the rat, where the distance between the "proximal injury" and the recipient nerve is extremely short [9]. In models where the donor and recipient nerves are close to each other, such as peroneal recipient nerves and tibial nerve donors, regenerating axons may originate from the proximal stump of the transected nerve. This stump may project axons within or along donor nerve fasicles or epineurium. Contamination of this type has been noted histologically [10–13] and efforts have been made to rule out contamination from proximal stump axons in a number of studies [14–17]. Double-labeling experiments in animals have been used to exclude the possibility of proximal stump contamination and provide evidence for collateral sprouting. The labeling of cell bodies in dorsal root ganglia (sensory) or the ventral horn (motor) can be achieved when different tracers are injected at the level of the donor nerve and distal to the coaptation site and allowed to be transported retrograde to the appropriate area of brain. This technique eliminates the proximal stump as a source of axons because the tracer is only injected into the donor and recipient nerve. However, the use of double-labeling techniques cannot remove the other potential source of false-positive results, namely, regenerative sprouts from inadvertent axonal injury. In fact, a double-labeled axon may be explained either by a spontaneous collateral sprout, or by a regenerating unit with multiple daughter axons traveling down various paths, each capable of transporting a retrograde tracer. As a result, in most published studies on ETS repairs currently available, ETS nerve repair with deliberate axotomy and may not be distinguishable as a separate procedure from ETS nerve repair without deliberate axotomy [5].

Regenerative sprouts from inadvertent or unintentional axotomy are a recognized source of regenerating axons. ETS repairs are commonly performed with the creation of an epinurial or perineurial window. In these procedures, no deliberate attempt to injure the nerve is made. However, evaluation of donor nerves and the muscles that they innervate after ETS repair with epinurial or perineurial window has shown histologic evidence of axonal degeneration [18] and denervated muscle fibers [19], suggesting inadvertent axotomy despite good technique.

Although some studies initially suggested that the conjunctival layers of peripheral nerve simply represent a barrier to regenerating axons [20–22], axonal injury after creation of an epineurial or perineurial window is well established. In 1975, Spencer and colleagues [23] demonstrated that a perineurial window resulted in a localized region of demyelination with a small degree of Wallerian degeneration. Further studies have characterized the histologic and functional evidence of injury following short (1 mm) and long (5 mm) perineurial windows [24]. The length of injury to the blood–nerve barrier and the presence of Wallerian degeneneration are more pronounced in the longer perineurial window, suggesting greater injury. Therefore, removal of the conjunctival layers of the nerve does not simply eliminate a physical barrier, but likely creates some form of inadvertent axonal injury that is a source of regenerating axons. Unless a truly atraumatic coaptation (fibrin glue, biologic coaptations) is used, inadvertent axon disruption can never be eliminated as a potential source of regenerating axons [10,25–27].

Sensory versus motor regeneration after end-to-side repair

Given the wide interest in ETS techniques since 1992, many experimental and clinical studies of the technique have been performed with differing results. Many of the published studies suffer from the various limitations already discussed in this article, namely that proximal contamination could not be ruled out or that true "de novo" collateral sprouting could not be excluded from nondeliberate axonal injury. Deliberate axonal injury in ETS techniques always induces axonal regeneration, but with varying, unpredictable morbidity to the donor nerve.

Histologic examination of the dorsal root ganglia and ventral horn after retrograde tracing of the terminal limb of an ETS repair shows tracer within dorsal root ganglia by 4 weeks after the repair [23,28,29]. When retrograde labeling techniques are employed, ventral horn (motor) staining was frequently noted to be reduced [30], variable [31], or nearly absent [32,33]. We recently compared regenerating motor axons versus sensory axons across ETS nerve repairs with varying degrees of axonal injury [34]. Retrograde labeling was essentially confined to sensory dorsal root ganglia neurons in ETS repairs without deliberate axonal injury. These findings suggest that sensory sprouts are more likely than motor sprouts

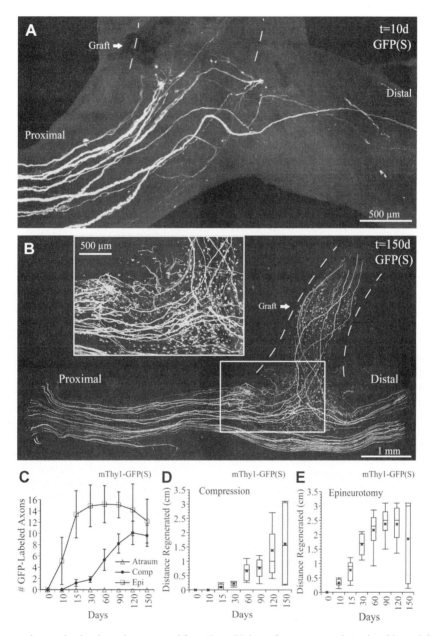

Fig. 1. No axonal sprouting has been demonstrated for at least 30 days after reconstruction using this noninjurious ETS technique in this green fluorescent protein (GFP) transgenic mouse line, suggesting the reliance of ETS repair on axotomy to produce axonal sprouting. (*A*) Ten days following epineurotomy, growth cones with clear injury-induced sprouting are shown. (*B*) At 150 days, the number of axons populating the terminal limb approximates the net donor nerve deficit. (*C*) Injury-induced sprouting occurs with a traumatic ETS repair only. (*D*) Box plots in compressive and (*E*) epineurotomy forms of ETS repair further illustrate the need for donor nerve injury to induce sprouting. (*From* Hayashi A, Pannucci C, Moradzadeh A, et al. Axotomy or compression are required for axonal sprouting following end-to-side neurorrhaphy. Exp Neurol 2008;211:544; with permission.)

following ETS repair. Several explanations for these findings are possible: (1) Retrograde tracers may be more efficiently transported or administered to sensory than to motor fibers; (2) sensory fibers are more abundant than motor fibers; or (3) spontaneous collateral sprouting can only occur at the nodes of Ranvier in myelinated axons (all motor nerves), but essentially anywhere along unmyelinated fibers (some sensory afferents) [29]. Few animal studies of functional sensory return have been conducted because of the difficulty characterizing functional recovery in animal models [20,35]. Several reports of upper extremity ETS repairs have shown return of protective sensation in the median [36–38], ulnar [39], and radial [39] nerve distributions. Mennen [40] notes two-point discrimination of 3 mm 2 years after ETS repair. Considering all available information regarding sensory recovery after ETS nerve repair, we concluded the clinical role for ETS nerve repair, without deliberate nerve injury, is limited and should currently only be used to reconstruct noncritical sensory deficits.

With one exception, virtually all published animal studies demonstrating motor regeneration after ETS used a model that likely included non-deliberate injury to axons [14,16,20,41–47]. That exception is Hayashi and colleagues [26]. Hayashi and colleagues report two noninjurious models of ETS coaptation using a sciatic nerve graft separated in the midline and reapproximated distally after enveloping the median nerve or using spinal aponeurosis in the coaptation of a nerve graft ETS to the median nerve. Both groups show regenerating axons in the graft not significantly different from the control ETS with a perineurial window group. Stimulation of the graft produced contraction of median nerve innervated muscles bilaterally, indicating dual innervation. Fluorescence staining to localize sprouting axons suggests collateral sprouting in the spinal aponeuosis group. The results of this study indicated particularly high axon counts in the recipient nerve. These counts were even higher than those noted in uninjured donor nerves. This study has recently been repeated using *Thy1-GFP(S)* mice. These mice express green fluorescent protein in 10% or less of motor axons [48], enabling serial imaging of regeneration in living animals [49]. No axonal sprouting has been demonstrated for at least 30 days after reconstruction using this noninjurious ETS technique in this transgenic mouse line (Fig. 1), suggesting the reliance of ETS repair on axotomy to produce axonal sprouting.

Clinical cases using ETS repairs have also been published [40,50–53]. In these cases, motor regeneration is reported as being present. However, overall, the functional results are questionable. Given a full review of the experimental literature and clinical experience, ETS repair without deliberate nerve injury should not be used to obtain useful motor recovery. ETS with deliberate axonal injury produces unreliable results and may cause unpredictable donor dysfunction.

Summary

Our evaluation of the literature suggests that the presence and degree of motor sprouting with ETS repair depends on the degree of motor nerve injury, while sensory sprouting is less dependent on nerve injury. Given this finding, we suggest that nerve transfers using carefully selected fascicles with well-defined nerve topography currently provide a more reproducible method of recruiting donor axons with less risk of donor nerve dysfunction and morbidity [54,55]. For sensory reconstruction, the clinical role for ETS nerve repair without deliberate nerve injury should be limited to the reconstruction of noncritical sensory deficits.

Future experimental studies should focus on animal models of noninjurious ETS coaptation. Such studies will help further clarify the mechanism of true collateral sprouting while eliminating false-positive results from contaminating axons. At present, experimental and clinical experience with ETS neurorrhaphy has rendered at best mixed results and more extensive clinical and laboratory experimentation is required before ETS neurorrhaphy can be included with the more established techniques of nerve repair.

References

[1] Ballance CA, Ballance HA, Stewart P. Operative treatment of chronic facial palsy of peripheral origin. Br Med J 1903;2:1009–13.

[2] Harris W, Low VW. On the importance of accurate muscular analysis in lesions of the brachial plexus and the treatment of Erb's palsy and infantile paralysis of the upper extremity by cross-union of the nerve roots. British Medical Journal 1903;24: 1035–8.

[3] Kennedy RA, McKendrick. On the restoration of co-ordinated movements after nerve-crossing, with interchange of function of the cerebral cortical centres. Philos Trans R Soc Lond B Biol Sci 1901; 194:127–62.

[4] Al-Qattan MM. Terminolateral neurorrhaphy: review of experimental and clinical studies. J Reconstr Microsurg 2001;17:99–108.

[5] Rovak JM, Cederna PS, Kuzon WM Jr. Terminolateral neurorrhaphy: a review of the literature. J Reconstr Microsurg 2001;17:615–24.

[6] Viterbo F, Trindade JC, Hoshino K, et al. Two end-to-side neurorrhaphies and nerve graft with removal of the epineural sheath: experimental study in rats. Br J Plast Surg 1994;47:75–80.

[7] Viterbo F, Trindade JC, Hoshino K, et al. Latero-terminal neurorrhaphy without removal of the epineural sheath. Experimental study in rats. Rev Paul Med 1992;110:267–75.

[8] Viterbo F, Trindade JC, Hoshino K, et al. End-to-side neurorrhaphy with removal of the epineurial sheath: an experimental study in rats. Plast Reconstr Surg 1994;94:1038–47.

[9] Al-Qattan M, Al-Thunayan A. Variables affecting axonal regeneration following end-to-side neurorrhaphy. Br J Plast Surg 1998;51:238–42.

[10] Matsumoto M, Hirata H, Nishiyama M, et al. Schwann cells can induce collateral sprouting from intact axons: experimental study of end-to-side neurorrhaphy using a Y-chamber model. J Reconstr Microsurg 1999;15:281–6.

[11] McCallister WV, Tang P, Smith J, et al. Axonal regeneration stimulated by the combination of nerve growth factor and ciliary neurotrophic factor in an end-to-side model. J Hand Surg [Am] 2001;26:478–88.

[12] McCallister WV, Tang P, Trumble TE. Is end-to-side neurorrhaphy effective? A study of axonal sprouting stimulated from intact nerves. J Reconstr Microsurg 1999;15:597–603 [discussion: 603].

[13] Tham SK, Morrison WA. Motor collateral sprouting through an end-to-side nerve repair. J Hand Surg [Am] 1998;23:844–51.

[14] Bontioti E, Kanje M, Lundborg G, et al. End-to-side nerve repair in the upper extremity of rat. J Peripher Nerv Syst 2005;10:58–68.

[15] Sanapanich K, Morrison WA, Messina A. Physiologic and morphologic aspects of nerve regeneration after end-to-end or end-to-side coaptation in a rat model of brachial plexus injury. J Hand Surg [Am] 2002;27:133–42.

[16] Goheen-Robillard B, Myckatyn TM, Mackinnon SE, et al. End-to-side neurorrhaphy and lateral axonal sprouting in a long graft rat model. Laryngoscope 2002;112:899–905.

[17] Rovak JM, Cederna PS, Macionis V, et al. Terminolateral neurorrhaphy: the functional axonal anatomy. Microsurgery 2000;20:6–14.

[18] Noah EM, Williams A, Fortes W, et al. A new animal model to investigate axonal sprouting after end-to-side neurorrhaphy. J Reconstr Microsurg 1997;13:317–25.

[19] Cederna PS, Kalliainen LK, Urbanchek MG, et al. "Donor" muscle structure and function after end-

[20] Bertelli JA, Soares dos Santos AR, Calixto JB. Is axonal sprouting able to traverse the conjunctival layers of the peripheral nerve? A behavioral, motor, and sensory study of end-to-side nerve anastomosis. J Reconstr Microsurg 1996;12:559–63.

[21] Zhang Z, Soucacos PN, Bo J, et al. Reinnervation after end-to-side nerve coaptation in a rat model. Am J Orthop 2001;30:400–6 [discussion: 407].

[22] Zhao JZ, Chen ZW, Chen TY. Nerve regeneration after terminolateral neurorrhaphy: experimental study in rats. J Reconstr Microsurg 1997;13:31–7.

[23] Spencer PS, Weinberg HJ, Raine CS, et al. The perineurial window—a new model of focal demyelination and remyelination. Brain Res 1975;96:323–9.

[24] Walker JC, Brenner MJ, Mackinnon SE, et al. Effect of perineurial window size on nerve regeneration, blood–nerve barrier integrity, and functional recovery. J Neurotrauma 2004;21:217–27.

[25] Yamauchi T, Maeda M, Tamai S, et al. Collateral sprouting mechanism after end-to-side nerve repair in the rat. Med Electron Microsc 2000;33:151–6.

[26] Hayashi A, Yanai A, Komuro Y, et al. Collateral sprouting occurs following end-to-side neurorrhaphy. Plast Reconstr Surg 2004;114:129–37.

[27] Gurney ME, Yamamoto H, Kwon Y. Induction of motor neuron sprouting in vivo by ciliary neurotrophic factor and basic fibroblast growth factor. J Neurosci 1992;12:3241–7.

[28] Mackinnon SE, Dellon AL, O'Brien JP. Changes in nerve fiber numbers distal to a nerve repair in the rat sciatic nerve model. Muscle Nerve 1991;14:1116–22.

[29] Sorkin LS, Wallace MS. Acute pain mechanisms. Surg Clin North Am 1999;79:213–29.

[30] Chen YG, Brushart TM. The effect of denervated muscle and Schwann cells on axon collateral sprouting. J Hand Surg [Am] 1998;23:1025–33.

[31] Kanje M, Arai T, Lundborg G. Collateral sprouting from sensory and motor axons into an end to side attached nerve segment. Neuroreport. 2000;11:2455–9.

[32] Tarasidis G, Watanabe O, Mackinnon SE, et al. End-to-side neurorrhaphy resulting in limited sensory axonal regeneration in a rat model. Ann Otol Rhinol Laryngol 1997;106:506–12.

[33] Tarasidis G, Watanabe O, Mackinnon SE, et al. End-to-side neurorraphy: a long-term study of neural regeneration in a rat model. Otolaryngol Head Neck Surg 1998;119:337–41.

[34] Brenner MJ, Dvali L, Hunter DA, et al. Motor neuron regeneration through end-to-side repairs is a function of donor nerve axotomy. Plast Reconstr Surg 2007;120(1):215–23.

[35] Kovacic U, Bajrovic F, Sketelj J. Recovery of cutaneous pain sensitivity after end-to-side nerve repair in the rat. J Neurosurg 1999;91:857–62.

[36] Kostakoglu N. Motor and sensory reinnervation in the hand after an end-to-side median to ulnar nerve

coaptation in the forearm. Br J Plast Surg 1999;52:
404–7.

[37] Ogun TC, Ozdemir M, Senaran H, et al. End-to-side
neurorrhaphy as a salvage procedure for irreparable
nerve injuries. Technical note. J Neurosurg 2003;99:
180–5.

[38] Ulkur E, Yuksel F, Acikel C, et al. Comparison of
functional results of nerve graft, vein graft, and
vein filled with muscle graft in end-to-side neurorrhaphy. Microsurgery 2003;23:40–8.

[39] Yuksel F, Peker F, Celikoz B. Two applications of
end-to-side nerve neurorrhaphy in severe upper-
extremity nerve injuries. Microsurgery 2004;24:
363–8.

[40] Mennen U. End-to-side nerve suture—a technique
to repair peripheral nerve injury. S Afr Med J
1999;89:1188–94.

[41] De Sa J, Mazzer N, Barbieri C, et al. The end-to-side
peripheral nerve repair: functional and morphometric study using the peroneal nerve of rats. J Neurosci
Methods 2004;136:45–53.

[42] Sundine MJ, Quan EE, Saglam O, et al. The use of
end-to-side nerve grafts to reinnervate the paralyzed
orbicularis oculi muscle. Plast Reconstr Surg 2003;
111:2255–64.

[43] Sato T, Konishi F, Kanazawa K. End-to-side
pudendal nerve anastomosis for the creation of
a new reinforcing anal sphincter in dogs. Surgery
2000;127:92–8.

[44] Lutz BS, Wei FC, Ma SF, et al. Effects of insu-
lin-like growth factor-1 in motor nerve regeneration after nerve transection and repair vs. nerve
crushing injury in the rat. Acta Neurochir 1999;
141:1101–6.

[45] Mennen U. End-to-side nerve suture in the primate
(chacma baboon). Hand Surg 1998;3:1–6.

[46] Oppenheim RW, Houenou LJ, Parsadanian AS,
et al. Glial cell line–derived neurotrophic factor
and developing mammalian motoneurons: regulation of programmed cell death among motoneuron
subtypes. J Neurosci 2000;20:5001–11.

[47] Palazzi S, Vila-Torres J, Lorenzo JC. Fibrin glue is
a sealant and not a nerve barrier. J Reconstr Microsurg 1995;11:135–9.

[48] Feng G, Mellor RH, Bernstein M, et al. Imaging neuronal subsets in transgenic mice expressing multiple
spectral variants of GFP. Neuron 2000;28:41–51.

[49] Myckatyn TM, Mackinnon SE, Hunter DA, et al.
A novel model for the study of peripheral-nerve
regeneration following common nerve injury para-
digms. J Reconstr Microsurg 2004;20:533–44.

[50] Mennen U. End-to-side nerve suture in the human
patient. Hand Surg 1998;3:7–15.

[51] Mennen U, van der Westhuizen MJ, Eggers IM.
Re-innervation of M. biceps by end-to-side nerve
suture. Hand Surg 2003;8:25–31.

[52] Viterbo F, Franciosi LF, Palhares A. Nerve graft-
ings and end-to-side neurorrhaphies connecting the
phrenic nerve to the brachial plexus. Plast Reconstr
Surg 1995;96:494–5.

[53] Amr SM, Moharram AN. Repair of brachial plexus
lesions by end-to-side side-to-side grafting neurorrhaphy: experience based on 11 cases. Microsurgery
2005;25:126–46.

[54] Tung TH, Mackinnon SE. Flexor digitorum superficialis nerve transfer to restore pronation: two case
reports and anatomic study. J Hand Surg [Am]
2001;26:1065–72.

[55] Tung TH, Novak CB, Mackinnon SE. Nerve transfers to the biceps and brachialis branches to improve
elbow flexion strength after brachial plexus injuries.
J Neurosurg 2003;98:313–8.

ELSEVIER
SAUNDERS

Hand Clin 24 (2008) 461–483

HAND
CLINICS

Nerve Fiber Transfer by End-to-Side Coaptation

Hanno Millesi, MD[a,*], Robert Schmidhammer, MD[a,b]

[a]Millesi Center, Vienna Private Clinic, Pelikangasse 15, A-1090 Vienna, Austria
[b]Austrian Cluster for Tissue Regeneration, Ludwig Boltzmann Institute for Experimental and Clinical Traumatology,
Research Center for Traumatology, Austrian Workers' Compensation Board, Vienna, Austria

In 1994, at a meeting in New York organized by Berish Strauch, Viterbo and colleagues [1] presented his experiments and first experimental results with end-to-side nerve coaptation, which had been published in 1992. In spite of great skepticism, the surgical community reacted quickly and a few years later a series of experimental papers appeared [2–5] confirming the occurrence of something like neurotization of a denervated peripheral stump coapted end-to-side to an innervated nerve. However, in subsequent years, disagreements among researchers emerged with all the passion of debates between religious fundamentalists.

In 1997, one of the authors of this article, Millesi, became interested in using end-to-side coaptation in brachial plexus surgery, and acquired clinical experience related to the procedure over the years. Both authors performed experiments with baboons to collect data and to find new applications because it was obvious that nerve fiber transfer using end-to-side coaptation would always yield results inferior to those with classical techniques of nerve repair.

To what degree "nerve specialists" were prejudiced against end-to-side coaptation is illustrated by a remark of a reviewer of the authors' first experimental paper. The reviewer noted: "I have a bias against end-to-side coaptation" and criticized the paper for using the term "Riche-Cannieu anastomosis." The paper was rejected for these and other minor reasons. Millesi was informed by the nerve specialist reviewing the paper that the term "anastomosis" should not be used in peripheral nerve surgery. Apparently the specialist had

no knowledge of well-established terms in the anatomic literature, such as Martin-Gruber anastomosis or anastomosis of Riche-Cannieu. To bring some light into the ongoing controversy, the authors organized a symposium in 2006 titled *How To Improve Peripheral Nerve Surgery*. The authors sought the participation of experienced surgeons and researchers who had made personal contributions in the field. This article contains information collected at this symposium.

This article also presents the authors' clinical results and ideas illustrating the potential of nerve fiber transfer by end-to-side coaptation.

Definitions

Before going into detail, it may be useful to clarify some terms.

The term *neurotization* means ingrowth of nerve fibers into a territory deprived of nerve fibers. After Wallerian degeneration, a distal stump of a transected peripheral nerve is denervated. After a neurorrhaphy, the distal stump becomes neurotisized again (nerve-to-nerve neurotization) by neurons supplying the original nerve.

If another donor nerve is used, one performs a neurotization by nerve transfer of axons from another zone of neurons to supply the end organs of the distal stump.

Neurotization of the denervated distal stump is the aim of the procedure, neurorrhaphy or nerve grafting is the procedure itself, and nerve transfer refers to the origin of the nerve fibers.

The precision of these terms is important because the term *neurotization* has been imprecisely used as a synonym for nerve transfer.

If a denervated muscle is in close contact with an innervated muscle without a fascia in between,

* Corresponding author.
E-mail address: millesi@wpk.at (H. Millesi).

0749-0712/08/$ - see front matter © 2008 Published by Elsevier Inc.
doi:10.1016/j.hcl.2008.04.007

nerve fibers sprout from the small branches of the innervated muscle to the denervated muscle (muscle-to-muscle neurotization). Muscle-to-muscle neurotization also works when a small segment of muscle tissue from the lower lip is transferred with preserved blood supply to the upper lip. Nerve fibers from the innervated left orbicularis oris superior are, however, not able to neurotisize the denervated right orbicularis oris superior muscle in a right facial nerve paralysis, an indication that factors we do not understand play an important role.

In an accessory nerve lesion, the major part of the trapezius muscle becomes paralyzed. If there is a ramus trapezius of the cervical plexus, the whole or an important part of the trapezius muscle may be neurotisized by axon sprouts from the small nerve branches of the ramus trapezius within the muscle (internal muscular neurotization).

In summary, neurotization can follow any of a number of actions. A surgeon can induce neurotization, but neurotization can also develop spontaneously if supported by the anatomy.

Nerve (fiber) transfer by end-to-side coaptation means in our context stimulation of the neurotization of a denervated nerve by coapting it end-to-side to an innervated nerve directly or via a graft to restore the function of this nerve and simultaneously preserve the function of the donor nerve.

The problems

When surgeons realized that nerve fiber transfer by end-to-side coaptation offers realistic potential, an enormous feeling of optimism arose. Millesi's first contact with end-to-side coaptation were cases originating outside of Austria of partial brachial plexus in whom the surgeon did not do complicated reconstructive procedures, such as nerve grafts, but simply created an epineurial and a perineurial window in an innervated trunk and coapted a denervated trunk end-to-side to it.

Brachial plexus surgery seamed to become a very simple surgical technique. All these cases operated upon elsewhere failed. It can be understood that a prejudice developed against this useless simplification.

Does end-to-side coaptation exist at all?

There is an outspoken group of surgeons respectively researchers who deny the existence of fiber sprouting after end-to-side coaptation. A pioneer of this group, Fernandez [6], holds the

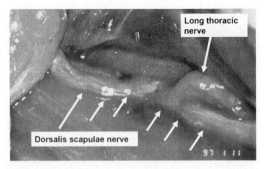

Fig. 1. This patient suffered a complete brachial plexus lesion with multiple avulsions. A multiple nerve grafting procedure was performed on January 11, 1997, involving nerve fiber transfer by end-to-side coaptation of the distal stump of the denervated long thoracic nerves to the innervated dorsalis scapulae nerve. The serratus anterior showed a function of M3 according to the Medical Research Council scale 13 months after surgery.

view that end-to-side coaptation without a perineurial window is impossible because the perineurium is too thick to be penetrated by axon sprouts. In his view, any injury to the perineurium may cause injury to nerve fibers and this causes axon sprouting as in a partial nerve lesion. Successful nerve fiber transfer by end-to-side coaptation represents, therefore, a partial end-to-end coaptation. Fernandez writes: "Such procedure appears justified only in an investigational setting."

Does end-to-side coaptation exist and does it provide useful recovery?

A second group of researchers and surgeons look to the example of Frey and colleagues [7], who successfully innervated a free functional muscle graft by end-to-side coaptation of the muscle

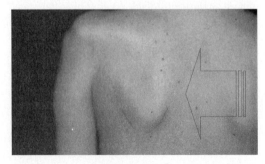

Fig. 2. The patient suffers from a brachial plexus lesion on the left side. Avulsion of the C5, C6, and C7 roots was found. A scapula alata on the left side (*arrow*) is shown preoperatively.

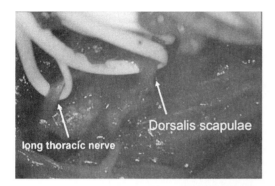

Fig. 3. Exploration of the brachial plexus reveals close proximity of the long thoracic nerve and the dorsal scapular nerve running parallel.

branch to an intact motor nerve with full preservation of the donor nerve. This group holds the view that mainly sensory nerve fibers sprout across an end-to-side coaptation [4,8–13].

Lutz and colleagues [10] reported that motor recovery in rats using a perineurial window was on average 70% greater than that with end-to-end neurorrhaphy. However, functional results were unpredictable. In research on rabbits, Jaberi and colleagues [14] reported recovery, but not sufficient enough to be functional.

Dahlin, who has been involved in many studies on end-to-side coaptation [15–18], also presented at the 2006 symposium [19]. He reported on experiments with rats where the musculocutaneous nerve was used as axon donor, and the radial nerve, ulnar nerve, and median nerve were used as recipient nerves creating an epineurial window [19]. For useful recovery, an injury of the donor nerve by the end-to-site coaptation is necessary.

End-to-side can initiate cell activation, such as nuclear translocation of the activating transcription factor 3 (ATF 3) [20] in sensory neurons in the dorsal root ganglion, in motor neurons in the spinal cord, and in nonneuronal cells, such as Schwann cells, in the donor nerve trunk [16]. ATF 3 is a marker of stress response in a cell and occurs in neurons that regenerate. Putting a piece of nerve alongside a nerve does not induce any activation. Creating an epineurial window with or without attachment of a piece of nerve alongside induces ATF 3 in neurons and nonneuronal cells. This indicates that Wallerian degeneration of such nerve fibers may occur [21].

Wiberg's group [22] experimented with baboons, coapting median to ulnar nerve and vice versa creating an epineurial window. Regeneration occurred but was very variable.

Battiston and colleagues [23] mixed peripheral nerves in humans. Useful regeneration occurred in 20% of cases.

The opinion of this second group can be summarized: Something happens but the functional results are unpredictable. The common feature of all these experiments is the execution with mixed nerve trunks.

Origin of the sprouts

The discussion varies between terminal and collateral sprouting.

Terzis observed, after end-to-side coaptation, that double-labeled neurons appeared as an expression of collateral sprouting in 50% of the fibers.

Lars Dahlin and colleagues [19] observed only few double-labeled neurons, but nevertheless

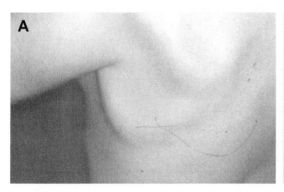

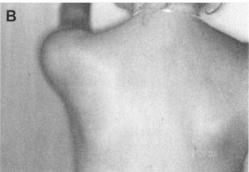

Fig. 4. (A) The movement of the inferior angle of the left scapula 3 months after nerve fiber transfer by end-to-side coaptation of the long thoracic nerve to the dorsal scapula nerve. (B) No scapula alata on the left side is seen 7 months after nerve fiber transfer.

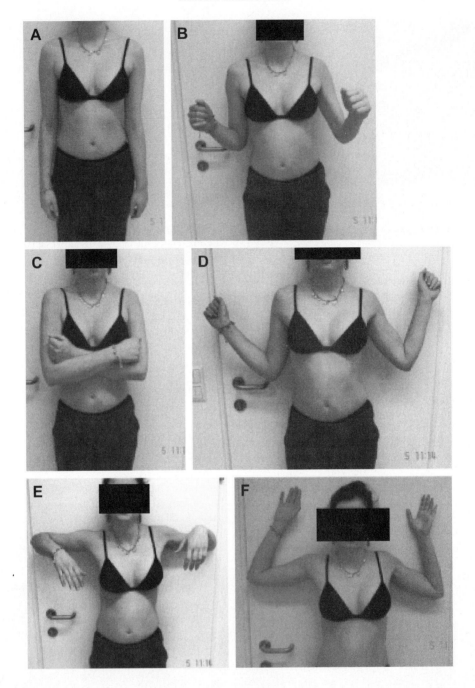

Fig. 5. (*A–S*) The chains of movements of the scapula during external rotation and elbow flexion, elbow flexion and internal rotation, abduction and external rotation, abduction and internal rotation, anteversion, anteversion, and pressing against a wall develop in a smooth and a more-or-less normal way. Minimal protrusion of the inferior angle of the scapula occurs only in certain phases.

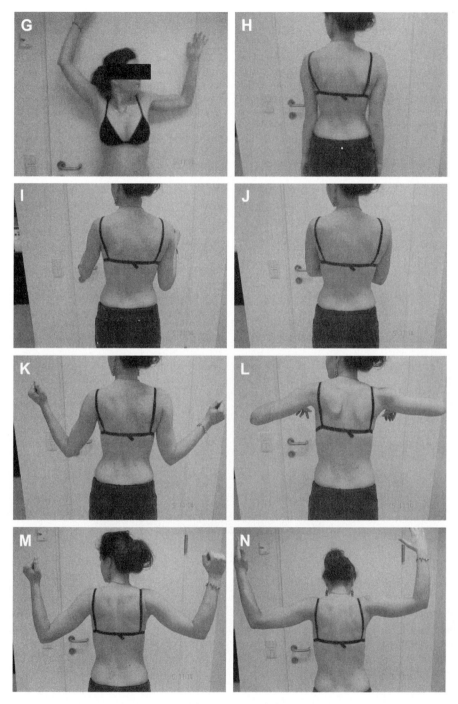

Fig. 5 (*continued*)

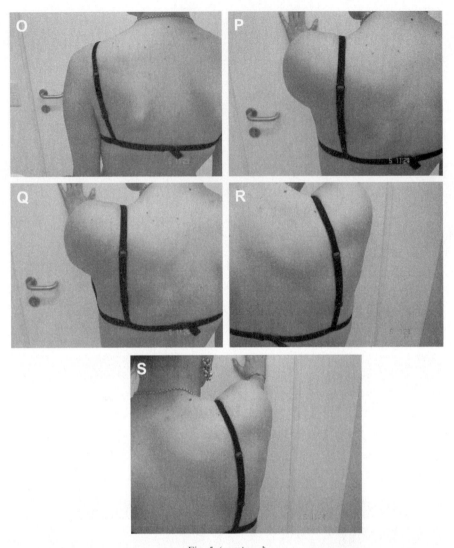

Fig. 5 (*continued*)

proved the presence of some. The difference between the observations of Terzis and Dahlin can be explained by timing. Terzis performed her studies very early after end-to-side coaptation procedures. Terzis [24] did double-labeling studies later after end-to-side coaptation. Many of the double-labeled neurons had apparently been removed by pruning [24].

Perineurial or epineurial window

Many investigators, such as Terzis and Dahlin, regard the creation of a perineurial window

mandatory [24]. Other investigators, such as Wiberg and colleagues, favor an epineurial window only [22].

Early personal clinical experience

In the experience of one of the authors of this article, Millesi, one of the problems in brachial plexus surgery is the control of the scapula, which is not possible if the serratus anterior muscle is paralyzed because of an avulsion lesion of the ventral branches of the spinal nerves C5, C6, and C7, denervating the three roots of the long

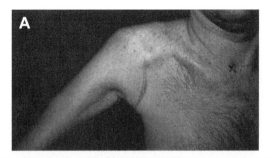

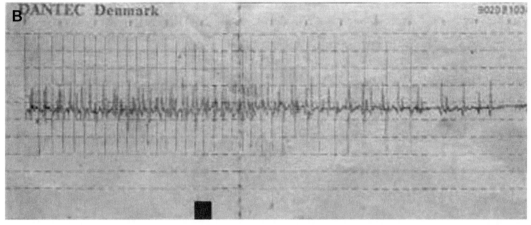

Fig. 6. (*A*) The result of nerve fiber transfer by end-to-side coaptation from the accessory nerve to the suprascapular nerve. (*B*) The electromyogram of the supraspinatus muscle after nerve fiber transfer by end-to-side coaptation from the accessory nerve to the suprascapular nerve.

thoracic nerve. Restoration of the serratus anterior function has therefore for many years been a top priority in cases of multiple root avulsions. Intercostal nerve transfer has provided some favorable results, but the intercostal nerves were needed for neurotization of, for example, the musculocutaneus or thoracodorsal nerve. The best results were achieved if the dorsalis scapulae nerve were transferred end-to-end to the long thoracic nerve. However, this sacrifices important functions. The best solution would be of course to preserve dorsalis scapulae nerve function and regain full serratus anterior function.

Because both nerves are anatomically very close together at the exit on the lateral surface of the scalenus medius muscle, a nerve fiber transfer was attempted by end-to-side coaptation from the innervated dorsalis scapulae nerve to the denervated long thoracic nerve.

The first case of this kind was operated upon on January 11, 1997 (Fig. 1). Unfortunately the photo documentation of this case is insufficient. For this reason one of the next cases is described in detail.

Case report 1

Case report 1 involves a female patient, 16 years old, who was involved in a car accident on July 21, 1998. The accident left a radicular lesion of C5, C6, and C7 on the left side. Physicians found total paralysis of the biceps brachii, brachialis, deltoid, supraspinatus, infraspinatus, and serratus anterior muscles (Fig. 2 shows the paralyzed serratus anterior muscle with scapula alata). The finger and forearm extensors, pectoralis major, latissimus dorsi, and teres major were partially paralyzed.

During surgery 2 months after the accident, a lesion of the root-nerve complex C5, C6, C7 was found. The very close location of the long thoracic nerve and the dorsal scapular nerve can be seen in Fig. 3.

The following nerve transfers were performed:

- Accessory via two nerve grafts (length 15 cm) to musculocutaneus nerve
- Phrenic nerve via two nerve grafts (each 16 cm in length) to axillary nerve (the accessory

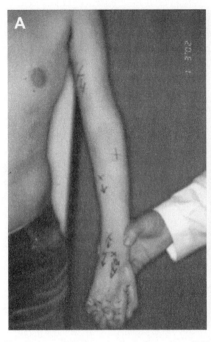
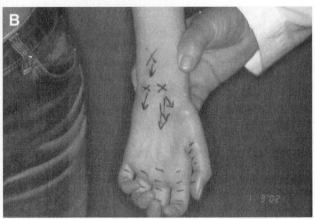

Fig. 7. (*A* and *B*) Restoration of some sensibility in the median and ulnar nerve territories by end-to-side coaptation of the distal stump of the ulnar nerve to the median nerve after harvesting the ulnar nerve as a pedicled vascularized nerve graft for the contralateral C7 transfer.

phrenic nerve was used for nerve fiber transfer by end-to-end coaptation)

- C4 via two nerve grafts (6 cm) to subscapular nerve
- Dorsalis scapulae (innervated) as donor and long thoracic nerve (denervated) as recipient coapted end-to-side by an epineurial window and fixed by two epineurial stitches as an end-to-side neurorrhaphy

Status of recovery and a follow-up after 8.5 years are illustrated in Figs. 4 and 5.

Case report 2

Case report 2 involves a male, born April 2, 1968, involved in a motorcycle accident resulting in a brachial plexus lesion. There was an avulsion of the roots C5, C6, C7, and C8. T1 showed

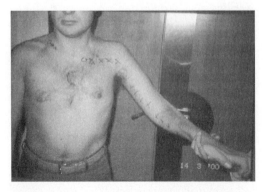

Fig. 8. An advancing Tinel sign after contralateral C7 transfer using nerve fiber transfer by end-to-side coaptation.

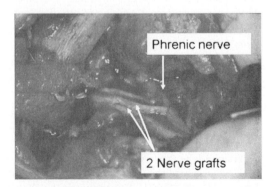

Fig. 9. The end-to-side coaptation site of the phrenic nerve with two nerve grafts using an epineurial window (incision only) at the supraclavicular region.

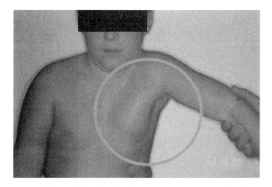

Fig. 10. This boy suffers from a traumatic avulsion of all roots of the brachial plexus on the left side. A multiple nerve grafting procedure, including a contralateral C7 transfer, was performed. Image shows the clinical result of major pectoralis muscle reinnervation by nerve fiber transfer via end-to-side coaptation from the phrenic nerve to the lateral and medial major pectoralis nerves 24 months after surgery.

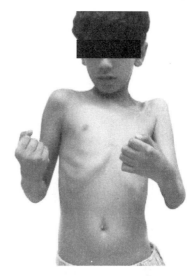

Fig. 11. This boy, 11 years old, suffers from a complete brachial plexus lesion with avulsion of all roots. Image shows the result of elbow flexion restored by nerve fiber transfer via end-to-side coaptation from the phrenic nerve to the musculocutaneous nerve using two nerve grafts 21 months after the procedure.

preserved continuity. The accessory nerve was destroyed.

Surgery was performed on November 15, 1997. Reinnervation of musculocutaneus nerve, median nerve, and radial nerve was performed by intercostal nerve transfer. In a later stage, a contralateral C7 transfer was projected. The last remaining axon donor for the moment was the phrenic nerve. The author Millesi felt a transection of the phrenic nerve as an axon donor was contraindicated because the authors had transferred the intercostal nerves 3, 4, 5, 6, and 7. For this reason, Millesi decided to transfer axons by end-to-side coaptation from the phrenic nerve via nerve grafts to the suprascapular (Fig. 6) and to

the lateral pectoral nerve. The distal ends of the grafts were coapted end-to-end with the above-mentioned nerve. In both instances, useful recovery occurred.

During this same period, the authors performed a series of contralateral C7 transfers. The ulnar nerve was used as a graft pedicled on the superior collateral ulnar artery and vein as a vascularized graft. The ulnar nerve was transected proximal of the wrist, mobilized on the pedicle, and transposed to the contralateral side to be

Table 1
Reinnervation of the lateral and medial pectoralis major nerve by end-to-side coaptation

Clinical results: Medical Research Council scale (M0–M5)	Number of cases	Average follow-up (mo)	Length of nerve graft (cm)
M4 or better	4	54	8–10
M3–M3+	4	48	8–10
M2	1	16	10

Results of nerve transfer by end-to-side coaptation for reinnervation of the major pectoralis muscle are shown. The donor nerve was the phrenic nerve. Nerve grafts were coapted end-to-side to the phrenic nerve and end-to-end to the medial or lateral pectoralis nerve. The length of the nerve grafts varied between 10 and 12 cm.

Table 2
Reinnervation of the musculocutaneus nerve by end-to-side coaptation

Medical Research Council scale	Number of cases	Months of follow-up after reinnervation
≥ M3	4	12–24
M2	1	12–24
M1	1	< 12

Six total cases. Nerve fiber transfer from the phrenic nerve to the musculocutaneous nerve via two nerve grafts. Medical Research Council scale shows strength of the muscles innervated by the musculocutaneous nerve. Most of cases revealed good recovery 12 months after the end-to-side coaptation. The length of the two nerve grafts in each patient was 15 cm on average.

Table 3
List of common nerve fiber transfers by end-to-side coaptation in brachial plexus lesion

Donor nerve	Nerve graft	Recipient nerve	Restored function
Dorsalis scapulae nerve	0	Long thoracic nerve	Movement and stabilization of scapula
Lateral pectoral nerve contralateral	1	Lateral pectoral nerve	Shoulder adduction, internal rotation
Phrenic nerve	2	Suprascapular nerve	Shoulder abduction
Phrenic nerve	2	Axillary nerve	Shoulder abduction
Phrenic nerve	2	Medial and lateral pectoral nerve	Shoulder adduction, internal rotation
Phrenic nerve	2	Musculocutaneous nerve	Elbow flexion
Accessory nerve	2	Musculocutaneous nerve	Elbow flexion

coapted end-to-end to the transected anterior or posterior division of contralateral C7. The distal coaptation was performed with the medius nerve. Because sensibility of poor quality returned in the median nerve area, the authors started to coapt the distal stump of the transected ipsilateral ulnar nerve end-to-side to the ipsilateral median nerve to be reneurotisized. In a series of these cases, some rudimentary feeling of touch and pain returned (case report 3).

Case report 3

This patient, born August 25, 1975, had complete brachial plexus lesion due to a motorcycle accident. Surgery was performed on July 14,

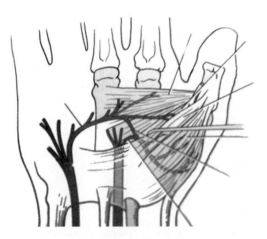

Fig. 12. Anatomy of a human hand. This is a variation in innervation of the thenar muscles by the deep branch of the ulnar nerve. These patients do not loose opposition of the thumb in complete median nerve lesion. (*From* Tackmann W, Richter H, Stöhr M. Kompressionssyndrome peripherer nerven. Berlin: Springer Verlag; 1989; with permission.)

2001. C5 and C6 were ruptured and continuity restored by nerve grafting.

A contralateral C7 transfer was performed in two steps on September 6 and 8, 2001. Coaptation was performed of the vascularized ulnar nerve to the posterior division of the medius trunk contralateral. Then coaptation was performed of the originally proximal end of the ulnar nerve with the distal stump of the median nerve at the level of the union of the two roots.

After isolation of the distal end of the ulnar nerve for the transfer, a distal stump several centimeters long was prepared and left in the area of the distal forearm. After creating an epineurial window to receive axon sprouts coming down from contralateral C7 along the median nerve, the distal stump was transferred to the median nerve at the wrist level and coapted end-to-side to the median nerve.

The follow-up on June 14, 2002, showed rudimentary sensibility against touch in the median as well as in the ulnar area of the hand (Fig. 7).

Only in one case of contralateral C7 transfer was the coaptation between the vascularized ulnar nerve graft and the anterior-posterior division performed in an end-to-side fashion. This was not done on purpose, but because the authors had no other choice.

Case report 4

Case report 4 involves a patient, born May 6, 1972, who suffered from a complete brachial plexus lesion due to a motorcycle accident and was operated on on July 14, 2001, in a hospital outside of Austria. A rupture of C5 and C6, and an avulsion of C7, C8, and T1 were diagnosed intraoperatively.

There was some regeneration in the upper roots (abduction 15°; biceps brachii muscle

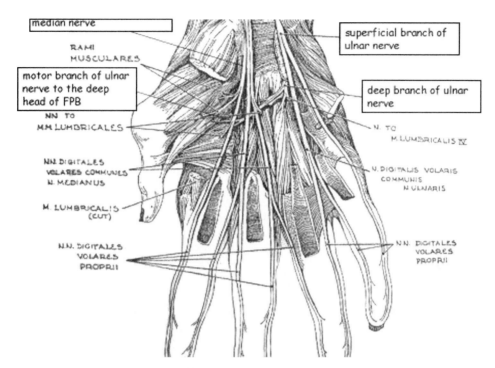

Fig. 13. Innervation of hand muscles in a baboon (a nonhuman primate). (*From* Swindler DR, Wood CD. Atlas of primate gross anatomy. Seattle (WA): University of Washington Press, 1973; with permission.)

showed an M1 according to the Medical Research Council scale). The lower roots were avulsed and a contralateral C7 transfer was suggested. There is fear in such cases that the patient might have a pre- or postfixation and the fiber distribution will not follow expectations. Of course, the authors do perform a control by electric stimulation intraoperatively but this is not always reliable and does not reveal abnormalities with sensibility. Therefore, the authors perform the contralateral C7 transfer in two stages. During the first stage, the authors explore the contralateral plexus and ligate the anterior and posterior division of the medius trunk. The following day the patient can be tested and, if the loss of function remains within the expected limits, the transfer itself is performed the following day. In this particular case, the patient showed some loss of function in the biceps and the deltoid muscle due to irregular innervations that were not detected during the intraoperative electric stimulation. It was decided to go on with the concept of contralateral C7 transfer but to open the ligature and perform the coaptation end-to-side without transection of the divisions. Fortunately, the biceps brachii and the deltoid muscle recovered perfectly in

a short time. Axons proceeded across the end-to-side coaptation site. A Tinel-Hoffmann sign proceeded along the nerve graft to the median nerve and along the median nerve to the hand (Fig. 8). There was, however, no useful recovery. In cases of avulsion of four or five roots, donors are in short supply. A strong muscle for external rotation of the shoulder is needed. The major pectoralis muscle would be such a muscle. Unfortunately, it is an internal rotator. This muscle is neurotisized with the intension to transfer it for external rotation in a second stage. Over a period of time, nerve fibers were recruited from the phrenic nerve, which is a strong donor for motor axons.

Millesi always hesitates to transect the phrenic nerve, especially if an intercostals nerve transfer is necessary as well. So the authors tried end-to-side coaptation of nerve grafts to the phrenic nerve at a proximal level. The distal ends of the grafts were coapted end-to-end to the medial and lateral pectoral nerves. The authors performed a follow-up study on a series of such cases (Figs. 9 and 10; Table 1).

The phrenic nerve has proven useful for elbow flexion as well. Two grafts are coapted end-to-side

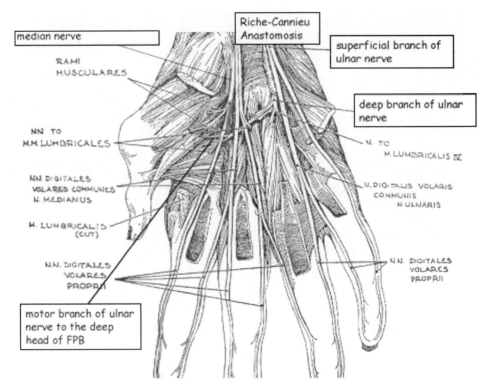

Fig. 14. Nerve fiber transfer via an artificial Riche-Cannieu anastomosis is created by end-to-side coaptation of a nerve graft to the terminal motor branch of the deep branch of the ulnar nerve and end-to-end coaptation of the nerve graft to the motor thenar branch of the median nerve. The donor nerve is the motor branch innervating the deep head of the flexor pollicis brevis muscle. (*From* Swindler DR, Wood CD. Atlas of primate gross anatomy. Seattle (WA): University of Washington Press, 1973; with permission.)

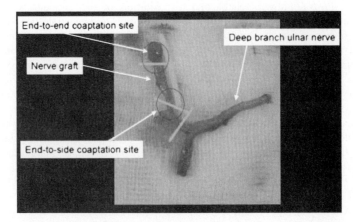

Fig. 15. Indication of nerve and nerve graft segments harvested for histologic and immunohistochemic studies: deep branch of ulnar nerve 5 mm proximal to the end-to-side coaptation site, nerve graft at the end-to-side coaptation site, nerve graft 2 mm proximal to the end-to-end coaptation site. Control: nonoperated left terminal deep branch of ulnar nerve.

Table 4
Assessment of anatomic innervations

	Latency (ms)	Amplitude (mV)	Compound nerve action potential (mV/ms)	Nerve conduction velocity (m/s)
Stimulation of median nerve distal: primarily superficial head of the flexor pollicis brevis muscle, control				
Mean	2.8	14.4	24.8	59.6
SD	0.3	1.4	3.0	4.8
Stimulation of ulnar nerve: primarily deep head of the flexor pollicis brevis muscle, control				
Mean	2.5	9.9	20.8	63.2
SD	0.3	3.6	6.8	10.9

Electrophysiological analysis during the primary procedure was performed for the assessment of anatomic innervation of thenar muscles, especially of different innervation of the superficial and deep head of the flexor pollicis brevis muscle. The needle electrode was placed into the abductor pollicis brevis muscle, and into the superficial and deep head of the flexor pollicis brevis muscle, according to the anatomic neural innervation. After the physiologic assessment of ulnar and median nerve thenar innervation, the median nerve was transected at distal forearm level, creating a defect of the nerve. The electrophysiological analysis of the median nerve thenar innervation was repeated for negative control. Data for negative control are not shown.

to the proximal segment of the phrenic nerve. The distal ends are coapted end-to-end to the musculocutaneous nerve (Fig. 11; Table 2).

As far as the major pectoralis is concerned, the authors were looking for another donor in multiple root avulsions. The authors followed a suggestion from Alain Gilbert and neurotizied the major pectoralis using the contralateral lateral pectoral nerve for the ipsilateral major pectoralis to save the phrenic nerve for the musculocutaneus.

Table 3 lists examples of common nerve fiber transfers by end-to-side coaptation in brachial plexus lesion.

In summary, the clinical results were very satisfying according to the authors' expectations. The authors never regarded that nerve fiber transfer by end-to-side coaptation to be equal to end-to-end coaptation and used it only in cases in which end-to-end coaptation was impossible. However, the authors are convinced that end-to-side coaptation represents a great option, provided the correct indications can be found. So the authors started an experimental study at a very distal level where nature has provided a link between two nerve territories.

Experimental study on synergistic nerve fiber transfer by terminal end-to-side coaptation

Connections may exist between branches of the deep branch of the ulnar nerve innervating the

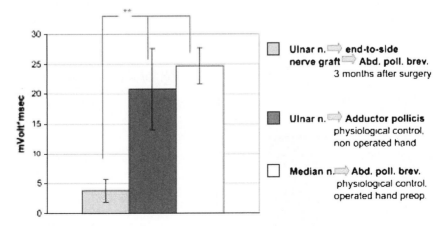

Fig. 16. Mean CNAP areas were 3.73 in the end-to-side nerve graft group, 22.85 mV/ms in uninjured ulnar nerve, and 25.13 mV/ms in uninjured median nerve. Mean CNAP area measured through the nerve graft reached only 14.8% to 16.2% of normal. This was significantly smaller than in uninjured nerves (**$P = .002$, *$P = .02$). abd. poll. brev., abductor pollicis brevis; n, nerve.

Table 5
Assessment of reinnervation in the abductor pollicis brevis muscle, which is now neurotisized by synergistic nerve fiber transfer via end-to-side coaptation

	Latency (ms)	Amplitude (mV)	CNAP (mV/ms)	Nerve conduction velocity (m/s)	Length of nerve graft (cm)
Animal 1	2.7	1.9	4.1	51.8	2.5
Animal 2	8.6	1.3	3.6	48.3	3.0
Animal 3	3.1	4.9	7.7	53.5	1.6
Animal 4	2.3	2.0	3.4	55.6	1.8
Animal 5	2.7	2.2	3.2	54.6	2.6
Animal 6	4.7	2.0	3.1	24.5	2.7
Animal 7	3.3	0.6	1.5	57.8	2.2
Mean	3.9	2.1	3.8	49.4	2.3
SD	2.2	1.3	1.9	11.4	0.5
Percent of normal	156.3%	21.4%	18.3%	78.3%	

Stimulation of right ulnar nerve at distal forearm level after end-to-side nerve graft. Electrophysiological analysis during the secondary procedure was performed 3 months after primary surgery. Latency, amplitude, CNAP, and nerve conduction velocity are given in each animal. The percentage to normal control is shown. The average length of the nerve graft was 2.3 cm.

deep head of the flexor pollicis brevis muscle. Such connections are called Riche-Cannieu anastomoses (Fig. 12) [25,26]. Therefore, in evaluating motor results in median nerve repair, the authors have always excluded such patients with a "mixed" innervation of thenar muscles. Such a mixed innervation was present in 29% of cases observed by one author, Millesi. These patients do not loose opposition in complete median nerve transection.

In this study, the authors tested the hypothesis that useful functional results can be achieved through such a very peripheral nerve fiber transfer by end-to-side nerve graft repair using terminal branches of the ulnar nerve with synergistic defined motor function to the median nerve innervated thenar muscles.

An end-to-side nerve graft repair bridging from the terminal motor branch to the deep head of the flexor pollicis brevis muscle (which is a branch of the deep branch of the ulnar nerve) to the thenar motor branch of the median nerve was performed in nonhuman primates (Figs. 13 and 14). The deep head of the flexor pollicis brevis muscle innervated by the ulnar nerve reveals a synergistic function to other thenar muscles for opposition of the thumb.

Material and methods

Seven adult baboons were used in this study. At baseline, the authors excluded electrophysiologically and by microsurgical dissection the variation in innervations of median and ulnar

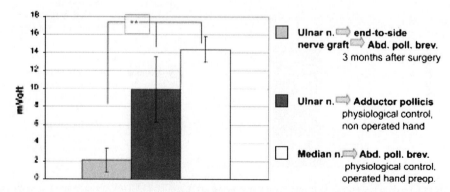

Fig. 17. Mean amplitudes were 2.1 mV in the end-to-side nerve graft group, 9.9 mV in the uninjured ulnar nerve, and 14.4 mV in uninjured median nerve. This was significantly smaller than in uninjured nerves (**$P = .002$ for ulnar nerve, *$P = .02$ for median nerve). abd. poll. brev., abductor pollicis brevis; n, nerve.

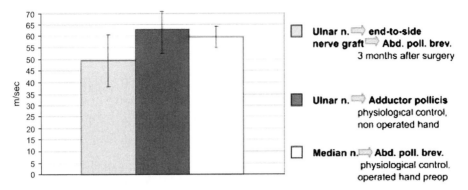

Fig. 18. Mean nerve conduction velocity was 49.03 m/s in the end-to-side nerve graft group , 56.81 m/s in the uninjured ulnar nerve, and 56.3 m/s in the uninjured median nerve. Mean NCV reached 86.3% (ulnar nerve) to 87.1% (median nerve) of uninjured nerves. This was not statistically significantly smaller than in the uninjured nerves. abd. poll. brev., abductor pollicis brevis; n, nerve.

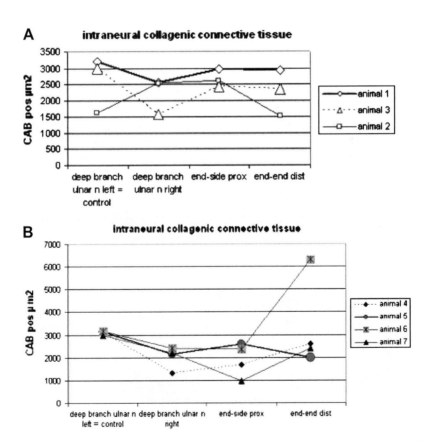

Fig. 19. (*A* and *B*) Neural collagenic connective tissue 3 months after surgery. Neural collagenic connective tissue was stained with CAB-chronotrope aniline blue. There were no statistically significant differences in the area of collagenic connective tissue between all nerve segments of end-to-side nerve graft repair animals and nonoperated control sites. However, the area of collagenic connective tissue was 6% larger 2 mm distal to the end-to-side repair site and 28% larger at the distal end of the nerve graft. Highest mean values were found at the distal site of the nerve graft because of a very strong collagenization of the nerve graft of animal number six.

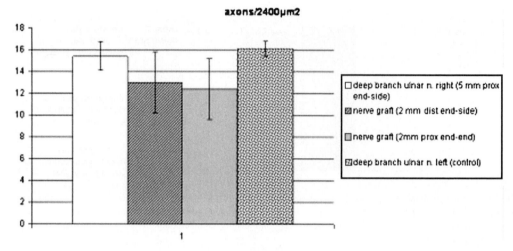

Fig. 20. Number of axons 3 months after surgery. The number of axons distal to the end-to-side repair site was smaller by 19% on average. Additionally, the authors found an average 23% decrease of axons 2 mm proximal to the end-to-end coaptation, compared with data of the deep branch of ulnar nerve (**P = .008). dist, distal; n, nerve; prox, proximal.

nerve–innervated thenar muscles. The median nerve was transected at forearm level, creating a nerve gap. Stimulation of the proximal stump of the median nerve and stimulation of the ulnar nerve was performed showing again no variation in innervation of the thenar muscles. Now a nerve graft was harvested from the dorsum of the hand using a branch of the superficial branch of the

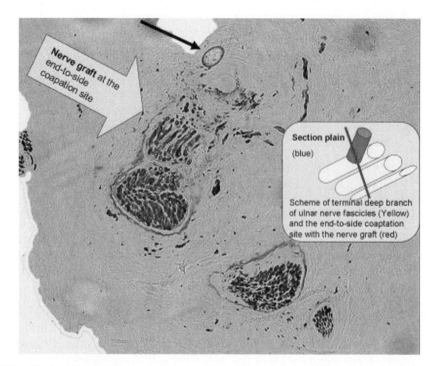

Fig. 21. S100 antibody staining of Schwann cells at the end-to-side nerve graft repair site 3 months after surgery. Image shows a transverse section of the terminal motor branch of the deep branch of ulnar nerve and longitudinal section of the end-to-side coaptation site. Black arrow indicates suture material of the end-to-side coaptation creating an epineurial window by incision only.

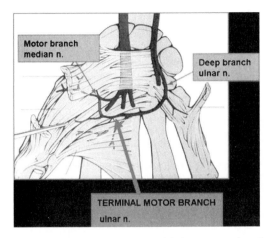

Fig. 22. Illustration of an artificial anastomosis of Riche-Cannieu, which is shown as a red connection between the motor branch to the deep head of the flexor pollicis brevis muscle and the thenar branch of the median nerve. n, nerve.

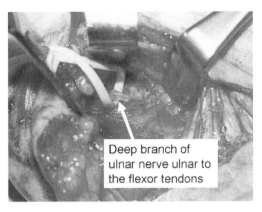

Fig. 24. The deep branch of the ulnar nerve is shown underneath the flexor tendons at the ulnar side. Flexor tendons are lifted by a Langenbeck hook.

radial nerve. End-to-side coaptation of a nerve graft to the synergistic part of the deep branch of the ulnar nerve (motor branch to the deep head of flexor pollicis brevis muscle), creating an epineurial window. End-to-end coaptation was performed between the nerve graft and the thenar motor branch of the median nerve.

Three months after surgery, functional recovery was assessed by electrophysiological evaluation, thenar muscle weight, and video slow-motion analysis. Specimens were harvested 3 months after surgery. Neural collagenic connective tissue, and

the number of Schwann cells were evaluated (Fig. 15).

Results

Hand function in the uninjured baboon with attention to opposition of the thumb

Preoperatively grasping patterns were studied in all animals.

As is well known, the thumb ray of the baboon hand is shorter than that of the human hand. Face-to-face position of the thumb with index, middle, ring, and small finger was not observed. However, when climbing inside their cages, all baboons grasped a thin rod by abduction, rotation, and flexion of the thumb, which we called opposition of the thumb, in a nonhuman primate

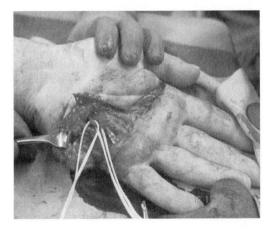

Fig. 23. After a y-shaped incision at the palm, the superficial and deep branch of the ulnar nerve are dissected ulnar to the flexor tendons.

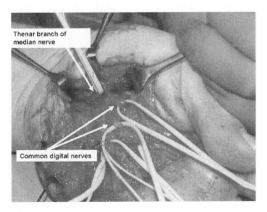

Fig. 25. The dissection of the more radial area of the palm. The common digital nerves and the motor thenar branch of the median nerve are indicated by nerve loops.

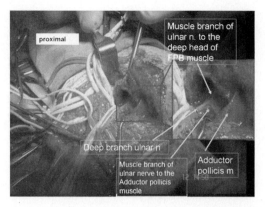

Fig. 26. The deep branch of ulnar nerve is dissected at a very terminal level at the radial region of the palm. Image shows the motor branch to the adductor muscle and the motor branch to the deep head of the flexor pollicis muscle. n, nerve.

fashion (short thumb-ray, full opposition, like in humans, is not possible). This was seen when the baboon approached the thin rod perpendicular to the length axis of the rod.

When the animals approached the thin rod from a position nearly parallel to the length axis of the rod, a different type of gripping was used. The length axis of the rod was now positioned between thenar and hypothenar, creating an increased shape of the palm arc. Baboons can easily grip in this way because they can use additional muscles of the metacarpus, called musculi contrahentes. The force of this gripping is increased by

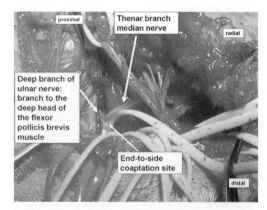

Fig. 27. Arrows indicate end-to-side coaptation site of the thenar branch of the median nerve to the motor branch of the ulnar nerve innervating the deep head of the flexor pollicis muscle. If the thenar branch of median nerve can be dissected retrograde sufficiently, no nerve graft is needed.

additional rotation and flexion of the thumb, which are both part of the opposition movement.

When grasping thicker rods, grasping was performed by flexion of fingers and adduction of the thumb only.

Intraoperative findings

Under the operation microscope, the authors did not find variations in innervated thenar muscles in operated baboons, and electrophysiogical evaluation confirmed these findings (Table 4).

In each animal, the thenar motor branch of the median nerve showed two or three terminal motor branches.

Postoperative functional results in the hand

The day after the primary procedure no animal displayed nonhuman primate opposition of the thumb.

Three months after surgery, all animals clinically showed nonhuman primate opposition of the thumb. Baboons preferred the left, nonoperated hand for such activities as scraping and fine grasping.

Electrophysiological analysis during the primary procedure and the nonsevered upper extremity

All baboons showed identical innervation of thenar muscles like that in humans (In humans, all thenar muscles are innervated by the median nerve except the deep head of flexor pollicis brevis muscle. This innervation is provided by the deep branch of the ulnar nerve) (see Table 4). The authors did not find any variation in innervation of the superficial and deep head of the flexor pollicis brevis muscle anatomically and electrophysiologically. The authors did not detect any electrophysiological signals into the abductor pollicis brevis muscle and the deep head of the flexor pollicis brevis muscle after transection of the median nerve.

Electrophysiological analysis 3 months after surgery

Compound nerve action potential area

Mean compound nerve action potential (CNAP) areas in the end-to-side nerve graft group were 3.8 mV/ms and 20.8 mV/ms in the uninjured ulnar nerve and 24.8 mV/ms in the uninjured median nerve (Fig. 16; Table 5). Mean CNAP area measured through the nerve graft reached only 15.3% to 18.2% of normal. This was significantly smaller

Electrode is located at the thenar region

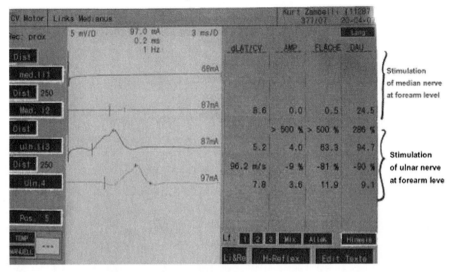

Fig. 28. The screen of an electromyogram machine during stimulation of the median nerve and ulnar nerve at forearm level in a patient who had a subtotal amputation at the proximal arm. The image was taken 21 months after synergistic terminal nerve fiber transfer from the ulnar nerve to the thenar branch of the median nerve. The electrode is located at the thenar region. The stimulation of the median nerve indicates no reinnervation. The stimulation of the ulnar nerve at forearm level shows reinnervation of thenar muscles by an artificial anastomosis of Riche-Cannieu.

than in uninjured nerves (**$P = .002$ for ulnar nerve, *$P = .02$ for median nerve).

Peak action potential amplitude

Mean amplitudes were 2.1 mV in the end-to-side nerve graft group, 9.9 mV in the uninjured ulnar nerve, and 14.4 mV in uninjured median nerve (Fig. 17). Thus, amplitudes were significantly smaller in the nerve graft group than in uninjured nerves (**$P = .002$ for ulnar nerve, *$P = .02$ for median nerve).

Nerve conduction velocity

Mean nerve conduction velocity (NCV) in the end-to-side nerve graft group was 49.4 m/s and 63.2 m/s in uninjured ulnar nerve, and 59.6 m/s in uninjured median nerve (Fig. 18). Mean NCV reached 78.2% (ulnar nerve) to 82.9% (median nerve) of uninjured nerves. There was no statistical difference in the NCV between the nerves in the end-to-side nerve graft group and the uninjured left hand nerves.

Onset latency (data not shown)

Mean nerve latency in the end-to-side nerve graft group was 3.9 ms and 2.5 ms in uninjured ulnar nerve, and 2.8 ms in uninjured median nerve. Mean latency reached 156% (ulnar nerve) to 139.3% (median nerve) of uninjured nerves.

Correlation length of nerve graft—NCV, CNAP area, amplitude and latency

No correlation between length of nerve graft and NCV, CNAP area, amplitude, and latency was found statistically.

Wet and dry thenar muscle weight of male baboons (data not shown)

On average, wet thenar muscle weight was 50.2% higher in the uninjured hand compared with reinnervated thenar muscles. Wet thenar muscle weight ranged from 2.5 g to 6.1 g in the uninjured hand and from 0.8 g to 3.4 g in reinnervated thenar muscles. The difference was statistically significant ($P = .02$). On average, dry thenar muscle weight was 55.3% higher in the uninjured hand compared with that of reinnervated thenar muscles. Dry thenar muscle weight ranged from 0.6 g to 1.4 g in the uninjured hand and from 0.2 g to 0.6 g in reinnervated thenar muscles. The difference was statistically significant ($P = .002$).

Correlation length of nerve graft—wet and dry thenar muscle weight

No statistical correlation between length of nerve graft and thenar muscle weight was found.

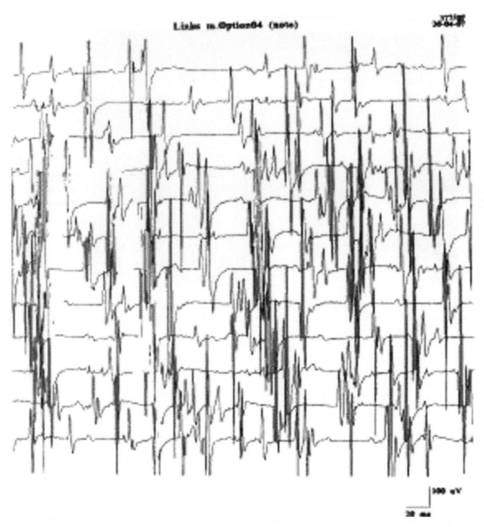

Fig. 29. Motion analysis of the thenar muscles during opposition of the thumb in a patient 21 months after creating an artificial anastomosis of Riche-Cannieu. Now thenar muscles are innervated by synergistic nerve fiber transfer by end-to-side coaptation from the deep branch of the ulnar nerve to the thenar branch of the median nerve.

Chronotype aniline blue staining—neural collagenous connective tissue 3 months after surgery

Chronotype aniline blue was used to stain neural collagenic connective tissue. There were no statistically significant differences in the area of collagenic connective tissue between all nerve segments of end-to-side nerve graft repair animals and nonoperated control sites (Fig. 19). However, the area of collagenic connective tissue was 6% larger 2 mm distal to the end-to-side repair site and 28% larger at the distal end of the nerve graft. Due to a very strong collagenization

of the nerve graft of animal number six, highest mean values were found at the distal site of the nerve graft (see Fig. 19B).

Neurofilament antibodies used to stain axons—number of neurofilaments positive axon 3 months after surgery

The number of axons distal to the end-to-side repair site was smaller by 19% on average (Fig. 20). Additionally, the authors found a decrease of axons of 23% on average 2 mm proximal to the end-to-end coaptation, compared with data of the deep branch of ulnar nerve ($P = .008$).

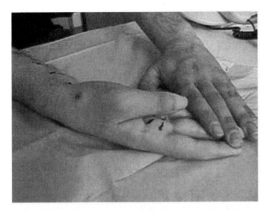

Fig. 30. Opposition of the thumb in a patient who had a subtotal amputation of the arm. Image was taken 21 months after synergistic nerve fiber transfer by end-to-side coaptation from the deep branch of the ulnar nerve to the thenar branch of the median nerve. There was a defect of the median nerve. The radial nerve was repaired. The ulnar nerve was uninjured.

S100 antibody–Schwann cells 3 months
after surgery (data not shown)

Schwann cell counts showed similar values within all nerve segments. There was no difference compared with the nonoperated control. Fig. 21 shows a transverse section of the very terminal

motor branch of the deep branch of ulnar nerve at the end-to-side coaptation site.

Conclusion of this experimental study

This nonhuman primate model demonstrated the functional efficacy of nerve fiber transfer by end-to-side nerve graft repair at the level of peripheral terminal motor branches. The authors concluded that end-to-side neurorrhaphy may present a viable alternative in conditions of unsuitable end-to-end coaptation and inappropriate nerve grafting procedures in humans.

Encouraged by the experimental results, the authors applied the technique in clinical cases.

Clinical application of synergistic nerve fiber transfer by end-to-side coaptation

The synergistic nerve fiber transfer by end-to-side coaptation procedure was performed in six patients with partial brachial plexus lesions (Fig. 22). None of these patients revealed regeneration of the median nerve. There was no opposition of the thumb. Median nerve innervated thenar muscles did not show reinnervation. Ulnar nerve innervated muscles were innervated.

Table 6
Examples of nerve fiber transfers by end-to-side coaptation using synergistic fibers for reinnervation of thenar muscles normally innervated by the median nerve

Initials; sex; age	Type of accident	Type of lesion	Primary procedure	End-to-side coaptation with or without nerve graft	Follow-up (months)	Medical Research Council scale
MM; male; 26 y	Traffic	Complete right brachial plexus lesion	Exploration brachial plexus and nerve graft	30-mm nerve graft	16	M4
MA; male; 25 y	Traffic	Subtotal amputation upper right arm	31-cm median nerve graft; 12-cm radial nerve graft	30-mm nerve graft	20	M4
AM; male; 9 y	Domestic	Median nerve transection right forearm	12-cm median nerve graft	30-mm nerve graft	12	M3+
ZK; male; 38 y	Labor	Subtotal amputation upper left arm	3 12-cm median nerve grafts; 2 13-cm musculocutaneus nerve grafts; 2 15-cm radial nerve grafts	No nerve graft	24	M4
CF; male; 23 y	Labor	Soft tissue defect right forearm	4 20-cm median nerve grafts	No nerve graft	18	M4
LS; male, 27 y	Traffic	Complete brachial plexus lesion	Neurolysis	10-mm nerve graft	4	M1

An artificial anastomosis of Riche-Cannieu was created.

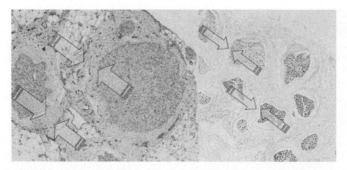

Fig. 31. The perineurium of the rat's sciatic nerve at thigh level shows high thickness (*thick arrows*) due to the multiple-layer structure that surrounds the fascicle. A very peripheral motor branch of the deep branch of ulnar nerve indicates a delicate structure of the perineurium (*narrow arrows*). The creation of a perineurial window without lesion of the axons seems to be impossible, even under the operating microscope.

Procedure

A y-shaped incision of the skin at the palm region was made to expose the superficial and the deep branch of ulnar nerve at the ulnar side of the flexor tendons (Figs. 23 and 24). The anatomic structures of the palm were defined, including the thenar motor branch of the median nerve (Fig. 25). Now the very terminal deep branch of ulnar nerve, including its motor branch to the deep head of the flexor pollicis brevis muscle (Fig. 26), was exposed. For nerve grafting, the authors used a branch of the medial cutaneous branch of the forearm. End-to-side coaptation of this terminal motor branch to the flexor pollicis brevis muscle (deep branch of the ulnar nerve) and the nerve graft was performed with two epineurial sutures after creating an epineurial window (incision of the epineurium only) under the surgical microscope. The nerve graft was placed into the prefabricated tunnel without any tension and end-to-end nerve repair was performed with the thenar motor branch of the median nerve.

In cases with a sufficient length of the thenar motor branch of the median nerve, no nerve graft was used and end-to-side coaptation to the muscle branch innervating the deep head of the flexor pollicis brevis muscle was performed (two cases) (Fig. 27). The length of the nerve graft was 3 cm on average (four cases). The wound was closed in layers.

The results of an electrophysiologic study 21 months after nerve fiber transfer by end-to-side coaptation is shown in Figs. 28 and 29. Opposition of the thumb 21 months after this surgery is illustrated in Fig. 30.

Table 6 shows an overview of clinical results of synergistic nerve fiber transfer by terminal end-to-side coaptation.

Discussion and future outlook

In retrospect, one can say that nerve fiber transfer by end-to-side coaptation certainly can work without damaging of nerve fibers. This was proven by the fact that sprouting starts in cases without any damage of the perineurium. Skeptics who have dismissed such transfers as impossible have reached conclusions too quickly. Researchers have found that, under the right experimental circumstances, regeneration of mainly sensible nerve fibers occurs, although results are unpredictable. Researchers have generalized their experience with main nerve trunks. They did not consider the possibility of the type of the nerve (large mixed nerve or small pure motor or sensory nerve) and the fact that the perineurium might not be the same in a proximal or a distal level (Fig. 31).

In the authors' hands, nerve fiber transfer by end-to-side coaptation yields consistently useful recoveries if small nerves with one main function are used as donors and recipients. The results are not as good as with end-to-end coaptation and therefore end-to-side coaptation should be applied only in cases in which end-to-end coaptation is impossible.

A new application was opened by transferring synergistic nerve fibers from one nerve, such as the ulnar nerve, to another nerve, such as the median nerve, with preservation of both functions within the same segment (C8 and T1). There are certainly several indications to use this method.

At present experimental studies are running to transfer nerve fibers under the same condition between nerves of different metamers. The authors still expect an expansion of indications.

References

[1] Viterbo F, Trindade JC, Hoshino K, et al. Latero-terminal neurorrhaphy without removal of the epineural sheath. Experimental study in rats. Rev Paul Med 1992;110:267–75.

[2] Dellon AL. Nerve grafting and end-to-side neurorrhaphies connecting phrenic nerve to the brachial plexus. Plast Reconstr Surg 1996;98(5):905.

[3] Tarasidis G, Watanabe O, Mackinnon SE, et al. End-to-side neurorrhaphy resulting in limited sensory axonal regeneration in a rat model. Ann Otol Rhinol Laryngol 1997;106:506–12.

[4] Tarasidis G, Watanabe O, Mackinnon SE, et al. End-to-side neurorraphy: a long-term study of neural regeneration in a rat model. Otolaryngol Head Neck Surg 1998;119:337–41.

[5] Noah EM, Williams A, Jorgenson C, et al. End-to-side neurorrhaphy: a histologic and morphometric study of axonal sprouting into an end-to-side nerve graft. J Reconstr Microsurg 1997;13:99–106.

[6] Fernandez E, Lauretti L, Tufo T, et al. End to side nerve neurorrhaphy: critical appraisal of experimental and clinical data. Acta Neurochir Suppl 2007; 100:77–84.

[7] Frey M, Giovanoli P. End-to-side neurorrhaphy of sensory nerves. Eur J Plast Surg 2003;26:85–8.

[8] Goheen-Robillard B, Myckatyn TM, Mackinnon SE, et al. End-to-side neurorrhaphy and lateral axonal sprouting in a long graft rat model. Laryngoscope 2002;112:899–905.

[9] Liu HJ, Dong MM, Chi FL. Functional remobilization evaluation of the paralyzed vocal cord by end-to-side neurorrhaphy in rats. Laryngoscope 2005; 115:1418–20.

[10] Lutz BS, Chuang DC, Hsu JC, et al. Selection of donor nerves—an important factor in end-to-side neurorrhaphy. Br J Plast Surg 2000;53(2):149–54.

[11] Matsumoto M, Hirata H, Nishiyama M, et al. Schwann cells can induce collateral sprouting from intact axons: experimental study of end-to-side neurorrhaphy using a Y-chamber model. J Reconstr Microsurg 1999;15:281–6.

[12] Robillard BG, Mackinnon SE. Invited discussion to: Okajima S, Terzis JK Ultrastructure of early axonal regeneration in an end-to-side neurorrhaphy model. J Reconstr Microsurg 2000;16:323–5.

[13] Voche P, Ouattara D. End-to-side neurorrhaphy for defects of palmar sensory digital nerves. Br J Plast Surg 2005;58:239–44.

[14] Jaberi FM, Abbas BP, Nezhad ST, et al. End-to-side neurorrhaphy: an experimental study in rabbits. Microsurgery 2003;23(4):359–62.

[15] Bontioti E, Dahlin LB, Kataoka K, et al. End-to-side nerve repair induces nuclear translocation of the activating transcription factor 3 (ATF3). Scand J Plast Reconstr Surg Hand Surg 2006; 40(6):321–8.

[16] Bontioti EN, Kanje M, Dahlin LB. Regeneration and functional recovery in the upper extremity of rats after various type of nerve injuries. J Peripher Nerv Syst 2003;8(3):159–68.

[17] Bontioti E, Kanje M, Dahlin LB. End-to-side nerve repair: attachment of a distal, compared with a proximal and distal, nerve segment. Scand J Plast Reconstr Surg Hand Surg 2006;40(3):129–35.

[18] Bontioti E, Kanje M, Lundborg G, et al. End-to-side nerve repair in the upper extremity of rat. J Peripher Nerv Syst 2005;10(1):58–68.

[19] Dahlin LB, Bontioti E, Kataoka K, et al. Functional recovery and mechanisms in end-to-side nerve repair in rats. Acta Neurochir Suppl 2007;100:93–5.

[20] Lindwall C, Dahlin L, Lundborg G, et al. Inhibition of c-Jun phosphorylation reduces axonal outgrowth of adult rat nodose ganglia and dorsal root ganglia sensory neurons. Mol Cell Neurosci 2004;27(3): 267–79.

[21] Cederna PS, Kalliainen LK, Urbanchek MG, et al. "Donor" muscle structure and function after end-to-side neurorrhaphy. Plast Reconstr Surg 2001; 107:789–96.

[22] Kelly EJ, Jacoby C, Terenghi G, et al. End-to-side nerve coaptation: a qualitative and quantitative assessment in the primate. J Plast Reconstr Aesthet Surg 2007;60(1):1–12 [Epub 2006 Jul 10].

[23] Battiston B, Tos P, Conforti LG, et al. Alternative techniques for peripheral nerve repair: conduits and end-to-side neurorrhaphy. Acta Neurochir Suppl 2007;100:43–50.

[24] Terzis JK. Discussion at the symposium PNS 2006, "How to improve the results of peripheral nerve surgery" held in Vienna from March 24–26, 2006.

[25] Schmidhammer R, Hausner T, Zandieh S, et al. Morphology after synergistic motor end-to-side nerve repair: investigation in a non-human primate model. European Surgery 2005;37(4):220–7.

[26] Schmidhammer R, Redl H, Hopf R, et al. End-to-side nerve graft repair based on synergistic peripheral terminal motor branches. Investigation in a non-human primate model. European Surgery 2005;37(5):308–16.

ELSEVIER
SAUNDERS

Hand Clin 24 (2008) 485

HAND
CLINICS

Erratum

Treatment of Thumb Metacarpophalangeal and Interphalangeal Joint Arthritis

Eon K. Shin, MD[a],*, A. Lee Osterman, MD[b]

[a]Thomas Jefferson University Hospital, The Philadelphia Hand Center, P.C., 834 Chestnut Street,
Suite G114, Philadelphia, PA 19107, USA
[b]Thomas Jefferson University Hospital, The Philadelphia Hand Center, P.C., 700 South Henderson Road,
Suite 200, King of Prussia, PA 19406, USA

The above article, which appeared in the August 2008 issue ("Thumb Arthritis"), erroneously credited Figs. 7 and 8 to Shin EK, Jupiter JB. Flap advancement coverage after excision of large mucous cysts. Tech Hand Up Extrem Surg 2007;11:159–62. These were original photographs. We apologize for the oversight.

ELSEVIER
SAUNDERS

Hand Clin 24 (2008) 487–490

HAND
CLINICS

Index

Note: Page numbers of article titles are in **boldface** type.

hand.theclinics.com